Textbook of Clinical Hemodynamics

Textbook of Clinical Hemodynamics

Michael Ragosta, MD, FACC, FSCAI

Associate Professor of Medicine,
Director, Cardiac Catheterization Laboratories,
University of Virginia Health System,
Charlottesville, VA

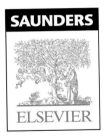

SAUNDERS

ELSEVIER

SAUNDERS
ELSEVIER

1600 John F. Kennedy Boulevard
Philadelphia, PA 19103

TEXTBOOK OF CLINICAL HEMODYNAMICS   ISBN: 978-1-4160-4000-2

Notice

Knowledge and best practice in this field are constantly changing. As new research and experience broaden our knowledge, changes in practice, treatment and drug therapy may become necessary or appropriate. Readers are advised to check the most current information provided (i) on procedures featured or (ii) by the manufacturer of each product to be administered, to verify the recommended dose or formula, the method and duration of administration, and contraindications. It is the responsibility of the practitioner, relying on their own experience and knowledge of the patient, to make diagnoses, to determine dosages and the best treatment for each individual patient, and to take all appropriate safety precautions. To the fullest extent of the law, neither the Publisher nor the Authors assumes any liability for any injury and/or damage to persons or property arising out of or related to any use of the material contained in this book.

The Publisher

Library of Congress Cataloging-in-Publication Data

Ragosta, Michael.
   Textbook of clinical hemodynamics / Michael Ragosta. – 1st ed.
      p. ; cm.
   Includes bibliographical references and index.
   ISBN 978-1-4160-4000-2
   1. Hemodynamics.   2. Cardiovascular system–Diseases–Diagnosis.   I. Title.
      [DNLM: 1. Hemodynamic Processes.   2. Heart Diseases–diagnosis.
   3. Heart Function Tests. WG 106 R144t 2008]
   RC670.5.H45R34 2008
   616.1'0754–dc22

                                                                    2007022989

Executive Publisher: Natasha Andjelkovic
Project Manager: Mary Stermel
Design Direction: Steve Stave
Marketing Manager: Todd Liebel

Printed in China.

Last digit is the print number: 9   8   7   6   5   4   3

Contributors

VISHAL ARORA, MD
Fellow, Interventional Cardiology
University of Virginia Health System
Charlottesville, VA

BRANDON BROWN, MD
Fellow, Interventional Cardiology
University of Virginia Health System
Charlottesville, VA

HOWARD P. GUTGESELL, MD
Professor of Pediatrics
University of Virginia Health System
Charlottesville, VA

D. SCOTT LIM, MD
Assistant Professor of Pediatrics
University of Virginia Health System
Charlottesville, VA

RAJAN A.G. PATEL, MD
Fellow, Cardiology
University of Virginia Health System,
Charlottesville, VA

MICHAEL RAGOSTA, MD, FACC, FSCAI
Associate Professor of Medicine
Director, Cardiac Catheterization
  Laboratories
University of Virginia Health System
Charlottesville, VA

Acknowledgments

This book originated from a desire to assemble the wisdom I gained from two of the most remarkable mentors I had as a cardiology fellow and young faculty member at the University of Virginia. Over the many years I worked with these talented individuals, first as a student and then as a colleague, Dr. Eric R. Powers and Dr. Ian J. Sarembock taught me a deep appreciation of the value of careful hemodynamic assessment in understanding cardiovascular pathophysiology, and I wish to thank them for all they taught me. My deepest gratitude goes also to the many patients suffering from cardiovascular disorders who I had the distinct privilege of serving and whose hemodynamic waveforms are included in this text from which future generations can learn. Most importantly, I want to thank my wife, Kiyoko, and my three marvelous children, Nick, Tony, and Sachi, for their support and patience and for the precious time I stole from them while writing this text.

Michael Ragosta, MD, FACC, FSCAI

Preface

Systematic analysis of pressure waveforms generated in the cardiac catheterization laboratory led to our current understanding of the pathophysiology of many valvular, congenital, myocardial and pericardial diseases. Assessment of hemodynamics has become an established component of cardiac catheterization protocols and, along with angiography, forms the basis of invasive cardiovascular diagnostic testing. However, many cardiologists and cardiology training programs currently neglect classic hemodynamic assessment, emphasizing instead the skills involved in angiography and intervention. Patients undergoing cardiac catheterization may be misdiagnosed or their condition mischaracterized because of errors in hemodynamic measurement or interpretation. In addition, recent advances in cardiovascular imaging and diagnostics have transformed the practice of cardiology to rely more heavily on echocardiograms, magnetic resonance images, and computed tomographic scans. Although these techniques offer unprecedented and exquisite anatomical details of the cardiovascular system, they have limitations regarding their ability to assess the physiologic impact of a specific disease entity. Thus, it is imperative for an astute cardiologist to be well versed in clinical hemodynamics and invasive physiologic assessment in order to correctly use and interpret diagnostic tests and to diagnose and treat many cardiac diseases.

It is the goal of this textbook to provide instruction in clinical hemodynamics from the analysis of waveforms generated in the cardiac catheterization laboratory. Normal physiology and common pathophysiologic states encountered in the cardiac catheterization laboratory and intensive care unit are covered extensively and illustrated with authentic hemodynamic waveforms collected in routine clinical practice demonstrating all important findings. This book is designed primarily as a resource for cardiologists in training, practicing cardiologists, and cardiac catheterization laboratory nurses and technicians, but may also prove useful for anyone involved in the care of cardiac patients, including cardiology nurse practitioners, physician assistants, coronary care unit nurses, and both internal medicine and critical care physicians.

Michael Ragosta, MD, FACC, FSCAI

Table of Contents

Introduction to Hemodynamic Assessment in the Cardiac Catheterization Laboratory

Michael Ragosta, MD

"Look into any man's heart you please, and you will always find, in every one, at least one black spot which he has to keep concealed."
Pillars of Society, act III
Henrik Ibsen, 1877

Despite the exhortations of poets and philosophers, the heart is, after all, simply a pump. The ability to "look into any man's heart" with the goal of understanding the function of this mysterious organ circumvented early generations of scientists and physicians. It would not take long, however, for science to garner the tools needed to peer into the hearts of men. Many of the major functions of the cardiovascular system important to our understanding of health and disease states are based on mechanical processes. Cardiac chambers contract and relax, valves open and close, and blood ebbs and flows based upon elementary principles of hydraulics. Contrast this with most other organ systems that exploit complex cellular and biochemical processes to accomplish their designated functions. For example, the kidneys balance fluid and electrolytes and excrete waste via an elaborate cellular array; the liver, pancreas, and intestinal cells digest food and absorb nutrients by a series of complicated biochemical steps, and muscle cells exert their cumulative toil through the elegant dance of complex protein molecules. The latter secrets eluded physicians and scientists, until only recently, when highly sophisticated tools became available to reveal the intricate and minute processes.

Many of the mechanical processes inherent to cardiac physiology can be understood by measuring changes in blood pressure and blood flow; the term *hemodynamics* refers to this discipline. Numerous brilliant investigators over many years applied the study of hemodynamics to collectively expand our knowledge of cardiovascular physiology in both normal and pathologic conditions. The lessons learned from these generations of researchers rapidly became assimilated into the contemporary practice of clinical cardiology. Currently, hemodynamics is considered indispensable to the clinician managing patients with cardiovascular disease and forms the foundation of invasive diagnostic cardiology.

A Brief History of Hemodynamic Assessment

All important human endeavors possess histories replete with colorful anecdotes and legendary characters. The saga of cardiac catheterization is no exception.

The practical measurement of hemodynamics in humans required several crucial developments. These included the invention of safe and reliable catheterization techniques to access and study the right and left sides of the heart, the ability to image catheter position, and the creation of devices to convert pressure changes into an interpretable graphic form.

Insertion of tubes into the bladders and rectums of living persons and the blood vessels of cadavers had been achieved since primitive times.[1] The first cardiac catheterization and pressure measurement performed on a living animal is attributed to the English physiologist Stephen Hales early in the 1700s and reported in the book *Haemastaticks* in 1733. By accessing the internal jugular vein and carotid artery of a horse, Hales performed his experiments using a brass pipe as the catheter connected by a flexible goose trachea to a long glass column of fluid. The pressure in the white mare's beating heart raised a column of fluid in the glass tube over 9 feet high.[1]

As early as 1844, the famous French physiologist Claude Bernard performed numerous animal cardiac catheterizations designed to examine the source of metabolic activity. Many prominent scientists theorized that "combustion" occurred in the lungs. Using a thermometer inserted in the carotid artery, Bernard[2] compared the temperature of blood in a living horse's left ventricle to blood in the right ventricle, accessed from the internal jugular vein, and showed slightly higher right-sided temperatures, indicating that metabolism occurred in the tissues, not in the lungs. Bernard[2] also appeared to

be the first to record intracardiac pressure using an early pressure recording system connected to the end of a glass tube inserted into a dog's right ventricle.

Later in the 1800s, in an attempt to address the controversy regarding the nature and timing of the cardiac apex beat, the French veterinarian Jean Baptiste Auguste Chauveau and physician Étienne Jules Marey performed catheterization using rubber catheters placed from a horse's jugular vein and carotid artery. These meticulous scientists recognized the importance of obtaining the highest quality data and recorded pressures in various cardiac chambers with clever mechanical devices invented by others but modified to suit their needs.[2] The graphic recordings obtained from these early transducers and physiologic recorders appear remarkably similar to those obtained in today's cardiac catheterization laboratories (Figure 1-1).

From these early explorations of cardiac pressure measurement evolved an interest to quantify blood flow. In 1870, the German mathematician and physiologist Adolph Fick[3] published his famous formula for calculating cardiac output

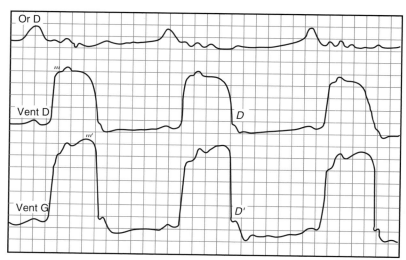

FIGURE 1-1. Early pressure recordings obtained from the cardiac chambers of a horse by Marey and Chauveau. (Reproduced with permission, Mueller RL, Sanborn TA. The history of interventional cardiology: Cardiac catheterization, angioplasty, and related interventions. *Am Heart J* 1995;129:146–172.)

(oxygen consumption divided by arterio-venous oxygen difference). However, Fick had more interest in the conceptual aspects of cardiac output determination than in its validation or application. The experiments necessary for validation of Fick's principle would fall to others more than 60 years later. Fick[3] also contributed to the emerging field of hemodynamics with his valuable work of refining early pressure recording devices.

Despite numerous animal studies over many years, the placement of a catheter into the deep recesses of a living human heart would have to wait for an accurate method to image the course and position of the catheter. This would, ultimately, be feasible only after Wilhelm Roentgen's discovery of X-rays in 1895 (Figure 1-2). The invention of an apparatus allowing us to peer inside the living human body for the first time represented one of the greatest medical advances in human history. At the start of the 20th century, it became possible to consider applying the lessons learned from animal research to humans. However, great trepidation remained among cardiovascular researchers because most considered the placement of a catheter into a living, beating human heart foolhardy with potentially deadly consequences.

Although the historical record bestows acclaim for the first human cardiac catheterization to Werner Forssmann (performed on himself in 1929), his accomplishment may have been trumped by the little known, often disputed, and poorly documented efforts of fellow Germans Fritz Bleichroeder, E. Unger, and W. Loeb[1,2] in 1905. In an effort to deliver therapeutic injections close to the targeted organ, these physicians attempted to place catheters, without radiologic guidance, into the central venous circulation via the basilic and femoral veins. During one attempt made on his colleague Bleichroeder, Unger may have actually gotten

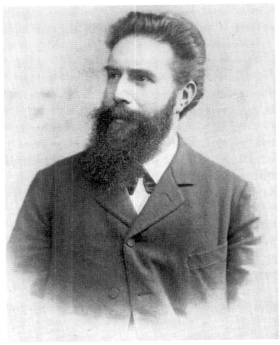

FIGURE 1-2. Wilhelm Konrad Roentgen, discoverer of the X-ray. (With permission, from Edward P, Thompson D: *Roentgen Rays and Phenomena of the Anode and Cathode.* VanNorstrand Co., NY, 1896.)

into the heart because Bleichroeder reported the development of chest pain. They could not prove this theory because they failed to document the catheter position by x-ray or pressure recording and never published their observations, attempting to gain credit only after Forssmann received his in 1929.[1]

The account of Forssmann's first cardiac catheterization on himself, for which he was awarded the Nobel Prize in Medicine and Physiology in 1956, along with André Frederic Cournand and Dickinson Woodson Richards,[2,4–7] has been recounted numerous times and with several versions, some more engaging and colorful than others. The consistently told elements of his narrative are nearly unimaginable to contemporary physicians familiar with the existing training, medicolegal, and practice environments.

The essential facts of Forssmann's story are as follows. After graduating medical school, Forssmann began training as a surgical intern at the Auguste-Viktoria Hospital in Eberswalde, Germany, a small community hospital outside Berlin (Figure 1-3). Forssmann's[6] motivation to pursue a means of instrumenting the right heart is unclear; he reported that it evolved from the desire to find a method of infusing lifesaving drugs into the heart safer than by direct intramyocardial injection. Forssmann discussed his interest with his chief, Dr. Richard Schneider, but Schneider banned the enthusiastic intern from pursuing this work, largely because he thought it unlikely that mainstream, German academic medicine would accept medical research from a community hospital. In addition, many considered placement of a catheter into the heart very dangerous; Schneider did not wish notoriety for his hospital in the event that these investigations ended poorly.

Undeterred by the prevailing lack of support, Forssmann first placed catheters into the heart of cadavers from an arm vein then, impressed with the ease at which the catheters advanced, decided to perform the experiment on himself. As he was forbidden to proceed with any

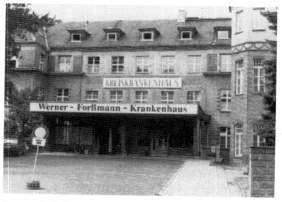

FIGURE 1-3. Werner Forssmann performed the first catheterization on himself at this hospital in Eberswalde, Germany. (Reproduced with permission, Forssmann-Falck R. Werner Forssmann: A pioneer of cardiology. *Am J Cardiol* 1997;79:651–660.)

human experimentation by Schneider, he decided to carry out his project in secret. Forssmann recruited a colleague, Peter Romeis, and a surgical nurse, Gerda Ditzen, to assist him. Forssmann's first attempt failed. Peter Romeis performed the cutdown on his cubital vein and advanced the catheter 35 cm, but he lost courage, believing it too dangerous to continue, and stopped the experiment even though Forssmann felt fine. A week later, Forssmann chose a quiet afternoon when most of the hospital staff napped, and together with his nurse accomplice gathered the surgical instruments in an empty room to perform the procedure. Gerda Ditzen insisted on being the first subject and Forssmann played along, fully intending to perform the procedure on himself. After restraining the nurse to the table and preparing her incision site with iodine, Forssmann turned from her, quickly performed the venous cutdown on his own left arm and inserted the ureteral catheter 65 cm. Ditzen became angry when she realized the deceit but quickly helped him walk down a corridor and two flights of stairs to the X-ray suite, where Forssmann confirmed the position of the catheter tip in his right atrium. Romeis apparently intercepted him in the X-ray suite to try to abort the experiment, but, according to one account, ". . . the only way Forssmann could hold him off was by kicking him in the shins."[4]

In his published account of his self-experimentation, Werner Forssmann[8] also describes a case where he used the catheter to deliver a solution of glucose, epinephrine, and strophanthin into the heart of a patient gravely ill with purulent peritonitis from a ruptured appendix. The patient died shortly after a brief period of improvement, and the autopsy confirmed the catheter position in the right atrium.

Forssmann's stunt did little to advance the field of cardiac catheterization beyond the bold demonstration that a catheter could actually be positioned safely in the human right atrium. No pressure measurements were made, and the catheter was not positioned in any other cardiac chambers. However, Forssmann had crossed the threshold and introduced the world to the potential of human cardiac catheterization.

Great turmoil and controversy followed Forssmann's publication. He failed to gain support from the medical community, and, while he continued investigations in cardiac catheterization (including at least six more self-experiments),[2] he became increasingly discouraged by the rigid, hierarchical nature of German academic medicine and became a urologist in private practice.

In the immediate years following Forssmann's success, a few isolated investigators dabbled in right-heart catheterization experiments.[1,2] However, nearly a decade would pass before there emerged a systematic discipline of right-heart catheterization exemplified by the classical work of André F. Cournand (Figure 1-4) and Dickinson W. Richards at Columbia University's First Medical Division of Bellevue Hospital. Development of right-heart catheterization arose out of Cournand and Richards's interest in pulmonary function, measurement of blood flow, and the interactions between the heart and lungs in both health and disease. In the early 1930s, the group desired to measure pulmonary blood flow using the direct Fick method; however, this would require measuring mixed venous blood from the right heart, a feat considered too dangerous. Aware of Werner Forssmann's act, the group first demonstrated safety in animals and then placed modified urethral catheters in the right atrium of humans, sampling blood for oxygen content and making determinations of blood flow using Fick's principle. By the early 1940s, a safe and valuable methodology of right-heart

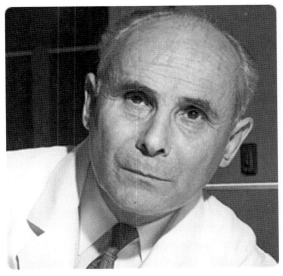

FIGURE 1-4. Winner André F. Cournand, MD, along with Dickinson W. Richards and Werner Forssmann, of the Nobel Prize in Medicine, 1956. (Reproduced with permission, Enson Y, Chamberlin MD. Cournand and Richards and the Bellevue Hospital Cardiopulmonary Laboratory. *Columbia Magazine,* Fall 2001.)

catheterization had been established and Columbia became recognized as the first "cardiopulmonary laboratory" capable of applying these techniques to the study of cardiac and pulmonary diseases. With the onset of worldwide hostilities and imminent war, the group first directed their efforts to the analysis of blood flow in traumatic shock, making important observations valuable in wartime. After the war, Cournand, Richards, and others from their group published many landmark articles describing the hemodynamic findings in congenital heart disease, cor pulmonale, valvular heart disease, and pericardial restrictive disease. Much of our current understandings of these conditions evolved from this important body of work.

Growing confidence and experience in right-heart catheterization techniques led to interest in catheterization of the left heart. Catheter access to the left heart offered unique challenges and a much greater concern about safety, and initial adventures in accessing the left heart proved highly dangerous. Proposed and attempted methods to access the left ventricle included direct apical puncture, retrograde access from puncture of the thoracic or abdominal aorta, and a sub-xiphoid entry first into the right ventricle and then followed by puncture of the interventricular septum. Methods to directly access the left atrium included a transbronchial approach via a broncho-scope and a direct, posterior paraverte-bral left atrial puncture. It is interesting that reports of experiments involving self-catheterization similar to Werner Forssmann's involving the left heart are noticeably absent from the literature.

Henry Zimmerman et al.[9] reported the first series of retrograde left-heart cathe-terizations from a left ulnar artery cut-down. This report noted failure to pass a catheter across the aortic valve from a retrograde approach in five normal sub-jects, theorizing that the normal aortic valve prevented "against the stream" passage of the catheter so they turned their attention to patients with aortic insufficiency. Zimmerman successfully entered the left ventricle in 11 patients with syphilitic aortic insufficiency. How-ever, in a single patient with rheumatic aortic insufficiency, the attempt proved fatal. Present-day cardiologists engaged in the regular performance of left-heart catheterization would find their account shocking. While attempting to pass the catheter into the left ventricle:

. . . the subject suddenly complained of substernal chest pain and the electrocardiogram which was being recorded showed the abrupt appearance of ventricular fibrillation. The catheter was immediately withdrawn. Nine cubic centimeters of 1 percent solution of procaine with 0.5 cc of a 1:1000 solution of adrenalin were injected directly into the heart without effect on the cardiac mechanism. The heart was then exposed

and massaged. This resulted in the restoration of a sinus rhythm, but the ventricular contractions were feeble and fifteen minutes after the onset of ventricular fibrillation the heart ceased beating.[9]

With a failure rate of 100% in normal patients and an initial procedural mor-tality of nearly 10%, it is a wonder that further attempts at retrograde left-heart catheterization were made. However, perseverance improved the safety and success at retrograde left-heart catheteri-zation to its currently recognized form. Additional advances included the devel-opment of trans-septal catheterization techniques, simultaneous right- and left-heart catheterization, and, of course, angiography. By the end of the 1950s, right- and left-heart catheterization had become firmly established clinical tech-niques for the evaluation of valvular, structural, and congenital heart disease.

With most of the basic elements of catheterization techniques in place, investigators turned to refinement in equipment and techniques. Catheter design represented one of the first impor-tant refinements. The stiff, unwieldy catheters available to earlier generations of cardiovascular researchers required substantial manipulative skill to position and often caused significant arrhythmia. The invention of the balloon flotation catheter exemplified by the Swan-Ganz catheter represented the innovation lead-ing to the universal acceptance and widespread practical application of hemo-dynamic assessment. The balloon flota-tion catheter became a clinical reality from the desire of Dr. Harold JC Swan, professor of medicine at the University of California, Los Angeles, and director of cardiology at Cedars-Sinai Medical Cen-ter, to apply cardiac catheterization tech-niques to study the physiology of acute myocardial infarction (Figure 1-5). In the early 1960s, cutting-edge hospitals began

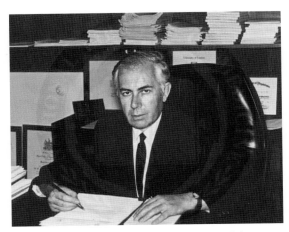

FIGURE 1-5. HJC Swan, MD, co-developer of the popular Swan-Ganz catheter. (Reproduced with permission from *U.S. National Library of Medicine.*)

to develop specialized coronary care units to care for patients with acute myocardial infarction. Designed primarily to monitor and treat arrhythmias, coronary care units also became an obvious place to study the physiology of acute myocardial infarction. Early efforts to measure hemodynamics in unstable patients with acute myocardial infarction with stiff catheters and the primitive techniques available at that time induced life-threatening arrhythmias. Cardiologists considered catheterization dangerous during the acute phase of infarction and that it carried an unacceptable risk.

Swan became aware of the work of Ronald Bradley,[10] who reported the use of very small tubing to safely instrument the pulmonary artery and measure pressures in "severely ill" patients. When Swan attempted this technique, however, he found little success in passing the flimsy, small-caliber catheters from a peripheral vein to the pulmonary artery. In addition to the dearth of techniques to access a central vein, the most likely explanation for Swan's lack of success related to the low output state of his patients compared to those of Bradley, preventing flotation of the catheter along the blood flow stream.

The answer to Swan's dilemma provides an entertaining and often told example of the near magical ability of the human mind to solve problems. Recalling this delightful story in his own words in 1991[11]:

In the fall of 1967, I had occasion to take my (then young) children to the beach in Santa Monica. On the previous evening, I had spent a frustrating hour with an extraordinary, pleasant but elderly lady in an unsuccessful attempt to place one of Bradley's catheters. It was a hot Saturday and the sailboats on the water were becalmed. However, approximately half a mile offshore, I noted a boat with a large spinnaker well set and moving through the water at a reasonable velocity. The idea then came to put a sail or a parachute on the end of a highly flexible catheter and thereby increase the frequency of passage of the device into the pulmonary artery. I felt convinced that this approach would allow for rapid and safe placement of a flotation catheter without the use of fluoroscopy and would solve the problem of arrhythmias.

Edwards Laboratories worked with Swan to create the first five prototype catheters that relied on a balloon to accomplish flotation rather than parachutes or sails. (Interestingly, an early form of a balloon flotation catheter was described by Lategola and Rahn and failed to gain the attention of cardiovascular investigators; it did, however, prevent Swan from obtaining a patent on the idea[11]).

Swan had previously hired William Ganz, an immigrant from the former Czechoslovakia and survivor of the World War II labor camps, to work in the experimental laboratory at Cedars of Lebanon Hospital. The first animal experiments performed by Ganz with the prototype catheters were a brilliant success. Once the catheter was advanced into the right atrium and the balloon inflated, the catheter quickly migrated across the tricuspid valve and out the pulmonary artery to the wedge position, confirming Swan's notion. The catheters were tried in humans with similar success and led to the landmark publication in the *New England Journal of Medicine.*[12] The group further refined the catheter's design, and Ganz added a thermistor to measure cardiac output by the thermodilution technique. Swan recognized that the catheter and procedure's success as a universally accepted bedside tool required that the technique be safe, easy to use, and not interfere with routine nursing care in the intensive care unit. According to Swan[11]:

. . . right heart catheterization became so routine and simple that the then Director of the Diagnostic Catheterization Laboratory, Dr. Harold Marcus, stated that he would ban the device because it was impossible to train the cardiac fellows in the appropriate manipulations of right heart catheters.

The core elements of diagnostic cardiac catheterization and hemodynamic assessment have changed little since the 1970s. Innumerable additional contributors have refined catheterization techniques and expanded our knowledge of hemodynamics in health and disease; the valuable contributions of these notable leaders will be presented in subsequent chapters of this book.

While the bulk of attention is paid to the colorful pioneers of cardiac catheterization, the important role of the unglamorous physiologic recorder in the advancement of the science of hemodynamics is often ignored. In fact, the development of accurate physiologic recording equipment provided substantial challenges. The contributions made by mostly anonymous geniuses are easily forgotten but were as crucial to the development of cardiac catheterization as

Roentgen's discovery of X-rays or Werner Forssmann's audacious self-experiments.

We take for granted the formidable task of translating a pressure wave sampled at the tip of the catheter to a graphic representation plotted as pressure versus time. The early pioneers of heart catheterization recorded intracardiac pressures in animals with primitive transducers consisting of elastic membranes attached to the catheter and using water-filled manometers that recorded pressure via a system of levers to a chart recorder *(sphygmograph).*[2] Springs and other clever mechanical adaptations to the devices improved their performance. Early in the 20th century, several individuals made key contributions in this field. Carl J. Wiggers[13] represents one of the key innovators in the development of high-fidelity pressure recording instruments. He is credited with the invention of the Wiggers manometer, the first optical manometer. The optical manometer was based on work originally conceptualized by Otto Frank. Wiggers spent time in Frank's Munich lab but was quite taken aback by Frank's secretive nature. Wiggers noted[13]:

Such a restrictive attitude in sharing newly developed apparatus was contrary to my scientific upbringing and threatened to frustrate my future use of them. Therefore, I connived with the laboratory mechanic who could use some extra money to make copies for me. In a sense, therefore, I smuggled the equipment I needed out of the laboratory.

The configuration of Wiggers's optical manometer consisted of the catheter attached to a fluid-filled chamber. At the end of small side arm from this chamber was an elastic membrane. A small mirror attached to this membrane reflected a light focused onto a light-sensitive recording paper. In this way, pressure changes from the catheter would be transmitted to the fluid-filled chamber and then to the membrane. The light beam essentially functioned as a weight-less lever arm and a very sensitive method of reproducing rapid pressure changes. This innovation allowed the first high-fidelity measurements of intra-cardiac pressure (Figure 1-6). Subsequent modifications by William F. Hamilton[14] provided the essential equipment used in Cournand and Richards's laboratory at Bellevue. Measuring and recording hemodynamics in that era required great patience and effort as demonstrated in this description[14]:

Once the catheter was in place, all lights in the room were turned off, and the Hamilton manometer (which focused a light on sensitive paper to record the pressure contour) was attached to the catheter and manipulated in absolute darkness so that its light output could be captured with a handheld mirror and adjusted to strike the paper. Researchers could then record intravascular pressures.

Advances in electronics changed the physiologic recorder. Oscilloscopes replaced the Hamilton manometer; the new systems converted catheter pressure to an electrical output displayed on cathode ray tubes. Many of us still recall the old-fashioned chart recorders that used mechanical stylets to trace the pressure contour onto heat-sensitive paper for later analysis and storage (Figure 1-7). These apparatuses have been replaced by tiny, cheap, and dis-posable table-mounted pressure transdu-cers capable of converting a mechanical force to an electrical one, with sub-sequent conversion of this electrical sig-nal in the "black box" of an advanced computer to the colorful graphic display to that we have become accustomed (Figure 1-8).

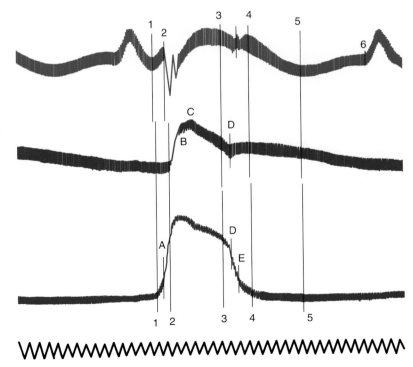

FIGURE 1-6. High-fidelity re-cordings obtained by Carl Wiggers in 1921 from the right atrium *(top)*, pulmonary artery *(middle)*, and right ventricle *(bottom)* of a dog, using the optical manometer. (Reproduced with permission, Reeves JT. Carl J. Wiggers and the pulmonary circulation: A young man in search of excellence. *Am J Physiol [Lung Cell Mol Physiol]* 1998;18:L467–474.)

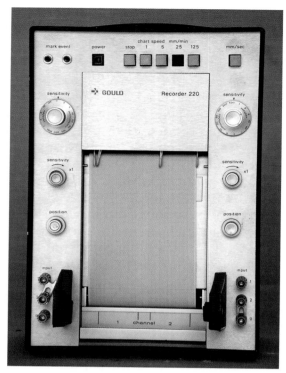

FIGURE 1-7. Mechanical recorder used to collect hemodynamics and popular in the 1980s and early 1990s.

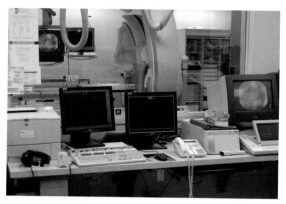

FIGURE 1-8. Modern cardiac catheterization laboratory outfitted with computerized hemodynamic monitoring systems used by the University of Virginia Cardiac Catheterization Laboratories, circa 2006.

Hemodynamic Assessment in Modern Clinical Practice

The ease at which we can now assess cardiovascular hemodynamics has established cardiac catheterization as a routine diagnostic procedure. Nearly all of the thousands of cardiac catheterizations performed each day in the United States measure left ventricular and aortic pressures; nearly a third of these also include assessment of right heart pressures and cardiac output. Many additional patients undergo right-heart catheterization alone in the cardiac catheterization laboratory. Medical, surgical, and coronary intensive care units contribute innumerable additional right-heart catheterization procedures performed at the bedside in critically ill patients, and anesthesiologists rely on right heart pressure monitoring during many high risk surgical procedures in the operating room. Thus, hemodynamic assessment has become an integral and established part of the daily practices of cardiologists, pulmonologists, anesthesiologists, surgeons, and intensivists.

There are many indications for invasive hemodynamic assessment. For patients referred to the cardiac catheterization laboratory, right- and left-heart catheterization is often performed for the evaluation and management of heart failure syndromes, shock, unexplained dyspnea, hypotension, respiratory failure, renal failure, edema, valvular heart disease, pericardial disease, hypertrophic cardiomyopathy, or congenital heart disease. Patients with unusual chest pain syndromes may require right-heart catheterization to exclude pulmonary hypertension. Most patients who undergo cardiac catheterization mainly for the evaluation of the coronary arteries, as seen in stable angina, abnormal stress tests, acute coronary syndromes, or uncomplicated myocardial infarction, require only measurement of left heart and aortic pressure. However, postmyocardial infarction patients who exhibit hypotension, serious arrhythmia, or heart failure, or in the case of a suspected complication such as right ventricular infarction, ventricular septal defect or mitral regurgitation should also undergo a careful right-heart catheterization. Patients under evaluation for heart or lung transplantation often undergo right-heart catheterization to identify pulmonary hypertension and, if present, a determination of reversibility by pharmacologic administration of a vasodilator agent.

Common indications for the bedside use of right-heart catheterization in patients with cardiac disease include the differentiation of cardiogenic from non-cardiogenic causes of pulmonary edema, profound hypotension or shock and the guidance of therapy in patients with heart failure, pulmonary edema, pulmonary hypertension or shock particularly if there is renal impairment. Detailed recommendations on the indications and use of bedside right-heart catheterization have been provided.[15]

Equipment

The essential components of a hemodynamic monitoring system include a catheter, a transducer, fluid-filled tubing to connect the catheter to the transducer, and a physiologic recorder to display, analyze, print, and store the hemodynamic waveforms generated.

A variety of catheters are available for pressure sampling (Figure 1-9). The optimal catheter for hemodynamic measurements is stiff to transmit the pressure wave to the transducer without absorption by the catheter, is easy and safe to position, and has a relatively large lumen opening to an end hole. The use of an end-hole catheter is especially important when sampling pressures within small chambers or when discerning pressure gradients over relatively small areas. An end-hole catheter may lead to damping or other artifact if the end-hole comes into contact with the wall of the cardiac chamber. The commonly used "pig-tail" catheter has multiple side-holes and samples pressure at each of these openings, resulting in a tracing representing a mixture of the pressure waves collected at each opening. Such catheters are adequate if sampling pressure in a large, uniform chamber such as the aorta or left ventricle. It will not, however, have the required resolution to discern pressure gradients within the left ventricle. Catheters with an end-hole and side-holes at

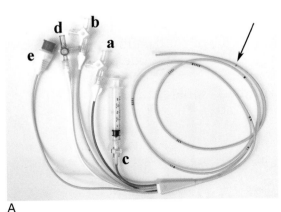
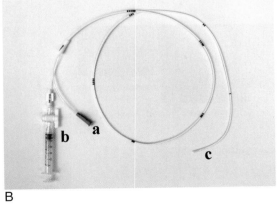

A   B

FIGURE 1-9. Catheters used for collecting hemodynamic measurements. **A,** The popular Swan-Ganz catheter. This model has four ports consisting of a proximal lumen *(a)*, a distal lumen *(b)*, and the balloon port *(c)*, which inflates the balloon mounted at the tip of the catheter. There is an extra infusion port *(d)* on this model. The thermistor for performance of thermodilution cardiac outputs connects to the computer via a connecting plug *(e)*. The catheter has 10-cm increments marked by lines *(arrow)*. **B,** Example of a Berman catheter. This is used for hemodynamics but also for angiography. There is a port connecting to the distal lumen *(a)* and a balloon inflation port *(b)*. There are multiple side-holes to allow angiography at the tip of the catheter *(c)*.

just the tip prevent damping or artifactual waveforms due to positioning of the catheter tip against the chamber wall and are useful for collecting samples for oxygen saturation. The Swan-Ganz catheter is the most commonly used catheter for measuring right-heart pressures. In addition to the balloon at the tip for flotation, it consists of an end-hole (distal port), a side-hole 30 cm from the catheter tip (proximal port), and a thermistor for measurement of thermodilution cardiac output. This catheter is used extensively in modern cardiac catheterization laboratories as well as at the bedside for invasive monitoring. Other balloon flotation catheters include the Berman catheter, which is constructed of multiple side-holes near the tip and no end-hole or thermistor and is used principally for performance of angiography, and the balloon-wedge catheter, which contains an end-hole similar to the Swan-Ganz catheter but no thermistor for cardiac output measurement or additional infusion or pressure monitoring ports. Other catheters rarely used today for pressure measurement or for blood sampling during right-heart catheterization do not use

balloon flotation to assist in catheter positioning and must be directed carefully through the cardiac chambers under fluoroscopic guidance by the operator. These include the Layman catheter and Cournand catheter consisting of an end-hole, the NIH catheter that contains multiple side-holes near the tip but no end-hole, and the Goodale-Lubin catheter consisting of an end-hole and two single side-holes near the tip and used mostly for blood sampling.

Transducers and tubing constitute the next important component of the hemodynamic measurement system. Table mounted, fluid-filled transducers currently used by most catheterization laboratories and intensive care units are inexpensive and disposable (Figure 1-10). The pressure wave is transmitted through the fluid-filled catheter to a membrane in the transducer and deforms the membrane resulting in a change in electrical resistance. This electrical signal is transmitted to the analyzing computer and converted to a graphic representation of the pressure wave. These relatively inexpensive transducers are factory calibrated but require "zeroing." They sometimes

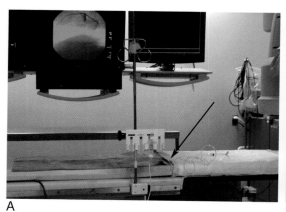
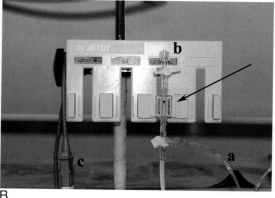

A   B

FIGURE 1-10. Setup for a table-mounted transducer used for pressure measurement in the cardiac catheterization laboratory. **A,** The general configuration. The catheter used to sample pressure is connected to a high-pressure tubing *(arrow).* A close-up view of the transducer is shown in **B** *(arrow).* The high-pressure tubing connecting to the patient attaches by a stopcock to the transducer *(a).* Another stopcock allows flushing and equilibration with air *(b).* The transducer connects by a cable to the hemodynamic computer *(c).*

do not hold calibration or a "zero" during use so should be replaced if suspicious or faulty data are obtained.

Fluid-filled systems are acceptable for clinical purposes but are subject to measuring artifact. The catheter and connecting tubing should be stiff; soft tubing will absorb the pressure wave, damping and distorting it. In addition, the catheter as well as the tubing connecting the catheter and transducer should be as short as possible, with as few connections as possible to prevent timing delays, pressure damping, and a potential source of air bubbles. Great care should be taken to prevent kinking of the catheter or introducing air or clot within the catheter or tubing because this will distort the waveform and lead to inaccuracies. Under certain circumstances, pressure may be measured directly in the cardiac chamber or vessel by use of a tiny transducer (micromanometer) mounted at the tip of a catheter, avoiding the limitations of a fluid-filled system. This is often the case when precise hemodynamic measurements are required as part of a research study but also form the basis of the pressure wire used for measurement of intracoronary pressure, which will be discussed in a later chapter.

Finally, a variety of proprietary computer systems are available for displaying, printing, and storing hemodynamic waveforms. The major systems in use are universally excellent and perform many of the analyses and calculations previously done manually. These systems analyze the waveforms and automatically identify systolic and diastolic pressure values. It is important to note, however, that the recognition algorithms in these systems occasionally misidentify waveforms, particularly if there is artifact in the waveform or on the electrocardiogram. For instance, left ventricular end diastolic pressure or pulmonary artery systolic pressure may not be properly identified if there is catheter whip or marked respiratory variation. It is important for the operator to compare his or her own interpretation of the waveforms with the numbers provided by the computer to ensure accurate reporting of these values.

Catheterization Protocols

During a complete right- and left-heart catheterization, the following routine is generally followed (Table 1-1). After obtaining arterial and venous access, the physician positions the Swan-Ganz catheter in the pulmonary artery and a pigtail catheter in the aorta. Thermodilution cardiac output is measured and blood sampled from the aorta and the pulmonary artery to calculate cardiac output using the Fick principle and to screen for an intracardiac shunt. Aortic and pulmonary artery pressures are measured and then the pigtail catheter advanced in a retrograde fashion across the aortic valve and into the left ventricle. The Swan-Ganz catheter is advanced to the

---

TABLE 1-1. Components of a Routine Complete Right- and Left-Heart Catheterization

1. Position pulmonary artery (PA) catheter.
2. Position aortic (AO) catheter.
3. Measure PA and AO pressure.
4. Measure thermodilution cardiac output.
5. Measure oxygen saturation in PA and AO blood samples to determine Fick output and screen for shunt.
6. Enter the left ventricle (LV) by retrograde crossing of the AO valve.
7. Advance PA catheter to pulmonary capillary wedge position (PCWP).
8. Measure simultaneous LV-PCWP.
9. Pull back from PCWP to PA.
10. Pull back from PA to right ventricle (RV) to screen for pulmonic stenosis and record RV.
11. Record simultaneous LV-RV.
12. Pull back from RV to right atrium (RA) to screen for tricuspid stenosis and record RA.
13. Pull back from LV to AO to screen for aortic stenosis.

pulmonary capillary wedge position and simultaneous left ventricular and pulmonary capillary wedge pressure measured to screen for the presence of mitral stenosis. Pressure recordings are obtained from each chamber as the right-sided catheter is withdrawn with careful attention paid as the catheter crosses the pulmonic and tricuspid valves to screen for valvular lesions. Simultaneous right ventricular and left ventricular pressure recordings are obtained to screen for restrictive/constrictive physiology. Finally, careful observation of the pressure waveform, as the left ventricular catheter is pulled back into the aorta, serves as a screen for aortic valve stenosis.

As in most procedures, there are few "absolute" contraindications to cardiac catheterization. The risk-benefit ratio should be carefully considered in each individual. Relative contraindications for invasive hemodynamic assessment relate to patient features that increase procedural risk. While generally considered safe, there are multiple, serious potential complications from right- and left-heart catheterization (Table 1-2). The most commonly observed complications relate to the access site, with hematoma, bleeding, and vessel injury not infrequent. Thus, significant coagulopathy or thrombocytopenia or treatment with anticoagulant or thrombolytic drugs increases the risk of the procedure. Careful consideration should be made in patients with active infections, particularly bacteremia. Left-heart catheterization is frequently avoided in patients with known left ventricular thrombus or active aortic valve endocarditis to minimize the risk of embolization. Arrhythmias are commonly seen during catheterization; most are due to catheter position, are transient, and of no clinical consequence. However, high-grade atrioventricular block can arise if the patient has underlying conduction

TABLE 1-2.   Some Potential Risks of Right- and Left-Heart Catheterization

1. Access site complications
   Bleeding
   Hematoma
   Vessel injury
   Nerve injury
   Infection
   Pseudoaneurysm formation
   Arteriovenous fistula formation
   Pneumothorax (for internal jugular vein puncture)
   Inadvertent arterial puncture
2. Arrhythmia
   Ventricular tachycardia, ventricular fibrillation
   Atrial arrhythmia, supraventricular tachycardia
   Transient bundle branch block
   Heart block
3. Myocardial infarction
4. Stroke
5. Infection
   Bacteremia
   Endocarditis
6. Pulmonary embolism/infarction
7. Pulmonary artery rupture
8. Vessel or cardiac chamber perforation
9. Catheter entrapment
10. Cholesterol embolization
11. Renal failure
12. Death

abnormalities. Catheter placement in the right ventricular outflow tract can lead to right bundle branch block; left bundle branch block may arise when the aortic valve is crossed. Thus, patients with existing left bundle branch block may develop complete block when right-heart catheterization is performed; similarly, patients with underlying right bundle branch block may develop complete heart block when the catheter crosses the aortic valve during a left-heart catheterization. Normal conduction is generally restored with prompt removal of the offending catheter but may persist for some time and even require placement of a temporary pacemaker. Catheterization should be postponed, if possible, in patients with serious electrolyte or metabolic disarray because these may predispose the patient to development of ventricular or atrial arrhythmias during catheterization.

References

1. Mueller RL, Sanborn TA. The history of interventional cardiology: Cardiac catheterization, angioplasty, and related interventions. *Am Heart J* 1995; 129:146–172.
2. Cournand AF. Cardiac catheterization. *Acta Med Scand* 1975;579(Suppl):7–32.
3. Acierno LJ. Adolph Fick: Mathematician, physicist, physiologist. *Clin Cardiol* 2000;23:390–391.
4. Fenster JM. *Mavericks, Miracles and Medicine. The Pioneers Who Risked Their Lives to Bring Medicine into the Modern Age.* Carroll and Graf Publishers, NY, 2003.
5. Fontenot C, O'Leary JP. Dr. Werner Forssman's self-experimentation. *Am Surg* 1996;62:514–515.
6. Steckelberg JM, Vlietstra RE, Ludwig J, Mann RJ. Werner Forssmann (1904–1979) and his unusual success story. *Mayo Clin Proc* 1979;54:746–748.
7. Forssmann-Falck R. Werner Forssmann: A pioneer of cardiology. *Am J Cardiol* 1997;79:651–660.
8. Forssmann W. Die Sondierung des rechten Herzens. *Klin wochenschr* 1929;8:2085–2087.
9. Zimmerman HA, Scott RW, Becker NO. Catheterization of the left side of the heart in man. *Circulation* 1950;1:357–359.
10. Bradley RD. Diagnostic right heart catheterization with miniature catheters in severely ill patients. *Lancet* 1964;284:941–942.
11. Swan HJC. The pulmonary artery catheter. *Disease-a-Month* 1991;37:478–508.
12. Swan HJ, Ganz W, Forrester J. Catheterization of the heart in man with use of a flow-directed balloon-tipped catheter. *N Engl J Med* 1970;283:447–451.
13. Reeves JT, Carl J. Wiggers and the pulmonary circulation: A young man in search of excellence. *Am J Physiol (Lung Cell Mol Physiol)* 1998;18:L467–474.
14. Enson Y, Chamberlin MD. Cournand and Richards and the Bellevue Hospital Cardiopulmonary Laboratory. *Columbia Magazine,* Fall 2001.
15. Mueller HS, Chatterjee K, Davis KB, et al. Present use of bedside right heart catheterization in patients with cardiac disease. *J Am Coll Cardiol* 1998;32:840–864.

CHAPTER 2

Normal Waveforms, Artifacts, and Pitfalls

MICHAEL RAGOSTA, MD

The proper collection and interpretation of hemodynamic waveforms are important components of cardiac catheterization often overshadowed by more glamorous aspects of invasive cardiology, such as angiography and coronary intervention. Accurate intracardiac pressure measurements provide invaluable physiologic information in both normal and pathologic states; poorly gathered or erroneously interpreted waveforms may lead to an incorrect diagnosis or a poor clinical decision. It is imperative that competent cardiologists understand normal and abnormal hemodynamic waveforms and are capable of troubleshooting problems and recognizing common artifacts and potential pitfalls during the collection of hemodynamic data.

Generation of Pressure Waveforms

The goal of a hemodynamic study is to accurately reproduce and analyze the changes in pressure that occur during the cardiac cycle within a cardiac chamber. These rapidly occurring events represent mechanical forces and require conversion to an electrical signal to be transmitted and subsequently translated into an interpretable, graphic format. The pressure transducer is the essential component that translates the mechanical forces to electrical signals. The transducer may be located at the tip of the catheter (micromanometer) within the chamber or, more commonly, the pressure transducer is outside of the body, and a pressure waveform is transmitted from the catheter tip to the transducer through a column of fluid. These transducers consist of a diaphragm or membrane attached to a strain-gauge-Wheatstone bridge arrangement. When a fluid wave strikes the diaphragm, an electrical current is generated with a magnitude dependent on the strength of the force that deflects the membrane. The output current is amplified and displayed as pressure versus time.

During the cardiac cycle, changes in pressure occur rapidly, corresponding with various physiologic events. The force wave created by these events generates a spectrum of wave frequencies. Consider, for example, the different events that occur within the aorta throughout a single cardiac cycle. Beginning with left ventricular ejection, the aortic valve opens, causing pressure to rise in the aorta, rapidly reaching a peak, then falling quickly following peak ejection. Closure of the aortic valve represents another event, marking the end of systole, and is associated with a slight rise in pressure followed by pressure decay during ventricular diastole until the next ventricular contraction. All of these events occur rapidly and are associated with varying wave frequencies. When the force wave strikes the transducer, it should precisely reproduce all of these events. The full range of frequencies needed to reproduce all of these force waves requires a sensing membrane capable of a rapid frequency response (0–20 cycles/second in the human heart). However, the physical properties of a membrane capable of such a wide frequency response might resonate, creating artifacts. This phenomenon is similar to the sound that a bell makes, continuing to oscillate after initially struck. Resonation artifact appears on the waveform as excessive "noise," but reverberations can also lead to harmonic amplification of the waveform overestimating systolic pressure and underestimating diastolic pressure (Figure 2-1). Therefore, hemodynamic measurement systems need to provide some level of "damping" to reduce resonation artifacts. Damping is a method of eliminating the oscillation; it may be done by the introduction of friction to reduce the oscillation of the sensing membrane, or it may be accomplished electrically by damping algorithms. However, note the importance that damping reduces the frequency response and may result in loss of information. Over-damping results in loss of rapid, high-frequency events (for example, the dicrotic notch on the aortic waveform), causing underestimation of the systolic pressure and overestimation of the diastolic pressure. The ideal pressure tracing has the proper balance of frequency response and damping.

Calibration, Balancing, and Zeroing

Previous generations of transducers required calibration against a mercury manometer; the factory-calibrated, disposable, fluid-filled transducers in clinical use today no longer need this. Table-mounted transducers do require balancing or "zeroing," which refers to the establishment of a reference point for subsequent pressure measurements. The reference or "zero" position should be determined before any measurements are made. By convention, it is defined at the patient's midchest in the anteroposterior dimension at the level of the sternal angle of Louis (fourth intercostal space) (Figure 2-2). This site is an estimation of the location of the right atrium and is also known as the *phlebostatic axis*. A table-mounted transducer is placed at this level and the stopcock is opened to air (atmospheric pressure) and set to zero by the hemodynamic system. The system is now ready for pressure measurements.

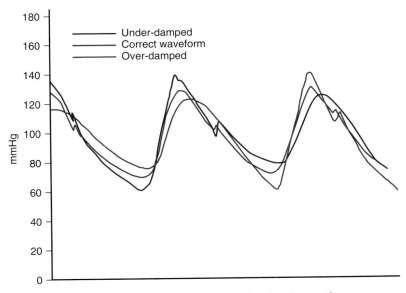

FIGURE 2-1. Schematic representation of the effects of over- or under-damping on the pressure waveform. An under-damped waveform will overestimate systolic pressure and underestimate diastolic pressure, whereas over-damping will have the opposite effects. In addition, the over-damped waveform obscures subtle hemodynamic findings, such as the dicrotic notch.

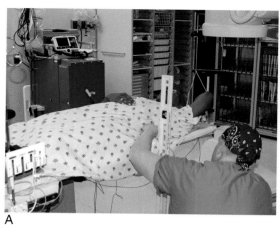 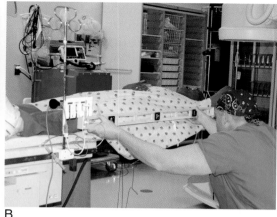

A   B

FIGURE 2-2. **A,** Demonstration of the "zero" position or phlebostatic axis representing a point midway in the antero-posterior chest dimension at the fourth intercostal space. **B,** Table-mounted transducers are positioned at this point using a level to ensure accuracy.

The tradition of using the midaxillary line as the zero position has been called into question. Because of the influence of hydrostatic pressure, in the supine position, and use of fluid-filled transducers, some physicians believe that setting the zero position as the upper border of the left ventricle is more accurate.[1] The difference between this location and the conventional location provides greatest accuracy in diastolic pressure measurements. However, most routine labs find this approach impractical because it requires the use of echocardiography to determine the precise location; it is more applicable to research investigations. A major advantage of the midchest position is that it has been shown to correlate with the position of the left atrium by magnetic resonance imaging studies regardless of the patient's age, gender, body habitus, or presence of chronic lung disease.[2] Frequently, busy catheterization laboratories might position the transducer at the same level for all patients or from a measured, fixed distance from either the table or from the top of the patient's chest, without taking into consideration the variations in patient position or body habitus. This practice will lead to marked inaccuracies, particularly in patients who are unable to lie flat or who are at the extremes of body weight. A transducer placed *above* the true zero position will furnish a measured pressure *lower* than the actual pressure; a transducer placed *below* the true zero position will result in a pressure measurement *higher* than the actual pressure. These small pressure changes caused by improper zeroing may lead to significant errors in diagnosis and, perhaps, inappropriate therapy.

Transducer *drift* refers to either the loss of calibration or loss of balance after initially setting the zero level. This is not uncommon. Many patients have been started on pressors for hypotension or a patient falsely diagnosed with mitral stenosis because of inaccurate transducer balancing, improper zero positioning, or transducer drifting. Careful attention to this aspect is important for proper interpretation.

Normal Physiology and Waveform Characteristics

Interpretation of pressure waveforms requires a consistent and systematic approach (Table 2-1). After confirming the zero level, the scale of the recording

TABLE 2-1.	A Systematic Approach to Hemodynamic Interpretation

1. Establish the zero level and balance transducer.
2. Confirm the scale of the recording.
3. Collect hemodynamics in a systematic method using established protocols.
4. Critically assess the pressure waveforms for proper fidelity.
5. Carefully time pressure events with the ECG.
6. Review the tracings for common artifacts.

is noted and a recording sweep speed is determined. Establishing standard protocols is helpful to ensure that all necessary information is collected in a systematic format (see Chapter 1). Careful scrutiny of the waveform ensures a high-fidelity recording without over- or under-damping. Each pressure event should be timed with the electrocardiogram (ECG). Finally, the operator should review the tracings for the presence of common artifacts that might lead to misinterpretation.

Note the importance of multiple events and their interrelationship to properly interpret pressure waveforms, particularly in disease states. Figure 2-3 demonstrates the three basic waveforms (atrial, ventricular, and arterial) and their relationships to key electrical and physiologic events during the normal cardiac cycle. Each waveform will be described in detail in the following sections.

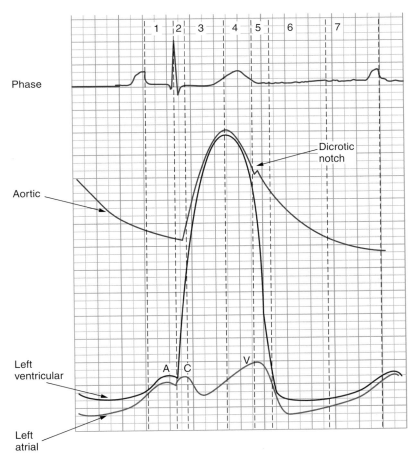

FIGURE 2-3. Timing of the major electrical and mechanical events during the cardiac cycle. Phase 1 = atrial contraction; Phase 2 = isovolumic contraction; Phase 3 = rapid ejection; Phase 4 = reduced ejection; Phase 5 = isovolumic relaxation; Phase 6 = rapid ventricular filling; and Phase 7 = reduced ventricular filling.

Right Atrial Waveform

The normal right atrial pressure is 2–6 mmHg and is characterized by *a* and *v* waves and *x* and *y* descents (Figure 2-4). The *a* wave represents the pressure rise within the right atrium due to atrial contraction and follows the *P* wave on the ECG by about 80 msec. The *x* descent represents the pressure decay following the *a* wave and reflects both atrial relaxation and the sudden downward motion of the atrioventricular (AV) junction that occurs because of ventricular systole. An *a* wave is usually absent in atrial fibrillation, but the *x* descent may be present because of this latter phenomenon (Figure 2-5). A *c* wave is sometimes observed after the *a* wave and is due to the sudden motion of the tricuspid annulus toward the right atrium at the onset of ventricular systole. The *c* wave follows the *a* wave by the same time as the PR interval on the ECG; the first-degree AV block results in a more obvious *c* wave (Figure 2-6). When a *c* wave is present, the pressure decay following it is called an x^1 descent.

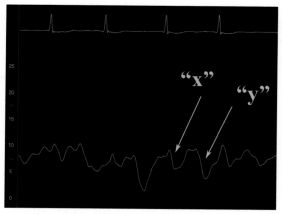

FIGURE 2-5. Right atrial waveform obtained in a patient with chronic atrial fibrillation, demonstrating persistence of the *x* descent despite loss of the *a* wave.

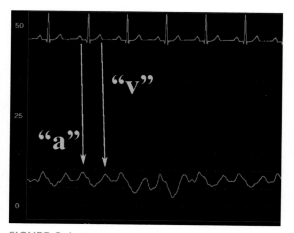

FIGURE 2-4. An example of a normal right atrial pressure waveform. Note the timing from the electrocardiographic *P* and *T* waves to the hemodynamic *a* and *v* waves, respectively.

The next pressure event is the *v* wave. A misunderstanding exists regarding the *v* wave. Although this event is occurring at the same time as ventricular systole, when the tricuspid valve is closed, the pressure rise responsible for the *v* wave is due to passive venous filling of the atrium, representing atrial diastole. Increased filling of the right atrium results in greater prominence of the *v* wave. The peak of the right atrial *v* wave occurs at the end of ventricular systole, when the atria are maximally filled and corresponds with the end of the T wave on the surface ECG. The pressure decay that occurs after the *v* wave is the *y* descent and is due to rapid emptying of the right atrium when the tricuspid valve opens. Atrial contraction follows this event and the onset of another cardiac cycle. In normal right atrial waveforms, the *a* wave typically exceeds the *v* wave. During inspiration, the mean right atrial pressure decreases due to the influence of decreased intrathoracic pressure, and there is augmentation of passive right ventricular filling; the *y* descents become more prominent (Figure 2-7).

FIGURE 2-6. Example of a right atrial waveform with prominence of the *c* wave due to the presence of first-degree AV block.

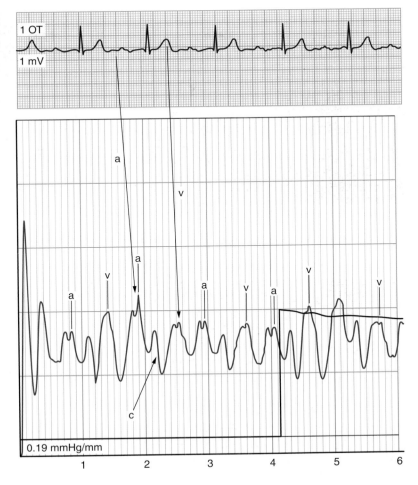

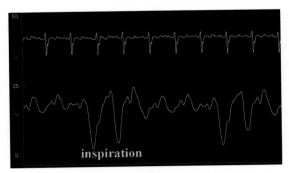

FIGURE 2-7. With inspiration, the *x* and *y* descents become more prominent on the right atrial waveform.

Right Ventricular Waveform

The normal right ventricular systolic pressure is 20–30 mmHg, and the normal right ventricular end-diastolic pressure is 0–8 mmHg. Right ventricular

tracings exhibit the characteristic features of ventricular waveforms with rapid pressure rise during ventricular contraction and rapid pressure decay during relaxation with a diastolic phase characterized by an initially low pressure that gradually increases (Figure 2-8). The right atrial pressure should be within a few mmHg of right ventricular end-diastolic pressure unless there is tricuspid stenosis. With atrial contraction, an *a* wave may appear on the ventricular waveform at end-diastole (Figure 2-9), which is not a normal finding because the normal, compliant right ventricle typically absorbs the atrial component without a significant pressure rise. Therefore, the presence of the *a* wave on a right ventricular waveform usually

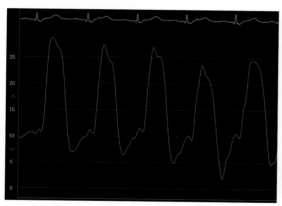

FIGURE 2-8. Example of a normal right ventricular waveform.

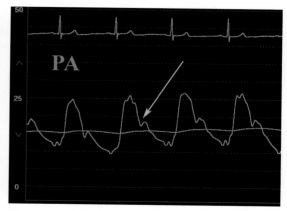

FIGURE 2-10. An example of a normal pulmonary artery waveform. Note the dicrotic notch *(arrow)*.

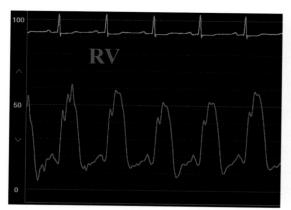

FIGURE 2-9. Right ventricular waveform obtained in a patient with pulmonary hypertension and right ventricular hypertrophy, demonstrating prominent *a* waves.

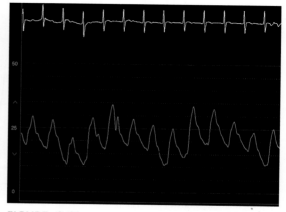

FIGURE 2-11. Respiratory variation in a pulmonary artery pressure wave.

indicates decreased compliance from pulmonary hypertension, right ventricular hypertrophy, or volume overload.

Pulmonary Artery Waveform

The normal pulmonary artery systolic pressure is 20–30 mmHg, and the normal diastolic pressure is 4–12 mmHg (Figure 2-10). A systolic pressure difference should not exist between the right ventricle and the pulmonary artery unless there is pulmonary valvular or pulmonary artery stenosis. The pulmonary artery pressure tracing is similar to

other arterial waveforms, with a rapid rise in pressure, systolic peak, a pressure decay associated with a well-defined dicrotic notch from pulmonic valve closure, and a diastolic trough. Peak systolic pressure occurs within the *T* wave on the surface ECG.

The pulmonary artery waveform, like other right heart chamber pressure waveforms, is subject to respiratory changes (Figure 2-11). Inspiration decreases intrathoracic pressure, and expiration increases intrathoracic pressure. The pressure changes associated with respiration transmitted to the cardiac chambers are often small and of little consequence.

However, patients on mechanical ventilators, with pulmonary disease or morbid obesity or in respiratory distress, may generate substantial changes in intrathoracic pressure, resulting in marked differences in pulmonary artery pressures during the respiratory phases (Figure 2-12). Most experts consider end-expiration to be the proper point to assess pulmonary artery (and other cardiac chamber) pressures because it is at this phase that intrathoracic pressure is closest to zero.[3] The pulmonary artery end-diastolic pressure is sometimes used as an estimation of the left atrial pressure; however, it is highly inaccurate, especially if the pulmonary vascular resistance is abnormal.[4]

Pulmonary Capillary Wedge Pressure Waveform

The normal mean pulmonary capillary wedge pressure, or PCWP, is 2–14 mmHg (Figure 2-13). A true PCWP can be measured only in the absence of anterograde flow in the pulmonary artery and with an end-hole catheter, such that pressure is transmitted through an uninterrupted fluid column from the left atrium, through the pulmonary veins and pulmonary capillary bed to the catheter tip wedged in the pulmonary artery. Under these circumstances, the PCWP is a reflection of left atrial pressure with *a* and *v* waves and *x* and *y* descents.

The PCWP tracing exhibits several important differences from a directly measured atrial pressure waveform. The *c* wave, sometimes identified in an atrial waveform, is absent because of the damped nature of the pressure wave. The *v* wave typically exceeds the *a* wave on the PCWP tracing. Because the pressure wave is transmitted through the pulmonary capillary bed, a significant time delay occurs between an electrocardiographic event and the onset of the corresponding pressure wave. The delay may vary substantially, depending on the distance the pressure wave travels.

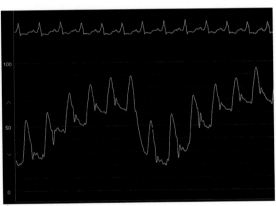

A

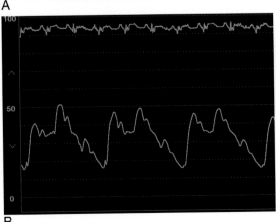

B

FIGURE 2-12. Marked respiratory variation in pulmonary artery pressure. **A,** A patient with marked pulmonary hypertension. **B,** A patient with morbid obesity.

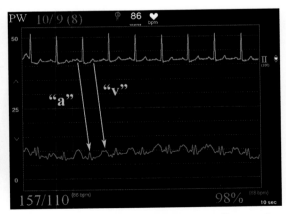

FIGURE 2-13. A normal pulmonary capillary wedge pressure waveform with distinct *a* and *v* waves.

Shorter delays are observed when the PCWP is obtained with the catheter tip in a more distal location. Typically, the peak of the *a* wave follows the *P* wave on the ECG by about 240 msec rather than 80 msec, as seen in the right atrial tracing.[5] Similarly, the peak of the *v* wave occurs after the T wave has already been inscribed on the ECG. The relation between a true left atrial pressure and the PCWP is shown in Figure 2-14. Note the time delay between the same physiologic events and the "damped" nature of the PCWP relative to the left-atrial (LA) waveform, with a pressure slightly lower than the left atrium it is meant

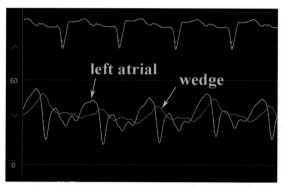

FIGURE 2-14. Relationship between the left atrial (LA) and pulmonary capillary wedge pressure (PCWP) waveforms. Note the time delay on the PCWP for the same events and the relatively "damped" appearance of the PCWP tracing with a slightly lower pressure compared with the LA pressure.

to reflect. In general, the mean PCWP is within a few millimeters of mercury of the mean left atrial pressure, especially if the wedge and pulmonary artery systolic pressures are low.[6] High pulmonary artery pressure creates difficulty in obtaining a true "wedge," falsely elevating the pulmonary capillary wedge pressure relative to the left atrial pressure.

Obtaining an accurate and high-quality PCWP tracing is not always easy or possible. An existing uninterrupted fluid column between the catheter tip and the left atrium is important. However, the lung consists of three distinct physiologic pressure zones with a different relation between the alveolar, pulmonary artery, and pulmonary venous pressures (the lung zones of West) (Figure 2-15).[7] Zone 1 is typically present in the apex of the lungs, where the alveolar pressure is greater than the mean pulmonary artery and pulmonary venous pressures. Zone 2 is located in the central portion of the lung, and pulmonary artery pressure exceeds alveolar pressure, which, in turn, is greater than the pulmonary venous pressure. These zones are not acceptable for estimation of the PCWP because capillary collapse is present based on these pressure relations, and a direct column of blood does not exist between the left atrium and the wedged catheter tip.

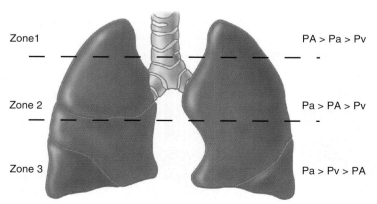

Zone 1   PA > Pa > Pv

Zone 2   Pa > PA > Pv

Zone 3   Pa > Pv > PA

FIGURE 2-15. Schematic representation of the three lung zones of West. PA = alveolar pressure, Pa = pulmonary artery pressure, Pv = pulmonary venous pressure. A true wedge pressure can be obtained only when an uninterrupted column of blood exists from the pulmonary vein to the pulmonary artery. In zone 1, alveolar pressure is the highest pressure compressing both vessels; in zone 2, although pulmonary arterial pressure exceeds pulmonary alveolar pressure, the pulmonary venous system is compressed by the higher alveolar pressures. Zone 3 is the only area where alveolar pressure is lower than pulmonary venous pressure and does not interfere with the column of blood, thus allowing an accurate wedge pressure.

Lung zone 3 is represented by the base of the lung, where alveolar pressure is lower than both pulmonary arterial and pulmonary venous pressure, allowing pressure transmission directly from the left atrium to the wedged catheter tip. Lung zone 3 is where PCWP accurately reflects left atrial pressure. Fortunately, in most patients in the supine position on a cardiac catheterization table, most of the lung is in zone 3. In addition, because most blood flows to that area, the catheter tip of a balloon flotation catheter usually ends up in zone 3. Situations associated with catheter tip location in a non–zone 3 location include the use of positive end expiratory pressure (PEEP), mechanical ventilation (alveolar pressure increased and less of lung is zone 3), and hypovolemia. Demonstrating that the catheter tip is below the level of the left atrium, however, ensures a zone 3 location and greater accuracy.[3]

Characteristics of a high-quality PCWP include (1) presence of well-defined *a* and *v* waves (note that the *a* wave is absent in atrial fibrillation and phasic waves may not be distinct at low pressures); (2) appropriate fluoroscopic confirmation with the catheter tip in the distal pulmonary artery and no apparent motion of the catheter with the balloon inflated; (3) an oxygen saturation obtained from the PCWP position is greater than 90%; and (4) a distinct, abrupt rise in mean pressure is observed when the balloon is deflated or the catheter is withdrawn from the PCWP position to the pulmonary artery. Of all these signs, obtaining an oxygen saturation greater than 90% from the catheter tip is the most confirmatory of a true PCWP. An "over-wedged" pressure occurs when the catheter tip is in a peripheral pulmonary artery and the balloon is over-inflated; this catheter position may lead to pulmonary artery rupture, a potentially

fatal complication of pulmonary artery catheterization. Over-wedging causes a false PCWP measurement without distinct *a* and *v* waves and a tracing that does not reflect left atrial pressure.

The mean PCWP is approximately 0–5 mmHg lower than the pulmonary artery diastolic pressure, unless there is increased pulmonary vascular resistance. Obtaining a suitable and accurate wedge pressure may be difficult or impossible in patients with pulmonary hypertension. Accordingly, if it is important to measure the left atrial pressure accurately, such as during evaluation of mitral stenosis, and if the operator is unable to confirm the wedge pressure, then a transseptal catheterization with direct measurement of the left atrial pressure is necessary. Similar to other right-sided pressure tracings, the end-expiratory wedge pressure is most representative of the true hemodynamic status if there is a great deal of respiratory variation.

Overall, a good correlation exists between the pulmonary capillary wedge, left atrial, and left ventricular end-diastolic pressures. The PCWP does not correlate with left ventricular end-diastolic pressures when there is mitral stenosis, severe mitral or aortic regurgitation, pulmonary venous obstruction, marked increase in positive end-expiratory pressure, left atrial myxoma, marked left ventricular noncompliance, or non–zone 3 location of the catheter tip.[8] In patients with large *v* waves, the trough of the *x* descent is the best predictor of the left ventricular end-diastolic pressure.[9]

Determination of the PCWP in patients on a ventilator with PEEP poses a common clinical dilemma. Positive end-expiratory pressure increases alveolar pressure, reducing the proportion of lung zone 3. In addition, the positive pressure is transmitted to the central circulation, directly affecting right-sided pressures and leading to an overestimation of the PCWP. The extent to which PEEP increases right-sided chamber pressures is not predictable and depends on such variables as compliance of the cardiac chamber, chest wall and lung, volume status, and existing filling pressures. The general consensus is that PEEP less than 10 cm H_2O does not significantly affect the PCWP. Still, debate exists on methods to correct the PCWP when PEEP exceeds 10 cm H_2O. The effect of PEEP on intrathoracic pressure can be determined by subtracting the esophageal pressure from the PCWP but this method is not practical in most coronary care units or cardiac catheterization laboratories. One suggested method for correction is based on the observation that PCWP rises 2–3 cm for every 5 cm H_2O increment in PEEP.[8]

Left Ventricular Waveform

The normal left ventricular systolic pressure is 90–140 mmHg, and the normal end-diastolic pressure is 10–16 mmHg. The left ventricular waveform is characterized by a very rapid upstroke during ventricular contraction, reaching a peak systolic pressure, and then the pressure rapidly decays (Figure 2-16). The pressure in early diastole is typically very low and slowly rises during diastole. Abnormalities in ventricular relaxation are apparent when early diastolic pressure is high and declines during diastole.[10] Similar to the right ventricular waveform, an *a* wave may be seen in the left ventricular tracing at end-diastole; however, this is usually abnormal and implies a noncompliant left ventricle. Left ventricular end-diastolic pressure is defined as the pressure just after the *a* wave and before the abrupt rise in systolic pressure coinciding with

ventricular ejection. However, identification of the left ventricular end-diastolic pressure (LVEDP) can sometimes be difficult. A late diastolic pressure rise may become incorporated into the left ventricular upstroke, obscuring the LVEDP (Figure 2-17). Again, in the presence of

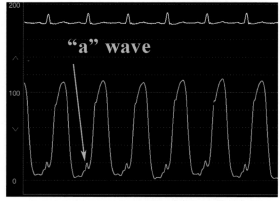

FIGURE 2-16. An example of a high-fidelity left ventricular pressure waveform. An *a* wave is present on this tracing, which is not always seen on left ventricular pressure waves, unless diminished compliance of the left ventricle is present.

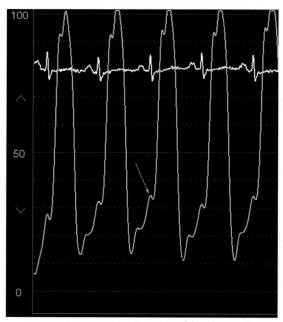

FIGURE 2-17. Marked elevation of the LVEDP *(arrow)* in a patient with heart failure.

large and prominent *a* waves, the pressure just after the *a* wave represents the LVEDP (Figure 2-18). Intrathoracic pressure changes due to the respiratory phases can also affect LVEDP, the pressure at end-expiration (Figure 2-19).

Central Aortic Pressure Waveform

The normal aortic systolic pressure is 90–140 mmHg, and the normal diastolic pressure is 60–90 mmHg. Central aortic waveforms have a rapid upstroke, a systolic peak, and a clearly defined dicrotic notch due to closure of the aortic valve during pressure decay (Figure 2-20). The peak systolic pressure equals the peak left ventricular systolic pressure, unless there is obstruction within the left ventricle, at the aortic valve, or within the proximal aorta. An anacrotic notch may be apparent during the systolic pressure rise (Figure 2-21), as a

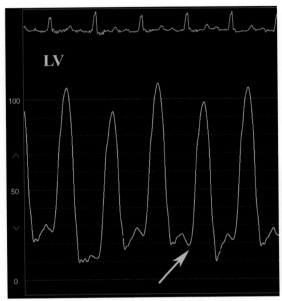

FIGURE 2-18. Large *a* wave on left ventricular pressure wave. When a large *a* wave is present, the LVEDP is identified as the pressure just after the *a* wave and before the LV systolic pressure rise *(arrow)*.

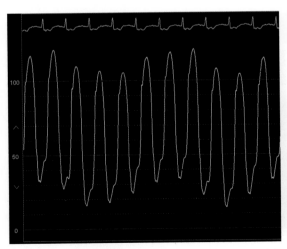

FIGURE 2-19. Marked respiratory variation on a left ventricular pressure wave. The LVEDP should be measured at end-expiration. In this case, the LVEDP is nearly 50 mmHg.

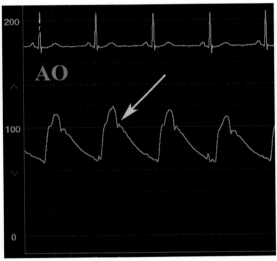

FIGURE 2-20. An example of a normal, high-fidelity aortic pressure waveform. Note the dicrotic notch *(arrow)*.

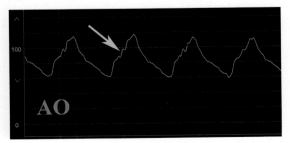

FIGURE 2-21. This waveform demonstrates an example of a prominent anacrotic "notch" or "shoulder" *(arrow)* in a patient with severe aortic regurgitation. An anacrotic notch may also be observed in patients with severe aortic stenosis and indicates turbulence during ejection.

result of turbulent flow during ejection, and indicates an abnormality in the aortic valve or proximal aorta.

The measured central aortic pressure is composed of two components: the pressure wave generated from forward flow from left ventricular ejection and the summation of pressure waves generated from "reflected" waves. Reflected waves result because as blood is ejected forward, it meets areas of resistance such as branch points or tortuous vessels. When the pressure wavefront strikes these areas, additional pressure waves are generated and directed back to the heart. These pressure waves strike the aortic valve, generating additional, forward-directed, smaller pressure waves. Therefore, the sampled pressure waveform represents a summation of all of the forward impulses.

This phenomenon is less apparent when pressure is sampled closer to the aortic valve. The effect increases further from the aortic valve but is usually negligible. Under some circumstances, however, the reflected waves may be of significant dimension. Factors that increase the effect of reflected waves include heart failure, aortic regurgitation, systemic hypertension, increased aortic stiffness from advanced age or peripheral vascular disease, aortic or ilio-femoral obstruction, or tortuosity and arterial vasoconstriction. Factors associated with diminished reflected waves include vasodilation, hypovolemia, and hypotension. The reflected wave is typically apparent late in the aortic waveform due to the time delay from its generation to its summation with the forward waves.

The effect of reflected waves is particularly notable in peripheral arterial waveforms (brachial, femoral, and radial) (Figure 2-22). Peak systolic pressure exceeds central aortic pressure by 10–20 mmHg due to peripheral amplification from reflected waves. The contour of the waveform changes further from the aortic valve, with a steeper upstroke, narrower systolic portion (spiked appearance), and markedly diminished or absent dicrotic notch.

Measurement of Simultaneous Pressures in Two or More Chambers

Cardiac catheterization protocols collect simultaneous pressure in two or more chambers for the purpose of screening for several specific conditions.

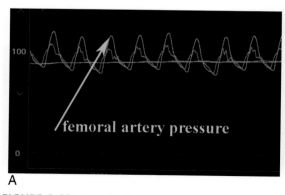
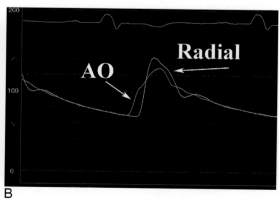

FIGURE 2-22. **A,** A simultaneous central aortic pressure and femoral artery sheath pressure obtained in a patient with aortic stenosis. Compared to the central aortic pressure, the femoral artery pressure wave exhibits a time delay, peripheral amplification with higher systolic pressure, and a "damped" appearance with loss of the dicrotic notch. **B,** A simultaneous central aortic and radial artery pressure showing the typical "spiked" appearance of a peripheral waveform.

Simultaneous left and right ventricular pressures and simultaneous left ventricular and PCWP recordings should be obtained on all patients who undergo a complete hemodynamic study that involves a right and left heart catheterization. The purpose of these two maneuvers is to screen for the presence of occult restrictive/constrictive physiology and mitral stenosis, respectively. Additional simultaneous pressure measurements include the collection of left ventricular and either central aortic or femoral arterial pressure when entertaining the diagnoses of aortic stenosis, left ventricular outflow tract obstruction, or coarctation of the aorta, and simultaneous right ventricular and pulmonary artery pressures collected if there is pulmonic valve or pulmonary artery stenosis. Simultaneous left atrial and left ventricular pressures are performed to assess for mitral stenosis when a PCWP is not adequate or possible.

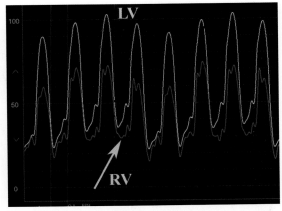

FIGURE 2-23. Simultaneous left and right ventricular waveforms in a patient with heart failure and pulmonary hypertension, showing the normal relationship between the two chambers. The systolic pressures rise and fall together during the respiratory cycle, and diastolic pressures are more than 5 mmHg apart.

Combination Left Ventricular and Right Ventricular Pressures

This maneuver is performed to screen for the presence of restrictive or constrictive physiology and should be a part of all complete, hemodynamic evaluations. Fairly complex interactions occur between the cardiac chambers, the pericardium, and the intrathoracic cavity during the respiratory cycle. In general, in patients without constrictive physiology, the net effect of these interactions causes left and right ventricular diastolic pressures to differ by at least 5 mmHg, with variation during the respiratory cycle. Peak systolic pressure changes during inspiration and expiration in the right and left ventricle parallel each other (Figure 2-23). Abnormalities in

these relationships are observed in constrictive pericarditis and restrictive cardiomyopathy. A detailed discussion of these interactions and the hemodynamic effects of pericardial and restrictive myocardial diseases is the subject of Chapter 8.

The hemodynamic effect of conduction abnormalities is often reflected in simultaneous right and left ventricular pressure tracings. Normally, the right ventricular waveform sits within the confines of the left ventricular wave (Figure 2-24, *A*). A right bundle branch block delays right ventricular contraction relative to left ventricular contraction, resulting in a delay in the right ventricular pressure wave and a shift to the right (Figure 2-24, *B*). The opposite occurs with a left bundle branch block (Figure 2-24, *C*).

Combination Pulmonary Capillary Wedge (or Left Atrial) and Left Ventricular Pressure

The purpose of this maneuver is to screen for the presence of mitral valve

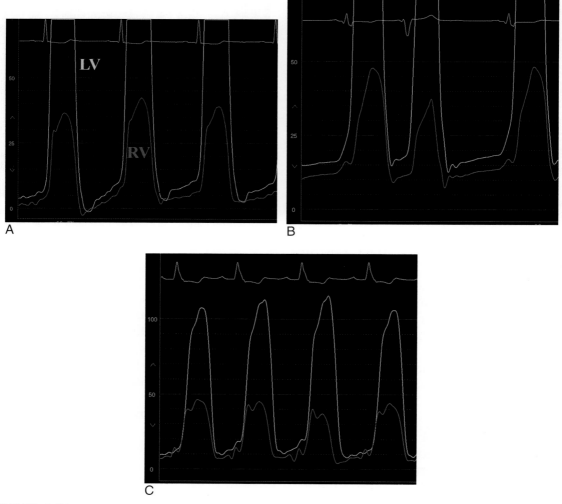

FIGURE 2-24. Effect of conduction abnormalities on simultaneous right and left ventricular pressure waveforms. **A,** Normally, the right ventricular pressure wave sits within the left ventricular pressure contour. **B,** In the presence of a right bundle branch block, the right ventricular wave is shifted to the right. Note how a premature ventricular contraction returns the right ventricular tracing to a more normal appearance. **C,** A left bundle branch block or intraventricular conduction delay interrupts left ventricular contraction relative to the right ventricle, causing the right ventricular waveform to shift to the left.

stenosis. In addition, simultaneous LV-PCWP is needed to determine the mitral valve orifice area in patients with known mitral stenosis. Normally, no gradient should exist between PCWP and LVEDP (Figure 2-25). A small gradient may be discernible only early in diastole. The time delay associated with the PCWP tracing causes the *a* and *v* waves to appear later in the left ventricular waveform. This

may be problematic if a large *v* wave exists, because it may be confused with a diastolic gradient (Figure 2-26). However, note the location of the *v* wave on a true left atrial waveform obtained by transseptal catheterization (Figure 2-27). The true position of the *v* wave as seen on the left atrial waveform is during ventricular systole and the *y* descent correlates with the decay in left ventricular pressure. Thus, if

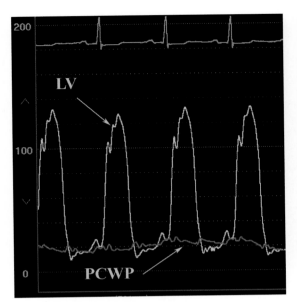

FIGURE 2-25. Simultaneous left ventricular and PCWP tracings obtained during a routine cardiac catheterization protocol as a screening test for mitral stenosis. As shown here, no pressure gradient normally exists late in diastole between the two chambers.

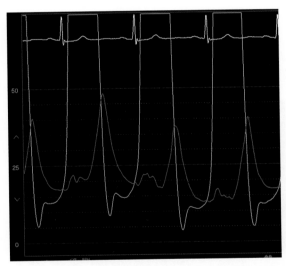

FIGURE 2-26. Simultaneous left ventricular and pulmonary capillary wedge pressure tracings obtained in a patient with severe mitral regurgitation, demonstrating a very large v wave. The time delay inherent to the wedge pressure waveform suggests the presence of a mitral gradient during diastole. Phase shifting the wedge tracing to the left corrects this false gradient.

there is a large *v* wave on the PCWP, the time delay can be corrected by shifting the PCWP to the left, allowing proper alignment with the left ventricular waveform.

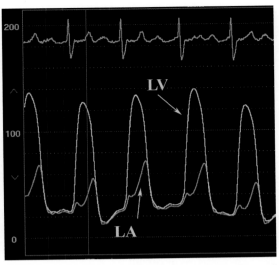

FIGURE 2-27. This simultaneous left ventricular and left atrial pressure tracing was obtained in a patient with significant mitral regurgitation using a transseptal approach to measure left atrial pressure. A prominent *v* wave is apparent, but no mitral gradient is present. Note the timing of the *v* wave on the left atrial pressure tracing relative to the left ventricular pressure waveform. As shown in Figure 2-26, the time delay inherent to PCWP recordings causes the *v* wave of a PCWP to appear later in diastole and may lead to a false diagnosis of a mitral gradient.

Combination Central Aorta (or Femoral Artery) and Left Ventricular Pressure

Simultaneous left ventricular and central aortic pressures are recorded in cases of known or suspected aortic stenosis as a method of determining the transvalvular gradient necessary to estimate valve area. Often, simultaneous left ventricular and femoral arterial sheath pressures are used for this purpose. However, discrepancies between central aortic and femoral arterial sheath pressures are commonly observed (see Figure 2-22, *A*). These include peripheral amplification resulting in a higher sheath than central aortic pressure, and peripheral vascular disease, catheter thrombosis, or kinking of the sheath resulting in higher central aortic than sheath pressure. Additional details regarding this assessment will be provided in a later chapter.

Common Errors and Artifacts

Most errors in the collection and interpretation of hemodynamic data are related to one of the reasons listed in Table 2-2. Erroneous data due to an improper zero level or unbalanced transducer might lead to patient mismanagement. With the commonly used fluid-filled systems, artifacts and errors may be caused by a small air bubble,

TABLE 2-2.	Common Sources of Error or Inaccuracy in Hemodynamic Assessment

1. Improper zero level or transducer balancing
2. Air bubbles, clots, or kinks in the system
3. Loose connections
4. Defective transducers
5. Tachycardia and loss of frequency response
6. Mechanical ventilators and excessive intrathoracic pressure changes
7. Artifacts:
   Over-damping
   Overshoot or "ring" artifact
   Catheter whip or "fling"
   Catheter entrapment
   Hybrid waveforms

kink, or blood clot anywhere along the line from the catheter tip to the sensing membrane. Similarly, a loose connection or stopcock can cause inaccuracy. Transducers may be defective or poorly calibrated, which should be considered when there is difficulty maintaining transducer balance or if the data obtained appear inconsistent. The frequency response of most clinically used systems may be exceeded in the presence of marked tachycardia, preventing the collection of high-fidelity tracings. Mechanical ventilators and extreme changes in intrathoracic pressure can make interpretation difficult. Finally, several artifacts frequently thwart an unsuspecting clinician.

Probably the most commonly observed artifacts relate to an improper degree of damping. The over-damped tracing (Figure 2-28) indicates the presence of excessive friction absorbing the force of the pressure wave somewhere in the line from the catheter tip to the transducer. The tracing lacks proper fidelity and

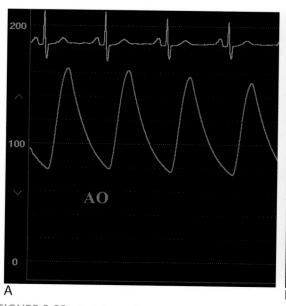 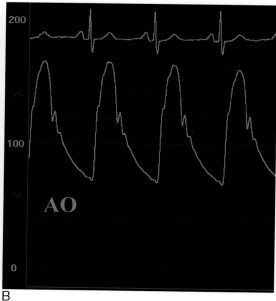

A B

FIGURE 2-28. **A,** A damped aortic pressure waveform due to the presence of an air bubble in the catheter. This tracing has poor fidelity, a smooth appearance, and lacks a dicrotic notch. **B,** Following vigorous flushing and removal of the offending air bubble, a high-fidelity tracing is apparent with return of a dicrotic notch.

appears smooth and rounded because of loss of frequency response. This will result in loss of data and will falsely lower peak pressures. Typically, the dicrotic notch on the aortic or pulmonary artery waveforms is absent, and the right atrial or PCWP waveforms will lack distinct *a* and *v* waves. The diastolic pressure tracing on an over-damped ventricular waveform will be smooth, preventing recognition of an *a* wave and making determination of end-diastolic pressure difficult. This artifact is usually caused by sloppy operators or air bubbles in the tubing, catheter, or transducer, or a loose connection anywhere in the system. The operator should also be aware that a thrombus or kink in the catheter may also cause this artifact as well as the presence of high viscosity radiographic contrast agents in the catheter. For the latter reason, hemodynamic data should always be collected with saline, and not contrast, in the catheter.

Under-damping causes *overshoot* or *ring artifact* (Figures 2-29 and 2-30). This artifact typically appears as one or more narrow "spikes" overshooting the true

pressure during the systolic pressure rise with similar, negatively directed waves overshooting the true pressure contour during the downstroke. This artifact may lead to overestimation of the peak

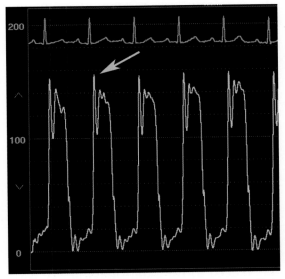

FIGURE 2-29. "Ring" artifact is a very common artifact, usually due to the presence of a small bubble somewhere in the system between the catheter tip and the transducer. The small bubble oscillates, causing the high-frequency, spiked artifact shown here *(arrow)*. This can usually be corrected by flushing the catheter or introducing a filter.

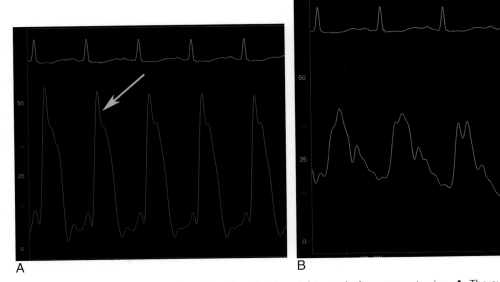

FIGURE 2-30. A commonly seen "overshoot" artifact in a right ventricular pressure tracing. **A,** The overshoot portion *(arrow)* may provide the false impression that **(B)** the right ventricular pressure exceeds pulmonary artery pressure, leading to an erroneous diagnosis of pulmonary artery or pulmonic valve stenosis.

pressure and underestimation of the pressure nadir. Tiny air bubbles that oscillate rapidly back and forth, transmitting energy back to the transducer, cause this artifact. Flushing the catheter or transducer often corrects this artifact; alternatively, introduction of a filter to the hemodynamic system may be necessary to eliminate this artifact. Figure 2-29 is an example of an overshoot artifact on a right ventricular waveform, resulting in a systolic pressure higher than the pulmonary artery pressure. If unrecognized, this might be falsely diagnosed as pulmonic stenosis.

Related to overshoot or ring artifact is *catheter whip* or *fling artifact* (Figure 2-31). This artifact is created by acceleration of the fluid within the catheter from rapid catheter motion and is commonly seen with balloon-tipped catheters in hyperdynamic hearts or balloon-tipped catheters placed in the pulmonary artery with extraneous loops. Similar to ring artifact, catheter whip causes overestimation of the systolic pressure and underestimation of the diastolic pressure. This artifact is difficult to remedy; eliminating the extra loops or deflation of the balloon can improve the appearance and limit this artifact.

Catheter malposition creates several interesting artifacts. *Catheter entrapment artifact* is sometimes observed, particularly when measuring left ventricular pressure with an end-hole catheter. Cardiac catheterization in patients with hypertrophic obstructive cardiomyopathy entails a search for an intraventricular pressure gradient. An end-hole catheter allows the operator to determine the precise location of a pressure gradient. Unfortunately, during these efforts the tip of the catheter may become buried or "entrapped" within the hypertrophied myocardium and reflect intramural rather than intracavitary pressure.

The resulting bizarre, spiked appearance to the left ventricular waveform may lead to a false diagnosis of a left ventricular outflow tract gradient (Figure 2-32). A *hybrid tracing* results when the sampled pressure represents a mixture of the waveforms from more than one cardiac chamber. Hybrid tracings are observed in two common clinical scenarios. In one scenario, a catheter such as a pigtail catheter, consisting of multiple side-holes, straddles two cardiac chambers. The pressure waveform conveyed to the transducer contains pressure elements from each chamber. For example, a pigtail may be improperly positioned within the left ventricle with side-holes lying above and below the aortic valve. The pressure waveform will contain both aortic and left ventricular pressure waveform elements, creating a hybrid of both chambers (Figure 2-33). Hybrid tracings may also be observed during attempts at obtaining a PCWP, particularly if there is pulmonary hypertension. In this case, the catheter may not completely occlude the pulmonary artery resulting in only partial wedging. The resulting waveform represents a mixture of a pulmonary artery and pulmonary capillary waveforms falsely elevating the wedge pressure. This artifact may be responsible for a false diagnosis of heart failure or mitral stenosis in patients with pulmonary hypertension. It may be difficult to detect because characteristic *a* and *v* waves may be observed (Figure 2-34). Confirmation of the PCWP position will require measurement of blood oximetry in such cases.

Finally, catheter malposition against a heart valve or wall of a blood vessel or cardiac chamber may create damping of the waveform when the catheter tip lies against a chamber wall (usually a low pressure chamber such as the right atrium) or a "spike" artifact when the catheter tip strikes a heart valve.

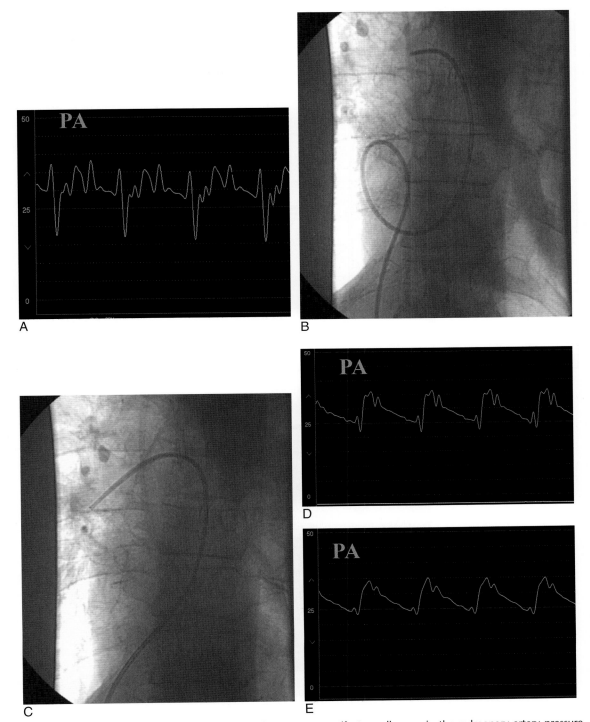

FIGURE 2-31. Catheter "fling" or "whip" is another common artifact usually seen in the pulmonary artery pressure waveform in patients with hyperdynamic hearts. In this case, **(A)** a pulmonary artery pressure waveform was nearly unrecognizable due to **(B)** excessive catheter whip from a prominent loop in the right atrium. **C,** Removal of the loop improved the appearance of the waveform, but **(D)** overshoot artifact remained. **E,** Addition of a filter resulted in further improvement in the appearance of the waveform.

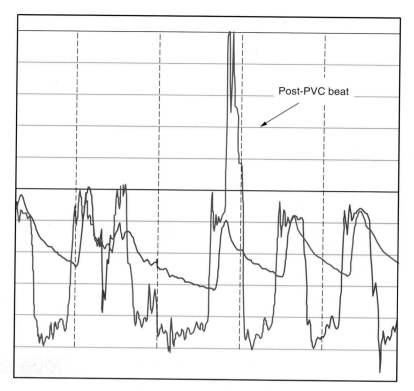

Post-PVC beat

FIGURE 2-32. Catheter entrapment artifact in a patient with marked left ventricular hypertrophy undergoing catheterization to determine the presence of a left ventricular outflow tract gradient. Note that the beginning phase of ventricular systole in the post-PVC beat appears similar to other beats but is then followed by a bizarre, spiked deflection representing intramyocardial pressure due to catheter entrapment.

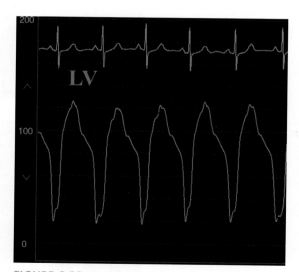

FIGURE 2-33. A hybrid waveform obtained from a pigtail catheter placed in the left ventricle. Some of the side-holes of the catheter are in the aorta, causing this peculiar waveform. More subtle versions of this artifact may not be recognized and lead the observer to falsely assume elevation of the LVEDP.

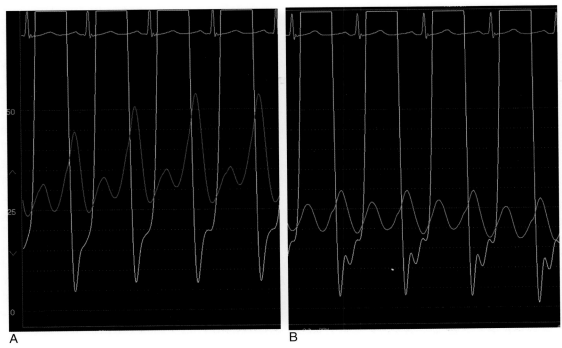

A   B

FIGURE 2-34. Hybrid tracings are very common during attempts to measure PCWP. In this example, elevated pulmonary artery pressure is present and measures 61/30 mmHg. **A,** With a balloon flotation catheter, the "wedge" pressure reveals distinct *a* and *v* waves and suggests the presence of a mitral valve gradient. However, the oxygen saturation from blood withdrawn from the catheter tip measures 72%. **B,** With the catheter positioned more distally, a better PCWP tracing is obtained with an oxygen saturation of 95%, thus confirming a true "wedge" position and absence of a mitral valve gradient.

References

1. Courtois M, Fattal PG, Kovacs SJ, et al: Anatomically and physiologically based reference level for measurement of intracardiac pressures. *Circulation* 1995;92:1994–2000.
2. Brown LK, Kahl FR, Link KM, et al: Anatomic landmarks for use when measuring intracardiac pressure with fluid filled catheters. *Am J Cardiol* 2000;86:121–124.
3. Swan HJ: The Swan-Ganz catheter. *Dis Mon* 1991;37:509–543.
4. Jenkins BS, Bradley RD, Branthwaite MA: Evaluation of pulmonary arterial end-diastolic pressure as an indirect estimate of left atrial mean pressure. *Circulation* 1970;42:75–78.
5. Sharkey SW: Beyond the wedge: Clinical physiology and the Swan-Ganz catheter. *Am J Med* 1987;83:111–122.
6. Walston A, Kendall ME: Comparison of pulmonary wedge and left atrial pressure in man. *Am Heart J* 1973;86:159–164.
7. West J, Dollery CT, Naimark A: Distribution of blood flow in isolated lung: Relation to vascular and alveolar pressures. *J Appl Physiol* 1964;19:713–724.
8. Summerhill EM, Baram M: Principles of pulmonary artery catheterization in the critically ill. *Lung* 2005;183:209–219.
9. Haskell RJ, French WJ: Accuracy of left atrial and pulmonary artery wedge pressure in pure mitral regurgitation in predicting left ventricular end-diastolic pressure. *Am J Cardiol* 1988;61:136–141.
10. Kern MJ, Christopher T: Hemodynamic rounds series II: The LVEDP. *Cathet Cardiovasc Diagn* 1998;44:70–74.

CHAPTER 3

Cardiac Outputs and Shunts

Vishal Arora, MD

We take for granted the relative ease that we are now able to measure the rate that the heart pumps blood, better known as the cardiac output. This was not always the case. Although Adolph Fick described the theoretical basis for cardiac output determination in man in 1870, more than 60 years elapsed before clinical application became possible. André Cournand[1] described the first set of cardiac output measurements in man in 1945 and noted:

The practical difficulty preventing the ready application of this (i.e., Fick's) principle in human subjects has been that of obtaining reliable samples of average or mixed venous blood. With the development of the technique of catheterization of the right heart, this difficulty has been largely overcome, and the experience of the last 3 years has led to a procedure for determining cardiac output in man which can be used in almost all forms of disease or injury, with safety and without discomfort to the patient beyond that attendant upon the insertion of a needle in the femoral artery, and cutting down on a median basilic vein both under novocaine anesthesia.

Currently, determination of cardiac output and the calculation of the magnitude of an intracardiac shunt are routine and integral parts of cardiac catheterization. The performance of these measurements, their limitations, and their role in modern catheterization will be discussed.

Measurement of Cardiac Output

Cardiac output can be determined by one of several techniques: Fick method, indicator-dilution method, thermodilution method, and angiography. Clinical catheterization laboratories and intensive care units rely primarily on the Fick and thermodilution methods. Cardiac output is expressed in liters/minute and is often corrected for patient size by dividing by the body surface area converting the measurement to the cardiac index in units of liters/minute/meter^2. The normal cardiac output at rest is 5–8 L/min, and the normal value for resting cardiac index is >2.4 L/min/m^2. With exercise, cardiac output increases substantially; elite athletes achieve cardiac outputs in excess of 30 L/min.

Fick Method for Cardiac Output Determination

Adolph Fick described the theoretical basis for cardiac output determination in 1870. Fick's principle states that the total uptake or release of a substance by an organ is the product of the *blood flow* to the organ and the *arteriovenous concentration difference* of the substance. Using the lungs as the organ and oxygen as the substance, blood flow to the lungs can be calculated by Fick's relationship, as follows:

$$\text{Pulmonary blood flow} = \frac{\text{Oxygen consumption}}{\text{Arteriovenous oxygen difference}}$$

In the absence of a shunt, because pulmonary blood flow equals systemic blood flow, the relationship can be used to calculate systemic output. The arteriovenous oxygen difference is the difference in oxygen content in the blood across the pulmonary circulation and is calculated as the arterial oxygen content minus the mixed venous oxygen content. Oxygen content is determined as the product of blood oxygen saturation, the hemoglobin concentration (in gram per deciliter), and the amount of oxygen carried per gram of hemoglobin (1.36 mL oxygen per gram of hemoglobin). This value is multiplied by 10 to correct the units. Thus, Fick's formula for determining cardiac output is

$$\text{Cardiac output} = \frac{\text{Oxygen consumption}}{(\text{Arterial saturation} - \text{Mixed venous saturation}) \times (\text{Hgb}) \times 13.6}$$

Fick's principle states that the arteriovenous oxygen (AV-O_2) difference is inversely proportional to the cardiac output. A normal AV-O_2 difference is about 20–50 mL/L. At low cardiac outputs, greater extraction of oxygen is present from the tissues and the mixed venous saturation is low, resulting in a high AV-O_2 difference. With high-output states, rapid extraction leads to high mixed venous saturations and low AV-O_2 difference. Note that the mixed venous saturation alone is a crude estimation of the cardiac output, with a low saturation indicating a low output and a high saturation indicating a high output. Furthermore, when cardiac output is low, AV-O_2 difference is large, making it easier to measure and therefore making it a more accurate method at low cardiac outputs.

The important variables measured in the cardiac catheterization laboratory are AV-O_2 content difference and the oxygen consumption. The AV-O_2 content difference is easily and accurately measured by simultaneously obtaining systemic arterial and mixed venous blood samples. Ideally, the arterial blood sample should be obtained from the pulmonary veins; however, in the absence of a right-to-left intracardiac shunt the central aortic, femoral, or radial artery oxygen content closely approximates pulmonary vein oxygen content. The pulmonary artery is the most reliable site for obtaining mixed venous blood as opposed to other proximal sites such as vena cava, right atrium, or right ventricle, where there may be significant variation in blood oxygen content within the chamber. Of course, this assumes the absence of an intracardiac shunt. These blood samples are analyzed for the percent oxygen saturation. To determine oxygen content, the AV-O_2 difference is multiplied by the measured hemoglobin, which is then multiplied by the oxygen-binding coefficient (1.36 mL O_2/g of hemoglobin). The product is multiplied by 10 to convert units from grams/deciliter to grams/liter.

The other important measurement used to calculate the cardiac output by Fick's method is the oxygen consumption. At steady state, oxygen consumption is the rate at which oxygen is taken up by the blood from the lungs and should ideally be measured directly in the catheterization laboratory. Various commercial systems are available and typically use a tight-fitting gas exchange mask that collects and measures the oxygen content of expired air. Measurement of oxygen consumption requires a steady state environment, cooperation of the patient, and technical personnel who are familiar and experienced with the equipment and methodology. This method is time-consuming and cumbersome and is rarely used clinically in the current era. Most catheterization laboratories use an "assumed" value for oxygen consumption based on the patient's age, gender, and body surface area. The assumed value is typically 125 mL/min/m^2 for average individuals and 110 mL/min/m^2 for elderly patients. Clearly, the obvious differences among patients who undergo cardiac catheterization would likely make these estimates inaccurate. Oxygen consumption varies greatly among adults at the time of cardiac catheterization, with large discrepancies between direct measurement of oxygen consumption and the assumed values.[2,3]

Although use of the "assumed" rather than the directly measured O_2 consumption is the major source of error in the Fick method, additional errors may be introduced because of improper collection of the mixed venous or arterial blood samples. Ideally, these blood samples should be collected simultaneously in a steady state environment. Errors may be present if, for instance, arterial blood is sampled early in the case and mixed venous blood is sampled at a later time in the procedure, when the patient may become oversedated, thereby causing the patient to hypoventilate and resulting in the lowering of the mixed venous oxygen content, falsely implying a lower cardiac output. In addition, care should be taken to ensure that the mixed venous sample is obtained from the pulmonary artery and that the pulmonary artery catheter has not migrated to a "wedge" position

that will falsely elevate the oxygen saturation. When the Fick method is performed correctly, the total error in determination of the cardiac output is about 10%.[4] Figure 3-1 shows an example of Fick's method for cardiac output calculation.

Indicator-Dilution Method for Cardiac Output Determination

Also based on Fick's principle, the cardiac output can be derived by studying the flow characteristics of an indicator substance. Upon injection of a substance into the circulation, the rate at which the indicator appears and disappears from a downstream point correlates directly with the cardiac output. For example, if the cardiac output is high, the indicator will rapidly appear and quickly wash out; if the cardiac output is low, the indicator will require a longer time to achieve its maximal concentration and a longer time to wash out. Therefore, the area under the time-concentration curve is related inversely

Body surface area	2.0 m²
Hemoglobin	15 gm/dL
Mixed venous saturation	60%
Aortic saturation	99%
Oxygen consumption (assumed)	125 mL/min/m²

Fick's formula:

$$\text{Cardiac output (L/min)} = \frac{O_2 \text{ consumption}}{\text{(A-V) } O_2 \text{ content difference}}$$

Where:

(A–V) O_2 content difference = (Arterial – Mixed venous saturation)(Hgb)(13.6)

$$\text{Cardiac output (L/min)} = \frac{(125 \text{ mL/min/m}^2) \times (2.0 \text{ m}^2)}{(0.99 - 0.60) \times (15)(13.6)}$$

$$\text{Cardiac output} = \frac{250}{79.56} = 3.14 \text{ L/min}$$

FIGURE 3-1. Example of the Fick method used to calculate cardiac output in a 61-year-old man with shortness of breath. Note how the assumed O_2 consumption is multiplied by the body surface area.

to the cardiac output. The Stewart-Hamilton formula for calculation of cardiac output takes into account the mean concentration of the indicator during the first passage and the duration of the extrapolated curve:

$$\text{Cardiac output (L/min)} = \frac{\text{Amount of indicator in mg} \times 60\,\text{sec/min}}{\text{Concentration of indicator (mg/mL)} \times \text{curve duration (sec)}}$$

Performance of this technique involves injection of a bolus of indicator into a systemic vein, the pulmonary artery, or the left atrium. The indicator mixes with the blood and its concentration is measured continuously as a function of time at a sampling site (generally, the aorta, radial, or femoral artery). Numerous indicators have been used, with indocyanine green dye representing the most commonly used indicator. The normal curve generated with this method has an initial rapid upstroke followed by slower downstroke and continued appearance due to recirculation of the tracer. This recirculation creates some uncertainty at the tail end of the curve, and extrapolation of the curve is necessary to correct for this distortion. The downslope of the primary curve is projected to the baseline to exclude indicator recirculation. Planimetry of the area under the curve yields the cardiac output.

This method has several limitations. Indocyanine green dye is unstable over time and can be affected by light. The indicator must mix well with blood before reaching the distal sampling site, and it must have an exponential decay over time so that extrapolation of the time/concentration curve can be accurately performed. This technique is not accurate in the presence of irregular rhythms, valvular regurgitation, or intracardiac shunts. Importantly, this method is inaccurate in low output

states in which the washout of the indicator is prolonged. In these cases, recirculation of the indicator begins well before an adequate decline in the indicator curve occurs, distorting the downslope of the curve before it reaches baseline and preventing correction for recirculation. When indicator-dilution measurements are compared with the Fick method, the disparity between the two measurements is increased in patients with low cardiac output and those with aortic and mitral regurgitation.[5] The disparity between the Fick method and indicator-dilution measurements is greater than the disparity between Fick and thermodilution measurements.[5] This technique has essentially been abandoned by clinicians and is primarily of historical interest.

Thermodilution Method for Cardiac Output Determination

Fegler[6] described the thermodilution method in 1954. This method is the easiest to perform and the most widely used method to measure cardiac output in catheterization laboratories and critical care units.

The thermodilution technique is a variation of the indicator-dilution technique, using blood temperature as the indicator. Saline at a known temperature is injected into the right atrium from the proximal port of a Swan-Ganz catheter. The saline mixes with blood and lowers its temperature. The temperature of blood is measured in the pulmonary artery by a thermistor mounted on the distal tip of the catheter. The thermistor is a variable resistor in which the resistance is proportional to the temperature. As the resistance changes, a change in voltage occurs. The measured change in voltage over time generates a temperature curve that is related to the cardiac output. Similar to the indicator-dilution method, cardiac output is inversely related to the area under the time-temperature curve. If the area under the curve is small, this means the temperature equilibrates rapidly with the ambient body temperature, indicating a high cardiac output. Conversely, if the area under the curve is large, it takes longer for the blood temperature to reach ambient body temperature, implying low cardiac output. The cardiac output is calculated using an equation that takes into account the temperature and specific gravity of injectate and blood and the injectate volume.

The thermodilution method is preferable to the indicator-dilution method because right-sided injection and right-sided sampling of the cold saline yields a curve that is less subject to recirculation-induced distortion than right-sided injection and left-sided sampling of indocyanine dye. Examples of a modern, computer-based system to measure cardiac output by thermodilution technique are shown in Figures 3-2 and 3-3. Note that the temperature plotted on the y axis decreases as the saline bolus

passes the thermistor on the pulmonary artery catheter. The curve of a patient with normal output shows a rapid drop in temperature, whereas patients with low output have a much slower drop in temperature.

Thermodilution cardiac output is very simple to perform, but several potential sources of error exist. After attaching the Swan-Ganz catheter to the measuring computer, the operator rapidly injects a 10-mL bolus of saline into the right atrium via the proximal port of the catheter. No infusions should be entering the right atrium from large peripheral or central lines. Ideally, the same amount of injectate at the same temperature should be used each time. Therefore, the operator must take great care to rapidly deliver each bolus, at a constant rate and with minimal contact with the syringe barrel to prevent warming and introduction of saline with widely varying temperatures with each injection. Using iced saline is not an advantage. The use of a dual thermistor catheter (located at both proximal and distal ports) improves the precision and accuracy of this technique.[7] While

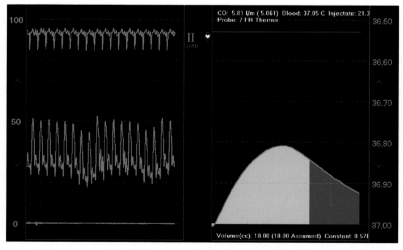

FIGURE 3-2. Thermodilution curves obtained from a patient with a normal cardiac output. The temperature is plotted on the y axis. In this case, the cardiac output measured 5.81 L/min.

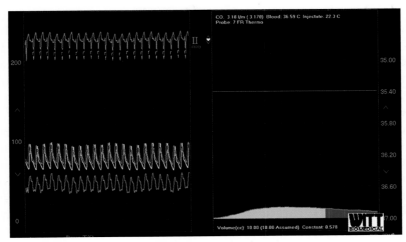

FIGURE 3-3. Thermodilution curves obtained in a patient with a profoundly depressed cardiac output from cardiogenic shock due to pump failure. Note the flattened shape of the curve compared to the normal curves obtained in Figure 3-2. The decrease in temperature over time is minimal because of slow flow. In this case, the cardiac output measured 3.18 L/min.

measuring cardiac output, the patient should be resting quietly without talking, laughing, or coughing because these will vary thoracic temperature and affect the measurement. The distal catheter tip should be in a stable position in the pulmonary artery, with avoidance of the "wedge" position. All redundancy or coiling of the catheter in the right atrium or right ventricle should be removed. Routinely, three to five cardiac output measurements are obtained and averaged. If wide variation in measured values occurs, numerous additional samples should be obtained and averaged.

The thermodilution method is inaccurate in the presence of intracardiac shunts, low flow states, marked respiratory variation, or cardiac arrhythmia. This method is likely inaccurate in severe tricuspid regurgitation because of the unpredictable mixing and loss of heat with regurgitation; however, studies have shown conflicting results regarding its accuracy in this condition when compared to other techniques.[8–10] In low cardiac output states, the thermodilution method overestimates cardiac output when compared to the Fick method. This overestimation is greatest (average difference of 35%) in patients with Fick cardiac outputs <2.5 L/min.[11]

Angiographic Method for Cardiac Output Determination

Cardiac output equals the product of stroke volume and heart rate. Left ventriculography can provide an estimation of stroke volume by tracing the contours of a high-quality ventriculogram and calculating the end-diastolic and end-systolic volumes. Stroke volume represents the difference between these values and is simply multiplied by the heart rate at the time of the ventriculogram. Obviously, this method is fraught with inaccuracies because of the inherent errors of calibrating chamber volumes by ventriculography and is particularly inaccurate in patients with valvular regurgitation and irregular heart rhythms, such as atrial fibrillation. This method is rarely used clinically.

Calculation of Shunts

In the absence of a shunt, blood flow through the pulmonary and systemic circulations is equal. The presence of an abnormal communication between intracardiac chambers results in shunting of blood either from the systemic to the pulmonary circulation (left-to-right shunt), the pulmonary to the systemic circulation (right-to-left shunt), or in both directions (bidirectional shunt). An intracardiac shunt is most commonly due to congenital heart disease, such as an atrial septal defect (ASD), ventricular septal defect (VSD), or patent ductus arteriosus (PDA). Shunts can also be acquired conditions—for example, as from an iatrogenic, a postsurgical fistula, or a postmyocardial infarction rupture of the interventricular septum.

Screening for Intracardiac Shunts and Performance of a "Shunt Run"

All routine right-heart catheterization procedures screen for the presence of a left-to-right shunt by measuring the oxygen saturation of blood from the pulmonary artery. Normally, pulmonary artery blood saturation should not exceed 75%; higher values indicate either a high cardiac output or a left-to-right shunt. Some variability in oxygen content in healthy people is observed if multiple samples are obtained from any particular chamber. For instance, the right atrium receives blood from the superior vena cava (SVC), the inferior vena cava (IVC), and the coronary sinus, all of which have varying degrees of oxygen saturation. Similarly, coronary venous blood, with its very low oxygen content, may directly enter the right ventricle by the Thebesian vessels. Therefore, oxygen saturation measured in blood samples obtained from the right atrium or right ventricle will vary depending on where blood is collected in this chamber relative to these sources.

A *significant step-up* is defined as one that exceeds the normal variability. Generally accepted criteria for a significant shunt are a mean absolute difference >7% at the atrial level and mean absolute difference >5% at the ventricular and great vessel levels.[12]

A better method of screening for a left-to-right shunt is to measure oxygen saturation in blood samples obtained from the SVC and the pulmonary artery. Again, these should be within 7% of each other; a variance of more than this indicates a left-to-right shunt, and a difference in oxygen saturation between these two samples of >9% provides excellent sensitivity, specificity, and predictive accuracy for identifying a large left-to-right shunt.[13] A right-to-left shunt is present when oxygen desaturation is discovered in arterial blood that does not correct with administration of 100% oxygen.

A full oxygen saturation run should be performed when an intracardiac shunt is suggested by the shunt screen or in cases of known or suspected shunts. A complete oximetry run involves obtaining samples in heparinized syringes from multiple levels within the heart (Figure 3-4). These include samples obtained from the left and right pulmonary artery; the main pulmonary artery; the midcavity of the right ventricle and right ventricular outflow and inflow tracts; the low, middle, and high right atrium; the low and high SVC; the low and high IVC; the left ventricle; and the distal aorta. The IVC saturation varies depending on where the sample is obtained, and the sampling site should be at the level of the diaphragm to ensure that hepatic venous blood is taken into account. If an ASD is discovered, the catheter should be placed across the atrial septum and a blood sample measured from both the left atrium and the pulmonary veins.

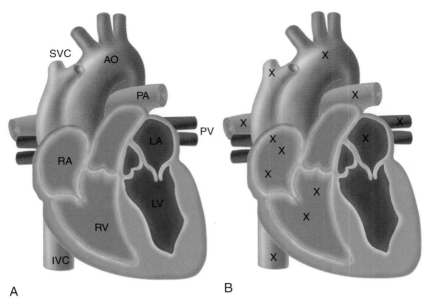

FIGURE 3-4. Locations for blood sampling when performing a complete saturation run. **A**, Various cardiac chambers. **B**, Optimal sites marked by an x. *AO*, Aorta; *IVC*, inferior vena cava; *LA*, left atrium; *LV*, left ventricle; *PA*, pulmonary artery; *PV*, pulmonary vein; *RA*, right atrium; *RV*, right ventricle; *SVC*, superior vena cava.

The typical catheter position across the atrial septum is confirmed by the catheter lying across the midline in the anteroposterior projection. Further confirmation can be obtained by the presence of a left atrial waveform and by obtaining an oxygen saturation exceeding 90%. These multiple samples allow a precise determination of the location of the anatomic shunt by identifying the site of the oxygen step-up within the heart. For example, if there is an isolated step-up in the low SVC or in the high right atrium, anomalous pulmonary venous drainage commonly associated with a sinus venosus ASD can be diagnosed.

Importantly, a shunt run should be performed in an expeditious manner, with all samples obtained quickly to ensure maintenance of a steady state; the entire oximetry run should take less than 7 minutes. Samples should be acquired with the patient breathing room air or ventilated with less than 30% oxygen using an end-hole catheter with its position confirmed by pressure waveforms and fluoroscopy.

Calculation of Shunt Size

The magnitude of a shunt can be expressed in terms of either absolute blood flow in liters/minute or, more commonly, a ratio of the pulmonary blood flow to systemic blood flow. A left-to-right shunt will cause an increase in the pulmonary blood flow relative to the systemic blood flow, whereas a right-to-left shunt causes increased systemic blood flow relative to pulmonary blood flow. Shunt-size calculation is based on the individual determination of systemic and pulmonary blood flow using Fick's principle, as described earlier. Therefore, systemic blood flow, or Qs, is determined, as follows:

$$Qs = \frac{\text{Oxygen consumption}}{(\text{Arteriovenous oxygen content difference across the body})}$$

The arteriovenous oxygen content difference across the body is first determined by measuring the oxygen saturation of aortic blood and subtracting the oxygen saturation of mixed venous blood. This value is then multiplied by the hemoglobin concentration, the amount of oxygen carried per gram of hemoglobin (1.36), and the number 10 to correct the units.

Importantly, in the presence of a left-to-right shunt, pulmonary artery blood *does not* represent mixed venous blood. The appropriate cardiac chamber that represents mixed venous blood depends on the location of the shunt. One method is to simply choose the chamber proximal to the shunt. For example, the right atrium can be sampled if there is a ventricular septal defect. This becomes more difficult if the shunt is located at the level of the right atrium (i.e., an ASD or anomalous pulmonary venous return). In these situations, both the SVC and the IVC sources are taken into account, as described by the Flamm[14] formula:

$$\text{Mixed venous oxygen content} = \frac{3(\text{SV } CO_2 \text{ content}) + 1(\text{IV } CO_2 \text{ content})}{4}$$

Similar to systemic blood flow, pulmonary blood flow, or Qp, can be determined by the relationship:

$$Qs = \frac{\text{Oxygen consumption}}{\text{(Arteriovenous oxygen content difference across the lung)}}$$

The arteriovenous oxygen content difference across the lung is determined by measuring the oxygen saturation of blood in the pulmonary vein and subtracting the oxygen saturation of pulmonary artery blood. This value is then multiplied by the hemoglobin concentration, the amount of oxygen carried per gram of hemoglobin (1.36), and the number 10 to correct the units.

In the case of a left-to-right shunt, once pulmonary and systemic blood flows are calculated, shunt flow can be determined by the relationship, as follows:

$$\text{Pulmonary blood flow (Qp)} = \\ \text{Systemic blood flow (Qs)} + \\ \text{left-to-right shunt flow}$$

In the case of right-to-left shunt:

$$\text{Systemic blood flow (Qs)} = \\ \text{Pulmonary blood flow (Qp)} + \\ \text{right-to-left shunt flow}$$

Determination of the absolute flow rates for pulmonary and systemic blood flow is important for calculation of pulmonary vascular and systemic vascular resistances. However, in most cases, the ratio Qp/Qs is used to determine the significance of the shunt. This ratio can be easily calculated by combining the equations for systemic and pulmonary flow equations and canceling all of the common terms (oxygen consumption, hemoglobin, and oxygen carrying capacity), as follows:

$$Qp = O_2 \text{ consumption}/ \\ \text{(pulmonary venous oxygen content} \\ - \text{pulmonary arterial oxygen content)}$$

$$Qs = O_2 \text{ consumption}/ \\ \text{(arterial oxygen content} \\ - \text{mixed venous oxygen content)}$$

Or, more simply,

$$Qp = \text{Systemic arterial saturation} \\ - \text{mixed venous saturation}$$

$$Qs = \text{Pulmonary venous saturation} \\ - \text{pulmonary arterial saturation}$$

The minimal detectable shunt by oxygen saturation method is a Qp/Qs ratio of 1.3 to 1. A Qp/Qs between 1.0 and 1.5 indicates a small left-to-right shunt, and a Qp/Qs >2.0 indicates a large left-to-right shunt. A Qp/Qs <1.0 indicates a net right-to-left shunt, as is seen in tetralogy of Fallot. An example of a calculation of the size of a left-to-right shunt is shown in Figure 3-5.

A

Hemoglobin (Hgb) 12 gm/dL
Body surface area (BSA) 1.8 m^2
O$_2$ consumption 125 mL/min/m^2
Oximetry Data:
Superior vena cava (SVC) 69%
Inferior vena cava (IVC) 73%
Low right atrium 79%
Mid right atrium 91%
High right atrium 69%
Right ventricle 93%
Left atrium (LA) 98%
Pulmonary vein (PV) 98%
Pulmonary artery (PA) 90%
Aorta (AO) 98%

Step 1: Determine mixed venous saturation

Step 2: Calculate pulmonary blood flow (Qp)

Step 3: Calculate systemic blood flow (Qs)

Step 4: Calculate shunt flow

Step 5: Determine Qp/Qs

B

Step 1: Determine mixed venous saturation:

$$\text{Mixed venous saturation} = \frac{3(\text{SVC}) + (\text{IVC})}{4} = \frac{3(.69) + (.73)}{4} = 0.70$$

Step 2: Calculate pulmonary blood flow (Qp)

$$Qp = \frac{O_2 \text{ consumption} \times BSA}{(\text{PV sat} - \text{PA sat})(\text{Hgb})(13.6)} = \frac{225}{(.98 - .90)(12)(13.6)} = 17.2 \text{ L/min}$$

Step 3: Calculate systemic blood flow (Qs)

$$Qs = \frac{O_2 \text{ consumption} \times BSA}{(\text{AO sat} - \text{MV sat})(\text{Hgb})(13.6)} = \frac{225}{(.98 - .70)(12)(13.6)} = 4.9 \text{ L/min}$$

C

Step 4: Calculate shunt flow

Shunt flow = Qp − Qs = 17.2 − 4.9 = 12.3 L/min

Shunt ratio = Qp/Qs = 17.2/4.9 = 3.5 to 1

Step 5: Determine Qp/Qs using simplified formula

$$\frac{Qp}{Qs} = \frac{(\text{AO sat} - \text{MV sat})}{(\text{PV sat} - \text{PA sat})} = \frac{28}{8} = 3.5 \text{ to } 1$$

FIGURE 3-5. Example of the calculation of the magnitude of a left-to-right shunt in a 42-year-old woman with a secundum atrial septal defect. **A,** The raw data for the calculations. **B** and **C,** Calculations.

Several limitations of the oximetric technique exist for quantifying a shunt. Measurement of oxygen saturation does not account for the dissolved form of oxygen. If, for example, a patient is mechanically ventilated with high fractions of inspired oxygen (>30%), a significant amount of oxygen may be present in dissolved form in the pulmonary venous sample, and saturation data may not provide accurate information regarding pulmonary blood flow for shunt calculation. The detection of a shunt by oximetry is dependent on the rate of systemic blood flow. For example, high systemic flow equalizes arteriovenous oxygen difference across the systemic bed, leading to higher mixed venous oxygen saturation. In this case, even a small increase in right heart oxygen measurements will indicate a significant left-to-right shunt. On the other hand, if systemic blood flow is reduced, the level of mixed venous oxygen saturation is low, and a larger increase must be detected to determine a significant left-to-right shunt.[12] Oximetrically derived Qp/Qs is subject to substantial intrapatient variability.[15] Small differences in pulmonary arterial saturations, for example, produce a substantial difference in the arteriovenous oxygen content difference across the lungs, which, in turn, lead to a sizable difference in calculated pulmonary blood flows and Qp/Qs ratios. The variability in Qp/Qs is greatly diminished by taking multiple blood samples from each chamber and averaging them before calculating the Qp/Qs.[16] Finally, the degree of shunting may vary. For example, the volume of blood shunting with an ASD depends not only on the size of the defect but also on the compliance of the left and right ventricles and is therefore subject to sympathetic tone and preload and afterload conditions.

Indicator-Dilution Method of Shunt Detection and Calculation

The indicator-dilution, or *dye curve*, method is a sensitive and accurate method for the detection and quantitation of intracardiac shunts, but this technique is time-consuming and cumbersome to perform and no longer routinely used for this purpose. An indicator (indocyanine green dye) is injected into a proximal chamber and a sample is taken from a distal chamber. Using a densitometer, the density of dye is displayed over time. To detect a left-to-right shunt, dye is injected into the pulmonary artery and sampling is performed in a systemic artery. The presence of a shunt is indicated by early recirculation of the dye noted on the downslope of the curve as a secondary rise in concentration. To detect a right-to-left shunt, dye is injected into the right side of the heart proximal to the location of the suspected shunt and blood samples obtained from a systemic artery. A right-to-left shunt is revealed by a distinct, early peak present on the upslope of the curve. The indicator-dilution method is more sensitive than the oximetric method in the detection of small shunts, but it cannot localize the shunt. Overall, the consensus is favorable between the two methods, especially concerning the pulmonary-to-systemic flow ratios.[17]

References

1. Cournand A, Riley RL, Breed ES, et al. Measurement of cardiac output in man using the technique of catheterization of the right auricle or ventricle. *J Clin Invest* 1945;24:104–116.
2. Kendrick AH, West J, Papouchado M, Rozkovec A. Direct Fick cardiac output: Are assumed values of oxygen consumption acceptable? *Eur Heart J* 1988;9:337–342.
3. Dehmer GJ, Firth BG, Hillis LD. Oxygen consumption in adult patients during cardiac catheterization. *Clin Cardiol* 1982;5:436.

4. Visscher MB, Johnson JA. The Fick principle: Analysis of potential errors in the conventional application. *J Appl Physiol* 1953;5:635.
5. Hillis LD, Firth BG, Winniford MD. Analysis of factors affecting the variability of Fick versus indicator dilution measurements of cardiac output. *Am J Cardiol* 1985;56:764–768.
6. Fegler G. Measurement of cardiac output in anesthetized animals by a thermodilution method. *Quart J Exp Physiol* 1954;39:153–164.
7. Lehmann KG, Platt MS. Improved accuracy and precision of thermodilution cardiac output measurement using a dual thermistor catheter system. *J Am Coll Cardiol* 1999;33:883–891.
8. Konishi T, Nakamura Y, Morii I, et al. Comparison of thermodilution and Fick methods for measurement of cardiac output in tricuspid regurgitation. *Am J Cardiol* 1992;70:538–539.
9. Hoeper MM, Maier R, Tongers J, et al. Determination of cardiac output by the Fick method, thermodilution, and acetylene rebreathing in pulmonary hypertension. *Am J Respir Crit Care Med* 1999; 160:535–541.
10. Balik M, Pachl J, Hendl J. Effect of the degree of tricuspid regurgitation on cardiac output measurements by thermodilution. *Intensive Care Med* 2002;28:1117–1121.
11. Van Grondelle AV, Ditchey RV, Groves BM, et al. Thermodilution method overestimates low cardiac output in humans. *Am J Physiol* 1983;245: H690.
12. Antman EM, Marsh JD, Green LH, Grossman W. Blood oxygen measurements in the assessment of intracardiac left to right shunts: A critical appraisal of methodology. *Am J Cardiol* 1980;46:265–271.
13. Hillis LS, Firth BF, Winniford MS. Variability of right-sided cardiac oxygen saturations in adults with and without left-to-right intracardiac shunting. *Am J Cardiol* 1986;58:129–132.
14. Flamm MD, Cohn KE, Hancock EW. Measurement of systemic cardiac output at rest and exercise in patients with atrial septal defect. *Am J Cardiol* 1969;23:258–265.
15. Cigarroa RG, Lange RA, Hillis LD. Oximetric quantitation of intracardiac left-to-right shunting: Limitations of the Qp/Qs ratio. *Am J Cardiol* 1989; 64:246–247.
16. Shepherd AP, Steinke JM, McMahan CA. Effect of oximetry error on the diagnostic value of the Qp/Qs ratio. *Int J Cardiol* 1997;61:247–259.
17. Daniel WC, Lange RA, Willard JE, et al. Oximetric versus indicator dilution techniques for quantitating intracardiac left-to-right shunting in adults. *Am J Cardiol* 1995;75:199–200.

CHAPTER 4

Mitral Valve Disorders

MICHAEL RAGOSTA, MD

Disorders of the mitral valve constitute a significant proportion of heart disease with a prevalence of 1%–2% among persons ages 26–84.[1] The decreasing incidence of rheumatic heart disease has made mitral stenosis increasingly rare, making mitral valve regurgitation the most common cause of mitral valve disease seen in the United States today. The hemodynamic abnormalities associated with both of these conditions provide interesting and significant challenges to physicians and will be discussed in the chapter.

Mitral Stenosis

Rheumatic heart disease is the most common cause of mitral stenosis; other etiologies are rare (Table 4-1). Although rheumatic heart disease has decreased dramatically in the United States, it continues to affect populations with substandard medical care, including Mexican Americans, Native Americans, and immigrants from developing nations. Pathologically, rheumatic mitral stenosis results from several mechanisms, including commissural fusion, cuspal fibrosis and thickening, and chordal fusion and thickening (Figure 4-1).[2]

The unobstructed, normal mitral valve orifice area measures approximately 4 cm^2. Symptoms become apparent when the valve area falls below 2 cm^2, and stenosis is deemed *critical* when valve area measures less than 1.0 cm^2. The natural history of mitral stenosis is characterized by a long latent period lasting many years, with patients experiencing either no or minimal symptoms.[2] Symptoms may arise insidiously over many years, leading to progressive disability from dyspnea or fatigue. Alternatively, a patient may experience the abrupt onset of symptoms from either the development of rapid atrial fibrillation or acute volume overload. Important complications that arise from the natural history of mitral stenosis include atrial fibrillation, cerebral and peripheral embolic events, hemoptysis, pulmonary hemorrhage, pulmonary hypertension and right-sided heart failure, endocarditis, and increased predisposition to infections.

Pathophysiology of Mitral Stenosis

Obstruction of the mitral valve causes a pressure gradient between the left atrium and left ventricle. The presence of this pressure gradient throughout diastole defines the hemodynamic hallmark of significant mitral valve stenosis. Very mild degrees of mitral stenosis have either an undetectable or very small diastolic gradient. With progressive narrowing of the mitral valve, left atrial pressure rises and the gradient becomes more pronounced. In addition to elevating left atrial pressure, incomplete emptying of the left atrium impairs filling of the left ventricle and diminishes cardiac output.

Because the left atrium is in series with the pulmonary circulation, elevated left atrial pressure passively elevates pressure in the pulmonary veins and arteries. Early in the course of the disease, pulmonary vascular resistance is normal with little effect on the right heart. As the condition progresses and becomes more chronic, the pulmonary artery pressures rise further. Pulmonary hypertension is due initially to reactive changes in the

TABLE 4-1.	Causes of Mitral Valve Stenosis

Rheumatic heart disease
Mitral annular calcification
Congenital mitral stenosis
Lupus
Infective endocarditis/vegetation
Carcinoid
Rheumatoid arthritis
Methylsergide therapy
Radiation-induced valve disease
Prosthetic mitral valve dysfunction

pulmonary arteriolar bed and is reversible. Marked pulmonary hypertension may result and reach systemic levels, obstructing blood flow through the lungs (the "second" stenosis of mitral stenosis), further decreasing cardiac output. Pulmonary vascular resistance increases substantially, causing enlargement of the right ventricle and right-sided heart failure. Although pulmonary hypertension is usually reversible following relief of mitral stenosis by either surgery or balloon valvotomy, with advanced, end-stage mitral stenosis, pulmonary hypertension may become fixed from permanent anatomic changes in the pulmonary arteries and arterioles.

The left atrial pressure and the cardiac output are the main determinants of symptoms in patients with mitral stenosis. Elevated left atrial pressure causes dyspnea, pulmonary edema, and hemoptysis. The low cardiac output associated with this condition causes fatigue. In addition to the mitral valve orifice area, left atrial pressure depends on the rate of flow across the valve (i.e., cardiac output), heart rate, size and compliance of the left atrium, and volume status; heart rate and volume status are particularly important. If given enough time, the left atrium will eventually empty even in the presence of severe mitral stenosis. Thus, for any given mitral valve area, bradycardia will result in lower left atrial pressures, and tachycardia will result in higher left atrial pressures. For this reason, the onset of rapid atrial fibrillation is poorly tolerated, leading to the abrupt onset of symptoms. Similarly, acute volume overload will rapidly increase left atrial pressure, leading to dyspnea or frank pulmonary edema.

Hemodynamics of Mitral Valve Stenosis

A wide spectrum of hemodynamic abnormalities is possible in patients with mitral stenosis, depending on the stage of their disease. Initially, the major hemodynamic abnormalities reflect solely the mitral valve obstruction and include (1) elevation of the left atrial or wedge pressure, typically to 20–25 mmHg with normal or low left ventricular end-diastolic pressure; (2) the presence of a pressure gradient that exists throughout diastole between the left atrium and left ventricle, usually ranging from 5–25 mmHg; (3) a reduction in cardiac output (3.5–4.5 L/min); and (4) abnormalities in the left atrial pressure tracing, affecting both *a* and *v* waves. In patients with normal sinus

FIGURE 4-1. Pathology of rheumatic mitral stenosis. **A,** Normal valve. **B,** A commissural fusion represents the most common pathologic mechanism of mitral stenosis, causing a "fish mouth" orifice. **C,** A noncommissural form in which there is extensive fibrosis and calcification at the leaflet tips, resulting in impaired opening of the valve and stenosis.

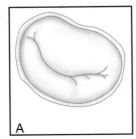
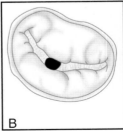
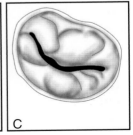

rhythm and mitral stenosis, the *a* wave on the left atrial or pulmonary capillary wedge pressure (PCWP) waveform may be accentuated because of the increased residual volume of the atrium at the onset of atrial systole (Figure 4-2). The *a* wave may be quite large, and values as high as 50 mmHg have been described.[3] A prominent *v* wave may also be observed in pure mitral stenosis because left atrial volume and pressure are already high, and any additional increase in volume that occurs during passive atrial filling results in a greater increase in pressure, generating a prominent *v* wave (Figure 4-3).[3,4] There also may be a contribution of reduced left atrial compliance from fibrosis. The presence of a large *v* wave correlates strongly with diminished exercise tolerance and is a significant predictor of pulmonary hypertension.[5,6] Furthermore, because mitral stenosis delays emptying of the left atrium, the slope of the *y* descent, representing the phase of early and rapid ventricular filling, is delayed (Figure 4-4) compared to the rapid descent seen in mitral regurgitation.

In early stages of the disease, pulmonary pressures are normal and then become only modestly elevated, despite the presence of severe mitral orifice narrowing. At this stage, the high pulmonary artery pressures reflect elevated left atrial pressure; the pulmonary vascular resistance is normal. Over time, however, the pulmonary vascular resistance increases due to reactive changes, and right ventricular enlargement occurs. Late stages of mitral stenosis are associated with marked pulmonary hypertension due to permanent anatomic changes in the arterioles, causing extreme

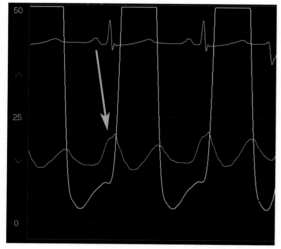

FIGURE 4-2. In patients with mitral stenosis and normal sinus rhythm, prominent *a* waves may be apparent on the left atrial or pulmonary capillary wedge pressure tracing (*arrow*).

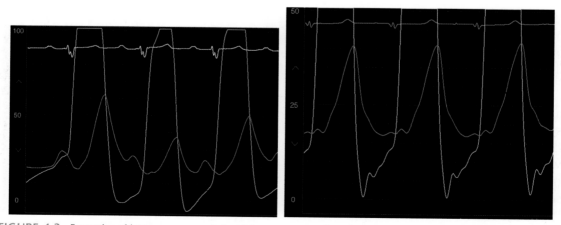

FIGURE 4-3. Examples of large *v* waves on left atrial pressure waveform in two patients with mitral stenosis.

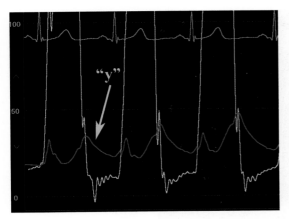

FIGURE 4-4. The *y* descent *(arrow)* is delayed in patients with mitral stenosis consistent with impaired emptying of the left atrium.

elevations in pulmonary vascular resistance, pronounced right ventricular failure, and severe secondary tricuspid regurgitation.

The existence of a pressure gradient between the left atrium and left ventricle during diastole both defines mitral stenosis and forms the basis of the hydraulic formula derived to calculate mitral valve orifice area. In patients without mitral stenosis, left atrial and left ventricular diastolic pressure curves appear nearly superimposable (Figure 4-5). In fact, a very small gradient must normally exist to allow blood to flow into the left ventricle, but this is usually not appreciable by the clinically used, fluid-filled transducers. In contrast, in mitral stenosis, a pressure gradient is present immediately upon opening of the mitral valve and persists in diastole so that diastasis is absent (Figure 4-4).[7]

The transmitral gradient is ideally assessed by obtaining simultaneous pressure waveforms from catheters positioned in the left atrium and left ventricle. However, most physicians are not facile at the performance of transseptal catheterization, and the PCWP is typically substituted for left atrial pressure. Although this practice may be acceptable in most cases, the potential for considerable error exists, and the limitations of this technique must be understood.

In general, the PCWP correlates well with left atrial pressure, which is particularly true when the PCWP is low (<25 mmHg), with no significant difference noted between left atrial and the PCWP.[8] When PCWP is >25 mmHg, considerable error may exist (variance in excess of 10 mmHg).

Although a good correlation exists between the mean left atrial pressure and PCWP, the transmitral gradient using the PCWP does not correlate as well with the gradient obtained using the left atrial pressure.[9-11] Major sources of error exist; first, the PCWP introduces a time delay (40–160 msec), depending on the position of the catheter; and second, dampening is present of the post–*v* wave descent, intrinsic to the generation of a PCWP waveform that will add to the gradient (Figure 4-6). In addition, in the presence of pulmonary hypertension (a common occurrence in patients with mitral stenosis), it may not be possible to obtain a true PCWP from the pulmonary artery position, and instead represent a hybrid between the two pressures and falsely elevate the "wedge."[11] These factors conspire to elevate the mean diastolic gradient compared to that obtained with left atrial pressure. Adjustment for the time delay by phase shifting the tracing relative to the left ventricular pressure provides a more accurate reflection of the left-atrial-left-ventricular pressure gradient.[10] However, several experts believe that these inaccuracies make the use of the PCWP an unreliable gauge of the transmitral gradient, and thus this method should not be used to make major decisions such as referral for mitral balloon valvuloplasty or repeat mitral valve surgery in patients with

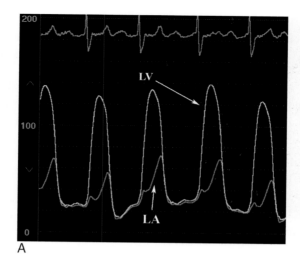

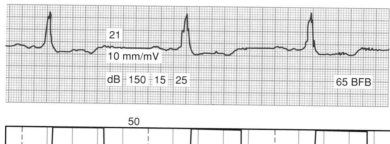

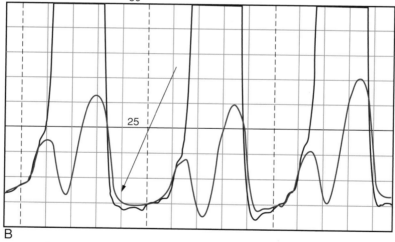

FIGURE 4-5. Normal left atrial and left ventricular relationship. **A,** A patient in atrial flutter with significant mitral regurgitation and a prominent *v* wave. Note that the *y* descent of the *v* wave is brisk and coincides with the downslope of the left ventricular pressure. The diastolic pressures are virtually superimposable. **B,** A small gradient between left ventricular diastolic pressure and the left atrial pressure may be apparent early in diastole *(arrow)*.

prosthetic mitral valves.[9,11] Importantly, if the PCWP is used, the operator must pay meticulous attention to detail and confirm the wedge pressure using oximetry sampling to demonstrate an arterial saturation >95%. Patients with evidence of significant gradient using the PCWP who have discrepant noninvasive studies, poor-quality wedge pressure waveforms, pulmonary hypertension, or

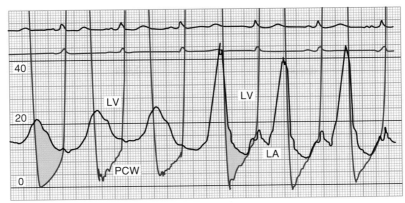

FIGURE 4-6. Use of the pulmonary capillary wedge pressure can overestimate the transmitral gradient compared to the left atrial pressure because there is a time delay with the pulmonary capillary wedge pressure and a dampening effect on the *v* wave, as shown here. (From Syed Z, Salinger MH, Feldman T. Alterations in left atrial pressure and compliance during balloon mitral valvuloplasty. *Catheter Cardiovasc Interv* 2004;61:571–579, with permission.)

prior prosthetic valve surgery should be considered for transseptal catheterization to confirm the gradient with a left atrial pressure measurement before making a major decision related to the mitral valve stenosis.

A transmitral gradient has several causes other than true mitral stenosis (Table 4-2). Severe mitral annular calcification may result in a transmitral gradient.[12] This may be seen in association with calcific aortic stenosis (Figure 4-7). A gradient may be present in patients with severe mitral regurgitation (averaging about 6 mmHg) because of the marked increase in flow across the valve,

but it is observed in early diastole only.[3] Other pathological conditions are rare.

More important are the hemodynamic artifacts resulting in an apparent transmitral gradient. Meticulous attention to detail is important when making these measurements, and pressure transducers should first be carefully leveled, calibrated, and zeroed. Because the pressures under consideration are relatively low, small errors in zeroing, transducer level or differences in frequency response between the two transducers may cause the false appearance of a transmitral gradient. Probably the most common artifact is due to the inability of the operator to achieve a true "wedge" position, particularly when severe pulmonary hypertension is present. In this scenario, the pressure wave represents a hybrid between the true wedge pressure and the pulmonary artery systolic pressure, falsely causing or elevating the gradient (Figure 4-8). Because of the time delay inherent to the generation of the PCWP waveform, the presence of large *v* waves will either cause or elevate the gradient. Phase shifting the tracing so that the *y* descent of the *v* wave coincides with the downslope of the left ventricular pressure waveform can improve or eliminate this artifact (Figure 4-9).

TABLE 4-2.	Causes of Gradient Between Pulmonary Capillary Wedge and Left Ventricular Diastolic Pressure

Mitral valve stenosis
Mitral annular calcification
Severe mitral regurgitation
Atrial myxoma (rare)
Cor triatriatum or pulmonary veno-occlusive disease (very rare)
Hemodynamic artifacts
   Improper zeroing, transducer balancing, or calibration
   Pulmonary artery catheter not in true "wedge" position
   Large *v* waves on pulmonary capillary wedge pressure

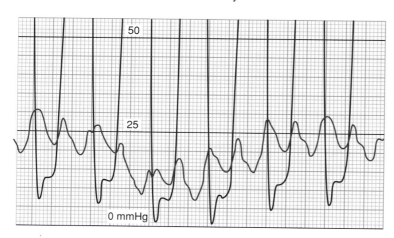

FIGURE 4-7. Example of a transmitral gradient from severe mitral annular calcification in a patient with calcific aortic stenosis.

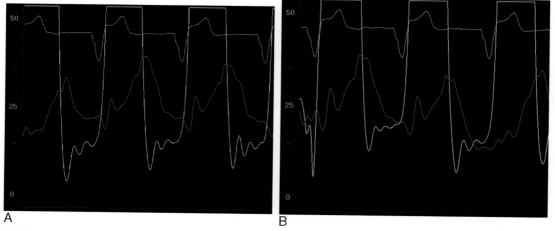

A B

FIGURE 4-8. A common source of error in the identification and quantification of a transmitral gradient when the pulmonary capillary wedge pressure is used instead of the left atrial pressure. **A,** A suitable wedge pressure and a significant *v* wave with an end-diastolic gradient of approximately 8 mmHg, suggesting mitral stenosis. However, a blood sample drawn from the catheter in this position revealed an oxygen saturation of 75%. **B,** The catheter was repositioned and wedge position was confirmed with an oxygen saturation of 95%; in this case, an end-diastolic pressure gradient is no longer present.

Calculation of Mitral Valve Area Using Gorlin's Formula

Richard Gorlin[13] and his father derived the Gorlin equation in 1951 based on the physics of hydraulic systems. First, Gorlin chose the hydraulic formula for determining the area of a "rounded edge" orifice:

$$F = Cc \, A \, V$$

where F = flow, A = orifice area, and V = the change in velocity of flow

across the orifice. The value Cc represents the coefficient of orifice contraction to allow for the contraction of the stream as it passes through the orifice. This formula is then combined with the relationship:

$$V = Cv\sqrt{2gh}$$

Where g = the gravitational constant (980 cm/sec²), and h = the height of the column of fluid and can be substituted for the pressure gradient across the orifice.

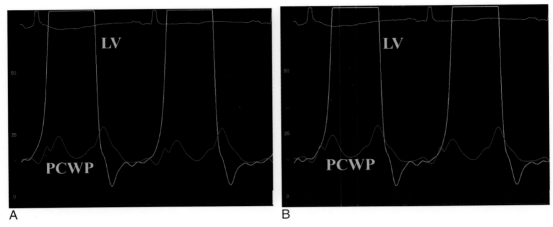

FIGURE 4-9. **A,** The time delay inherent to the generation of the pulmonary capillary wedge pressure tracing results in the impression of an early diastolic gradient due to the position of the *v* wave. **B,** A correction is made by phase shifting the pulmonary capillary wedge pressure tracing to the left.

The value Cv represents the coefficient of velocity to account for loss of energy through friction and turbulence. The two formulas are then combined and simplified and a single empiric constant C created to account for the various coefficients to create the essence of the Gorlin formula, which states:

$$\text{Valve Area} = \frac{\text{Valve Flow}}{C(44.5)(\sqrt{\text{Pressure Gradient}})}$$

Mitral valve flow is defined as the flow that occurs during diastole (diastolic filling period). Gorlin determined the empiric constant as 0.7 by collecting the hemodynamics from a single patient with mitral stenosis and then measuring the actual valve area by autopsy after the patient died, and solving the formula for *C*. Because Gorlin had no method to measure left ventricular end-diastolic pressure, he assumed a value of 5 mmHg and determined the diastolic filling period from the brachial artery tracing as the beginning of the dicrotic notch to the beginning of the upstroke of the next pressure pulse. Validation consisted of measurements obtained in 11 patients (6 autopsy and

5 surgical cases) with good correlation. Once left ventricular end-diastolic pressure could be measured routinely, the Gorlin constant was corrected from 0.7 to 0.85, and the Gorlin formula evolved into its present form[14]:

Mitral Valve Area
$$= \frac{\text{Cardiac Output}}{\dfrac{(\text{Diastolic Filling Period})}{(\text{Heart Rate})(37.9)(\sqrt{\text{Pressure Gradient}})}}$$

The pressure gradient represents the mean gradient and, in the current era, is typically measured with automated, computer-based hemodynamic systems. In normal sinus rhythm, five cardiac cycles are averaged. Because of the marked variation in the gradient with varying R-R intervals, at least ten cardiac cycles are required for patients in atrial fibrillation (Figure 4-10, *A*). If the patient is in sinus rhythm and the PCWP is used instead of left atrial pressure, the tracing should be phase shifted to the left to account for the time delay, as noted earlier.

A much simplified version of Gorlin's formula for calculating valve area has been proposed.[15] The formula is easy to remember and eliminates the heart

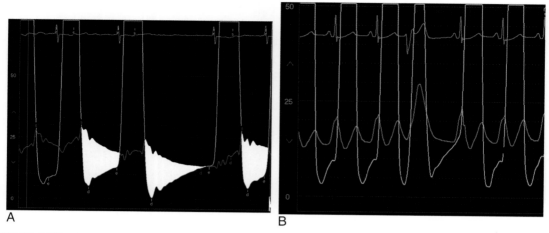

FIGURE 4-10. The heart rate greatly impacts the transmitral gradient. **A,** In atrial fibrillation varying R-R intervals occur and the transmitral gradient is greatest when there is a short R-R interval; longer R-R intervals allow more time for the atrium to empty and thus diastasis is achieved. **B,** In patients of normal sinus rhythm, the compensatory pause following a premature ventricular beat will prolong the R-R interval and diminish the end-diastolic pressure gradient, also allowing for diastasis.

rate, diastolic filling period, and the empiric constant:

$$\text{Valve Area} = \frac{\text{Cardiac Output}}{\sqrt{\text{Pressure Gradient}}}$$

When compared to the traditional Gorlin formula, the simplified formula may lead to significant disparity, especially if tachycardia is present (heart rate >100 beats/min).[16] Therefore, the simplified formula should be used with great caution.

Gorlin's formula for valve area calculation has several well-known criticisms and limitations. The formula is based on idealized relationships between flow across valves and orifice area and makes many assumptions and oversimplifications to create a tidy mathematical formula. The formula works best if normal sinus rhythm is present and is within the normal physiological range of flows. Co-existing mitral regurgitation represents a significant limitation of this method because Gorlin's formula underestimates the true valve area because the cardiac output entered in the numerator

is the forward flow and does not account for the regurgitant fraction included in the total transmitral diastolic flow.

The severity of mitral valve stenosis is routinely evaluated noninvasively. Echocardiographic techniques include use of 2D echocardiography with planimetry of the mitral valve area and use of Doppler echocardiographic techniques, including the pressure half-time and continuity equation methods. Although these techniques correlate reasonably well with the invasively determined techniques that rely on Gorlin's formula, considerable variability may exist between the methods in patients with symptomatic and significant mitral stenosis.[17,18] This case is particularly true in patients with lower transmitral gradients and higher cardiac outputs. Importantly, clinicians should not fixate on the absolute value generated by these "high tech" studies or rely solely on a single determination of the severity of stenosis. One series found that 12% of patients who underwent mitral valve surgery with severe symptoms and mitral stenosis had relatively small gradients (<10 mmHg) and only modest narrowing by calculated valve area (1.6 cm^2) yet improved dramatically with surgery, emphasizing the point that nothing substitutes for clinical judgment.[19]

Prosthetic Mitral Valves

Evaluation of prosthetic mitral valves represents a unique challenge. Small gradients are present across most mechanical and biological mitral valve prostheses. The pressure gradient across normally functioning prosthetic valves depends upon both the size of the prosthesis as well as its profile. The expected pressure gradient for many of the commonly used prosthetic valves has been reported and is based primarily upon noninvasive techniques, using Doppler echocardiography[20] (Table 4-3). These

guidelines can provide the cardiologist with a rough estimate regarding the expected transvalvular gradient when evaluating a prosthetic mitral valve invasively in the cardiac catheterization laboratory. Use of the Gorlin formula to describe a prosthetic valve area is problematic given the earlier described limitations of the method. In the setting of the aortic valve, the Gorlin formula inaccurately predicts prosthetic valve area[21]; similar inaccuracies in predicting mitral valve area are likely. In addition, the PCWP will tend to overestimate the transvalvular gradient, particularly if pulmonary hypertension is present; and many noted authorities recommend transseptal catheterization and direct measurement of left atrial pressure in this setting, particularly if a decision regarding reoperation is entertained.[11]

TABLE 4-3.	Expected Gradients Across Common Mitral Valve Prostheses		
VALVE	**SIZE**	**MEAN GRADIENT**	**ORIFICE AREA**
Mechanical			
Starr-Edwards (ball and cage)	28	7 ± 3 mmHg	1.9 ± 0.6 cm^2
	30	7 ± 3 mmHg	1.7 ± 0.4 cm^2
	32	5 ± 3 mmHg	2.0 ± 0.4 cm^2
Bjork-Shiley (single tilting disc)	27	5 ± 2 mmHg	1.8 ± 0.5 cm^2
	29	3 ± 1 mmHg	2.1 ± 0.4 cm^2
	31	2 ± 2 mmHg	2.2 ± 0.3 cm^2
St. Jude (bileaflet tilting disc)	27	5 ± 2 mmHg	1.7 ± 0.2 cm^2
	29	4 ± 2 mmHg	1.8 ± 0.2 cm^2
	31	4 ± 2 mmHg	2.0 ± 0.3 cm^2
Carbomedics (bileaflet tilting disc)	25	4 ± 1 mmHg	2.9 ± 0.8 cm^2
	27	3 ± 1 mmHg	2.9 ± 0.8 cm^2
	29	3 ± 1 mmHg	2.3 ± 0.4 cm^2
	31	3 ± 1 mmHg	2.8 ± 1.0 cm^2
Bioprosthesis			
Carpentier Edwards (pericardial)	29	5 ± 2 mmHg	—
	31	4 ± 1 mmHg	—
Hancock II (porcine)	27	—	2.2 ± 0.1 cm^2
	29	—	2.8 ± 0.1 cm^2
	31	—	2.8 ± 0.1 cm^2
	33	—	3.2 ± 0.2 cm^2

From Rosenhek R, Binder T, Maurer G, Baumgartner H. Normal values for Doppler echocardiographic assessment of heart valve prostheses. *J Am Soc Echocardiogr* 2003;16:116–127, with permission.

Hemodynamics of Mitral Balloon Valvuloplasty

Percutaneous mitral balloon valvuloplasty, using the double balloon technique or Inoue balloon, is considered the procedure of choice for treatment of symptomatic, severe mitral stenosis, assuming anatomy is favorable and no contraindications exist, such as significant mitral regurgitation or atrial thrombus.[22] The hemodynamic improvements are apparent immediately.[22–26] Both the left atrial pressure and the transmitral gradient fall and the cardiac output increases. Mitral valve orifice area increases on average from a baseline of 1.0 to 2.2 cm^2 and is similar to the results of open surgical commissurotomy.[23] An early improvement in pulmonary hypertension is augmented over time, although most patients with severe pulmonary hypertension will continue to have elevations of pulmonary artery pressure. Significant regression of tricuspid regurgitation has been reported even in the presence of a structural abnormality of the tricuspid valve.[25] The long-term results are favorable. The restenosis rate at 3 years is about 10% and similar to open commissurotomy.[23] The 10-year survival, free of death, repeat procedure on the mitral valve, or class III or IV symptoms, is 56%.[24]

Mitral Regurgitation

Regurgitation of the mitral valve occurs with greater prevalence than stenosis. The term *primary mitral regurgitation* refers to regurgitation caused by an abnormality of the valve leaflets, annulus, or mitral apparatus. The term *secondary mitral regurgitation* is used to describe valvular regurgitation in the setting of reduced ventricular function, with left ventricular dilatation causing distortion of an otherwise normal mitral

TABLE 4-4. Causes of Mitral Valve Regurgitation

PRIMARY MITRAL VALVE REGURGITATION

Myxomatous degeneration
Spontaneous chordal rupture
Papillary muscle rupture post-MI
Rheumatic valve disease
Endocarditis
Collagen vascular diseases
Hypertrophic obstructive cardiomyopathy (systolic anterior motion)
Mitral annular calcification
Prosthetic mitral valve dysfunction
Prosthetic valve paravalvular leak

SECONDARY MITRAL VALVE REGURGITATION

Mitral annular dilatation due to poor LV function
Ischemic mitral regurgitation

MI, Myocardial infarction; *LV,* left ventricular.

valve and apparatus and incomplete closure leading to regurgitation. Table 4-4 lists the most common etiologies of mitral regurgitation with the most common cause in the current era due to myxomatous mitral valve disease. Although ischemia may cause infarction and subsequent avulsion of the papillary muscle and acute severe mitral regurgitation, the most likely mechanism of mitral regurgitation in the setting of ischemia is from secondary mitral regurgitation due to incomplete mitral leaflet closure from associated left ventricular dysfunction and not from *papillary muscle dysfunction.*[27]

A variety of methods to quantify the degree of mitral regurgitation has been proposed. Several Doppler echocardiographic methods are commonly used to quantitate mitral regurgitation (Table 4-5). Each of these methods has limitations and drawbacks.[28] In the cardiac catheterization laboratory, mitral regurgitation is quantified by contrast ventriculography, using a semiquantitative scale (Table 4-6). This method is clinically useful but dependent on obtaining a high-quality ventriculogram. Emphasis on several important

TABLE 4-5.	Echocardiographic Methods of Quantifying Mitral Valve Regurgitation

Visual estimation of jet size
Flow mapping
Proximal isovelocity surface area (PISA) method
Vena contracta method
Quantified Doppler method

TABLE 4-6.	Grading the Severity of Mitral Valve Regurgitation

1+	Contrast clears with each beat, never filling the left atrium
2+	Contrast faintly fills the left atrium, but not as densely as the left ventricle, and does not clear with each beat
3+	Contrast completely opacifies the left atrium, ultimately, as densely as the left ventricle
4+	The left atrium becomes as densely opacified as the left ventricle, with the first beat becoming progressively denser with each beat and filling the pulmonary veins

technical issues can improve the physician's ability to grade mitral regurgitation with this technique. Careful attention to proper catheter position will limit the degree of artifactual mitral regurgitation either from provocation of a ventricular arrhythmia or from entanglement of the pigtail catheter into the mitral apparatus, causing the operator to overestimate the true degree of regurgitation. Underestimation of the degree of regurgitation may occur if the catheter is placed too high in the left ventricular outflow tract, underfilling the ventricle or in the presence of chronic mitral regurgitation and/or chronic atrial fibrillation when there is marked enlargement of the left atrium. In such cases, contrast may not opacify the giant left atria, despite severe regurgitation and thus leading the operator to define a lower grade of regurgitation. The use of larger volumes of contrast than normally used (i.e., 50–60 mL) may remedy the problem. Finally, inadequate right anterior oblique angulation may superimpose the left atrium

over the descending aorta, making it difficult to accurately grade the degree of regurgitation.

Pathophysiology of Mitral Regurgitation

Severe, acute mitral regurgitation (often due to spontaneous chordal rupture or avulsion of a papillary muscle head from acute infarction) typically occurs in the presence of a small, unadapted left atrium. The acute increase in volume rapidly raises left atrial and pulmonary venous pressures, transmitting to the lungs and causing pulmonary edema. With a large proportion of the left ventricular stroke volume deposited into the left atrium, forward flow is diminished and hypoperfusion and shock may ensue. Compensatory mechanisms are minimally effective and include tachycardia, in an effort to maintain cardiac output in the face of a diminished forward stroke volume and peripheral vasoconstriction to maintain perfusion of vital organs. Acute, severe regurgitation represents a medical emergency with urgent surgical repair often indicated.

Some patients with acute mitral regurgitation may stabilize and enter a chronic, well-compensated phase. Alternatively, mitral regurgitation may begin as mild or moderate in extent and slowly progress, allowing for chronic compensation. Importantly, mitral regurgitation tends to be progressive; thus, moderate degrees of regurgitation often worsen because the additional stress on the mitral apparatus changes left ventricular geometry, worsening regurgitation over time.

Chronic compensatory mechanisms allow for a prolonged asymptomatic state, despite severe mitral regurgitation. These mechanisms include the development of an increase in left ventricular volume with the preservation of the ejection fraction to allow for a greater stroke volume to maintain forward flow, despite the regurgitant volume.[28] Eccentric hypertrophy balances wall stress from increased ventricular size; however, diastolic function remains normal to allow the increase volume to occur without increasing left ventricular diastolic pressures. Another important compensatory mechanism is the increase in left atrial size to accommodate the regurgitant volume at lower filling pressures.

Over time, however, compensatory mechanisms fail. For poorly explained reasons, deterioration in contractile function occurs, resulting in myocardial dysfunction and a fall in ejection fraction. Although this phenomenon may be asymptomatic, it is often associated with symptoms of dyspnea from increased PCWP and/or fatigue from diminished cardiac output. Mitral valve repair or replacement is clearly indicated either upon arrival of symptoms or with the onset of ventricular dysfunction. Ultimately, if untreated or allowed to advance, decompensation leads to left heart failure and its consequences, including secondary pulmonary hypertension and right heart failure.

Hemodynamics of Mitral Regurgitation

The classically taught hemodynamic abnormality of mitral regurgitation is the presence of a prominent v wave on the PCWP or left atrial pressure tracing. However, prominent v waves are often absent, despite severe mitral regurgitation, and are frequently observed in conditions other than mitral regurgitation.

Recall that a v wave is a normal physiological event due to atrial filling at the end of ventricular systole when the mitral valve is closed. An abnormal or prominent v wave has been variably defined as a peak v wave in excess of 40 mmHg, a difference between the peak v wave and mean PCWP >10 mmHg or the ratio of the peak v wave to mean PCWP >2.[29] Some have proposed that a v wave height three times the mean PCWP is virtually diagnostic of severe, acute mitral regurgitation.[30]

It has been long recognized that the presence or absence of an abnormal v wave fails to correlate with either the presence or severity of mitral regurgitation, which is particularly true in the setting of chronic mitral regurgitation. As far back as 1963, Braunwald[31] observed that severe, chronic mitral regurgitation could exist with normal left atrial pressure and a normal-sized v wave. Several investigators have reported that about one third of patients with prominent v waves had no mitral regurgitation.[32,33] In one study of over 900 patients who underwent both ventriculography and right heart catheterization, using a large lumen catheter and performance of an oximetrically confirmed wedge pressure measurement, the presence of a prominent v wave was insensitive and had a poor positive predictive value for the presence of moderate or severe mitral regurgitation.[29] Interestingly, these investigators found that the *absence* of a prominent v wave was 94% specific and had a 93% negative predictive value for the *absence* of severe mitral regurgitation. This study consisted mostly of patients with chronic mitral regurgitation; the correlation might differ with acute mitral regurgitation, in which the v wave is more likely to be prominent.

The poor correlation between the presence or extent of mitral regurgitation and the height of the v wave likely relates to the numerous physiological factors involved in determining the v wave. These include (1) the rate and volume of blood that enter the left atrium during ventricular systole, (2) the volume and pressure of blood that exist within the left atrium, (3) systemic afterload that influences atrial emptying, (4) left ventricular contractile force that affects both left ventricular end-diastolic volume and pressure, and (5) left atrial compliance. Accordingly, abnormal *v* waves are seen in mitral regurgitation and in ventricular septal defects because of the increased volume that enters the left atrium. Similarly, large *v* waves are a prominent feature of both mitral stenosis and congestive heart failure (Figures 4-3 and 4-11) because the left atrial volume and pressure are high, and small additional increase in volume results in a greater increase in pressure, thereby generating a more prominent *v* wave. Tachycardia may result in *v* waves due to the shorter diastolic emptying period. Perhaps the most important variable, however, is left atrial compliance. The small, noncompliant atria of most patients with acute, severe mitral regurgitation explain why prominent *v* waves are more commonly

seen in these patients as compared to those with chronic mitral regurgitation, in which the left atrium may be more compliant. Conditions other than mitral regurgitation associated with diminished compliance of the left atrium are also associated with prominent *v* waves, including the postoperative state, rheumatic heart disease, and ischemia.

Patients with acute mitral regurgitation exhibit markedly abnormal hemodynamics. Hypotension, tachycardia, and a low cardiac output are often present (Figure 4-12). A marked elevation occurs of the PCWP, often with a very prominent *v* wave (Figure 4-13). In fact, because the left atrium is typically small and noncompliant, the *v* wave may reach giant proportions and, in some dramatic cases, may even be apparent on the pulmonary artery waveform (Figure 4-14). The transmission of this pressure wave from the pulmonary veins to the pulmonary artery also explains the occasional phenomenon of a false elevation in the pulmonary artery saturation, in some cases of severe mitral regurgitation.

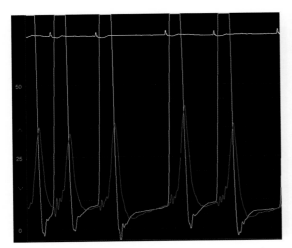

FIGURE 4-11. Example of a large *v* wave on a pulmonary capillary wedge pressure in the complete absence of mitral regurgitation. This patient had heart failure as the cause of the large *v* wave.

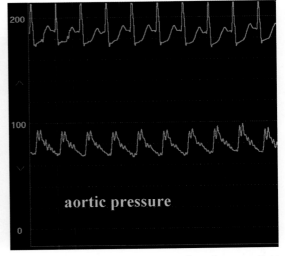

FIGURE 4-12. Aortic pressure waveform from a patient in cardiogenic shock from acute, severe mitral regurgitation due to papillary muscle rupture in the setting of an acute, inferior wall myocardial infarction.

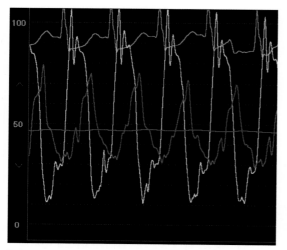

FIGURE 4-13. Simultaneous left ventricular and pulmonary capillary wedge pressure tracings obtained in the same individual, as depicted in Figure 4-12, with acute, severe mitral regurgitation. A prominent *v* wave is present on the pulmonary capillary wedge pressure tracing and hypotension. A difference of only about 30 mmHg exists between the peak of the *v* wave and the peak left ventricular systolic pressure.

In acute mitral regurgitation, the systolic murmur of mitral regurgitation may be absent or diminished, which is represented hemodynamically by the observation of minimal gradient between peak left ventricular systolic pressure and the height of the *v* wave on the PCWP tracing (Figure 4-15). An interesting hemodynamic finding is

due to the constraining effect of the intact, normal pericardium in the presence of acute volume overload from acute mitral regurgitation, resulting in hemodynamic abnormalities similar to constrictive pericarditis, with elevated and equalized right and left ventricular diastolic pressures.[34]

The hemodynamics seen in patients with chronic mitral regurgitation may, in fact, be entirely normal or only mildly abnormal at rest if ventricular function remains normal and they are well compensated (Figure 4-16). As mentioned earlier, the height of the *v* wave is an unreliable indicator of the severity of mitral regurgitation, with one third of patients with chronic mitral regurgitation demonstrating trivial *v* waves, despite severe mitral regurgitation[32] (Figure 4-17). A small diastolic pressure gradient may be observed across the mitral valve; however, unlike mitral stenosis, the gradient is present during early diastole only. In addition, the slope of the *y* descent in mitral regurgitation is steep rather than delayed, as seen in mitral stenosis.

Importantly, hemodynamic measurements in the cardiac catheterization

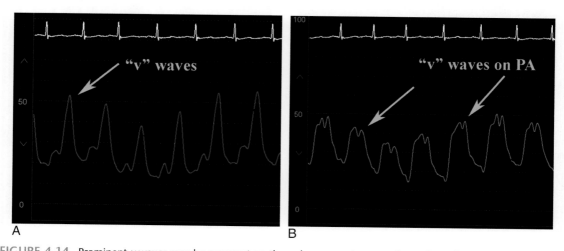

FIGURE 4-14. Prominent *v* waves may be apparent on the pulmonary artery waveform. **A,** In this case of severe acute mitral regurgitation, the pulmonary capillary wedge pressure demonstrated *v* waves that exceed 50 mmHg in height. **B,** Waves transmitted to the pulmonary artery systolic pressure waveform *(arrows)*.

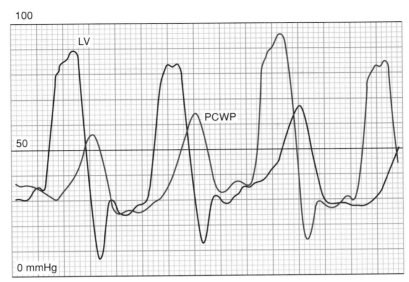

FIGURE 4-15. Severe acute mitral regurgitation with cardiogenic shock, large *v* waves, and minimal pressure difference between the height of the *v* wave and the peak left ventricular systolic pressure. In this case, no systolic murmur was appreciated.

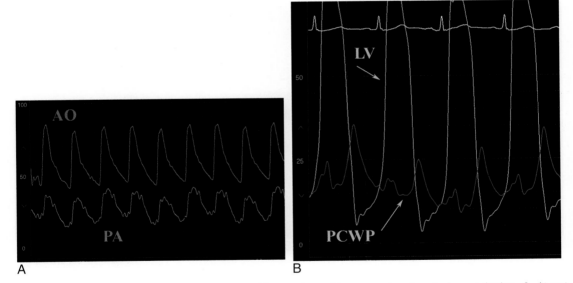

FIGURE 4-16. Example of hemodynamics obtained in a patient with severe, chronic mitral regurgitation. **A,** At rest, elevation of the pulmonary artery systolic pressures is moderate. The mean wedge pressure is normal, averaging 15 mmHg, and, **B,** the *v* wave reaches about 30 mmHg. This patient has symptoms with exertion when the pulmonary artery and pulmonary capillary wedge pressure likely exceed these resting values.

laboratory are obtained under resting conditions. Many patients with chronic mitral regurgitation experience symptoms with exertion. Hemodynamics obtained during dynamic exercise during cardiac catheterization may be more revealing. A dramatic rise in the wedge pressure or pulmonary artery systolic pressure during exercise may be revealing. In one study, about 20% of patients with normal resting PCWP developed *v* waves >50 mmHg with exercise.[35]

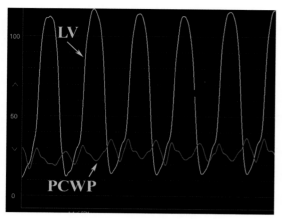

FIGURE 4-17. Severe, chronic mitral regurgitation that demonstrates a normal-sized *v* wave on the pulmonary capillary wedge tracing.

With the onset of symptoms and the development of decompensation, hemodynamic abnormalities become prominent and include the development of elevated left atrial and pulmonary artery pressures. Again, a *v* wave may or may not be present. Over time and similar to other conditions that cause chronic elevations in the pulmonary venous pressure, secondary pulmonary hypertension with high pulmonary vascular resistance and subsequent right-sided heart failure may develop (Figure 4-18). In this setting, secondary tricuspid regurgitation may arise from right ventricular enlargement and annular dilatation.

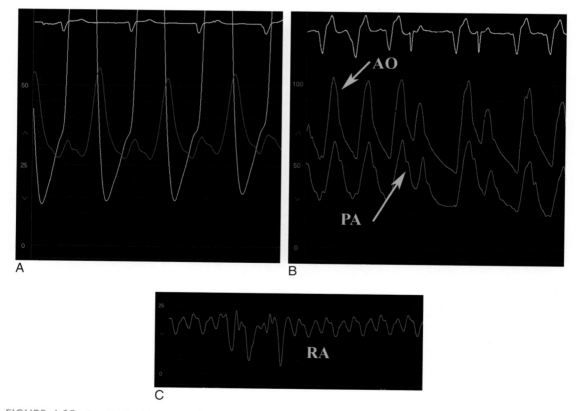

FIGURE 4-18. A patient with severe, chronic mitral regurgitation with evidence of decompensation and right-sided heart failure. **A,** Marked elevation of the pulmonary capillary wedge pressure with large *v* waves and, **B,** elevated pulmonary artery pressure in excess of 60 mmHg. **C,** Right atrial pressure is high, which is consistent with right-sided heart failure.

References

1. Thom T, Haase N, Rosamond W, et al. Heart disease and stroke statistics—2006 update: A report from the American Heart Association Statistics Committee and Stroke Statistics Subcommittee. *Circulation* 2006;114:e630.
2. Selzer A, Cohn KE. Natural history of mitral stenosis: A review. *Circulation* 1972;45:878–890.
3. Musser BG, Bougas J, Goldberg H. Left heart catheterization II. With particular reference to mitral and aortic valvular disease. *Am Heart J* 1956;52:567–580.
4. Morrow AG, Braunwald E, Haller JA, Sharp EH. Left atrial pressure pulse in mitral valve disease: A correlation of pressures obtained by transbronchial puncture with the valvular lesion. *Circulation* 1957;16:399–405.
5. Park S, Ha JQ, Ko YG, et al. Magnitude of left atrial *v* wave is the determinant of exercise capacity in patients with mitral stenosis. *Am J Cardiol* 2004; 94:243–245.
6. Ha JW, Chung N, Jang Y, et al. Is the left atrial *v* wave the determinant of peak pulmonary artery pressure in patients with pure mitral stenosis? *Am J Cardiol* 2000;85:986–991.
7. Braunwald E, Moscovitz HL, Amram SS, et al. The hemodynamics of the left side of the heart as studied by simultaneous left atrial, left ventricular, and aortic pressures; particular reference to mitral stenosis. *Circulation* 1955;12:69–81.
8. Walston A, Kendall ME. Comparison of pulmonary wedge and left atrial pressure in man. *Am Heart J* 1973;86:159–164.
9. Hildick-Smith DJ, Walsh JT, Shapiro LM. Pulmonary capillary wedge pressure in mitral stenosis accurately reflects mean left atrial pressure but overestimates transmitral gradient. *Am J Cardiol* 2000;85:512–515.
10. Lange RA, Moore DM, Cigarroa RG, Hillis LD. Use of pulmonary capillary wedge pressure to assess severity of mitral stenosis: Is true left atrial pressure needed in this condition? *J Am Coll Cardiol* 1989;13:825–831.
11. Schoenfeld MH, Palacios IF, Hutter AM, et al. Underestimation of prosthetic mitral valve areas: Role of transseptal catheterization in avoiding unnecessary repeat mitral valve surgery. *J Am Coll Cardiol* 1985;5:1387–1392.
12. Hammer WJ, Roberts WC, de Leon AC. "Mitral stenosis" secondary to combined "massive" mitral annular calcific deposits and small, hypertrophied left ventricles. Hemodynamic documentation in four patients. *Am J Med* 1978;64:371–376.
13. Gorlin R, Gorlin G. Hydraulic formula for calculation of the area of the stenotic mitral valve, other cardiac valves, and central circulatory shunts. *Am Heart J* 1951;41:1–29.
14. Cohen MV, Gorlin R. Modified orifice equation for the calculation of mitral valve area. *Am Heart J* 1972; 84:839–840.
15. Hakki AH, Iskandrian AS, Bemis CE, et al. A simplified formula for the calculation of stenotic cardiac valve areas. *Circulation* 1981;63:1050–1055.
16. Brogan WC, Lange RA, Hillis LD. Simplified formula for the calculation of mitral valve area: Potential inaccuracies in patients with tachycardia. *Cathet Cardiovasc Diagn* 1991;23:81–83.
17. Klarich KW, Rihal CS, Nishimura RA. Variability between methods of calculating mitral valve area: Simultaneous Doppler echocardiographic and cardiac catheterization studies conducted before and after percutaneous mitral valvuloplasty. *J Am Soc Echo* 1996;9:684–690.
18. Wang A, Ryan T, Kisslo KB, et al. Assessing the severity of mitral stenosis: Variability between non-invasive and invasive measurements in patients with symptomatic mitral valve stenosis. *Am Heart J* 1999;138:777–784.
19. Rayburn BK, Fortuin NJ. Severely symptomatic mitral stenosis with a low gradient: A case for low technology medicine. *Am Heart J* 1996;132:628–632.
20. Rosenhek R, Binder T, Maurer G, Baumgartner H. Normal values for Doppler echocardiographic assessment of heart valve prostheses. *J Am Soc Echocardiogr* 2003;16:116–127.
21. Cannon SR, Richard KL, Crawford MH, et al. Inadequacy of the Gorlin formula for predicting prosthetic valve area. *Am J Cardiol* 1988;62:113–116.
22. Feldman T. Core curriculum for interventional cardiology: Percutaneous valvuloplasty. *Catheter Cardiovasc Interv* 2003;60:48–56.
23. Reyes VP, Raju S, Wynne J, et al. Percutaneous balloon valvuloplasty compared with open surgical commissurotomy for mitral stenosis. *N Engl J Med* 1994;331:961–967.
24. Iung B, Garbarz E, Michaud P, et al. Late results of percutaneous mitral commissurotomy in a series of 1024 patients. Analysis of late clinical deterioration: Frequency, anatomic findings and predictive factors. *Circulation* 1999;99:3272–3278.
25. Hannoush H, Fawzy ME, Stefadouros M, et al. Regression of significant tricuspid regurgitation after mitral balloon valvotomy for severe mitral stenosis. *Am Heart J* 2004;148:865–870.
26. Syed Z, Salinger MH, Feldman T. Alterations in left atrial pressure and compliance during balloon mitral valvuloplasty. *Catheter Cardiovasc Interv* 2004;61:571–579.
27. Kaul S, Spotnitz WD, Glasheen WP, Touchstone DA. Mechanism of ischemic mitral regurgitation. An experimental evaluation. *Circulation* 1991;84: 2167–2180.
28. Carabello BA. Progress in mitral and aortic regurgitation. *Prog Cardiovasc Dis* 2001;43:457–475.
29. Snyder RW, Glamann B, Lange RA, et al. Predictive value of prominent pulmonary arterial wedge *v* waves in assessing the presence and severity of mitral regurgitation. *Am J Cardiol* 1994;73:568–570.
30. Grossman W, Baim DS. *Cardiac Catheterization, Angiography and Intervention*, 4th ed. Philadelphia: Lea and Febiger, 1991.
31. Braunwald E, Awe WC. The syndrome of severe mitral regurgitation with normal left atrial pressure. *Circulation* 1963;27:29–35.
32. Fuchs RM, Heuser RR, Yin FC, Brinker JA. Limitations of pulmonary wedge *V* waves in diagnosing mitral regurgitation. *Am J Cardiol* 1982;49:849–854.
33. Pichard AD, Kay R, Smith H, et al. Large *v* waves in the pulmonary wedge pressure tracing in the absence of mitral regurgitation. *Am J Cardiol* 1982;50:1044–1050.
34. Bartle SH, Hermann HJ. Acute mitral regurgitation in man. Hemodynamic evidence and observations indicating an early role for the pericardium. *Circulation* 1967;36:839–851.
35. Holm S, Frithiof D, Teien D, Karp K. Invasive evaluation of mitral regurgitation: The importance of hemodynamic measurements during exercise. *J Heart Valve Dis* 1997;6:383–386.

CHAPTER 5

Aortic Valve Disease

MICHAEL RAGOSTA, MD

Clinical decisions in patients with aortic valve disease rely heavily upon an accurate estimation of the severity of the valve lesion, which, in turn, often depends upon a correct understanding of the hemodynamic derangements associated with the disorder. Cardiac catheterization provides valuable hemodynamic data in patients with aortic regurgitation and aortic stenosis; however, potential sources of error and limitations of hemodynamic techniques present formidable challenges to the clinician. The adage, *"Bad data are worse than no data at all,"* is particularly relevant for aortic stenosis, in which errors in orifice area estimation may lead to an entirely wrong conclusion regarding the need for surgery. This chapter reviews the hemodynamic features of aortic regurgitation and valvular aortic stenosis emphasizing potential errors in data collection and interpretation.

Aortic Valve Regurgitation

Regurgitation of the aortic valve may be caused by a variety of conditions (Table 5-1). Currently, in the United States, aortic regurgitation is most commonly due to aortoannular ectasia from hypertension or a congenitally bicuspid aortic valve. The pathophysiology and hemodynamic abnormalities observed in aortic regurgitation depend upon several variables, including the severity of the regurgitation, whether regurgitation is acute or chronic and the compensatory response to volume overload intrinsic to this lesion.

Chronic Versus Acute Aortic Regurgitation

Hemodynamic consequences of severe aortic insufficiency differ depending on whether regurgitation is acute or chronic. In chronic aortic regurgitation, the gradual onset of progressive valve regurgitation leads to several important compensatory changes allowing a prolonged state of adaptation and a clinically asymptomatic state. Progressive left ventricular dilatation ensues with stroke volume increasing to maintain forward flow. Both end-diastolic and end-systolic volumes increase, maintaining ejection fraction. With enlargement of the left ventricular chamber, ventricular wall thickness must increase to maintain normal wall stress, as dictated by LaPlace's law stating that wall stress is proportional to the product of transmural pressure and radius divided by wall thickness. Traditionally, chronic aortic regurgitation has been considered to be an example of pure chronic volume overload. However, systolic pressure also rises in association with the augmented stroke volume, and thus the left ventricle in chronic, severe aortic regurgitation is both volume and pressure overloaded with compensation that consists of both ventricular dilatation and hypertrophy.[1,2] Chronic aortic regurgitation tops the pathological conditions, causing ventricular enlargement that generates the largest heart sizes clinically observed *(cor bovinum)*. Symptoms often develop with the onset of a decompensated state manifest by increased wall stress, diminished contractility, and decreased ejection fraction.

The physiologic benefits of vasodilators in chronic, severe aortic regurgitation relate primarily to improved left ventricular function and diminished afterload, especially when systolic hypertension is present. Vasodilator agents

TABLE 5-1.	Causes of Aortic Valve Regurgitation

Dilatation of the ascending aorta (aortoannular
   ectasia)
Prolapse or incomplete closure of a congenitally
   bicuspid valve
Endocarditis
Rheumatic valvular disease
Ankylosing spondylitis
Rheumatoid arthritis
Ehlers-Danlos syndrome
Marfan's disease
Syphilis
Aortic arch aneurysm
Aortic dissection
Ventricular septal defect (prolapsing cusp)
Subaortic membrane

do not reduce the regurgitant volume, unless associated diastolic hypertension is present, because the amount of regurgitation is based both on the regurgitant orifice area (unaffected by vasodilators) and the mean gradient between the aorta and the left ventricle during diastole. Because aortic diastolic pressures are already low, vasodilators cannot diminish this gradient further without compromising coronary blood flow.

Many of the interesting physical examination findings of chronic, severe aortic regurgitation parallel the hemodynamic findings and are consequences of the compensatory mechanisms that reflect primarily the increased left ventricular size and stroke volume. These include a wide arterial pulse pressure that may exceed 100 mmHg, a carotid "shudder" from increased stroke volume, the presence of a diffuse and hyperdynamic apical impulse with lateral displacement, and numerous, named signs for various peripheral manifestations (Table 5-2). Auscultation of the heart sounds reveals a soft or absent aortic component of the second heart sound and a characteristic decrescendo diastolic murmur. In chronic, compensated aortic regurgitation, the severity of regurgitation correlates with the duration rather than the intensity of the murmur; the murmur is holodiastolic in severe aortic regurgitation and is heard only in early diastole with mild aortic regurgitation. A systolic ejection murmur reflects the increased stroke volume. In some cases of chronic, severe aortic regurgitation, the regurgitant stream strikes the mitral valve and the elevations of the left ventricular diastolic pressure may cause early and partial closure of the mitral valve, resulting in a *functionally stenotic* mitral valve with an associated diastolic rumble (the Austin Flint murmur).

Acute aortic regurgitation behaves entirely differently. None of the compensatory mechanisms involved in the adaptation of chronic severe regurgitation, such as progressive left ventricular dilatation and hypertrophy, are possible with the acute onset of severe regurgitation. Instead, severe, sudden regurgitation causes a dramatic rise in left

TABLE 5-2.	Peripheral Manifestations of Chronic, Severe Aortic Valve Regurgitation

FEATURE	FINDING
Hill's sign	Systolic pressure in popliteal artery exceeds pressure in brachial artery
Corrigan's pulse	"Water hammer" or collapsing pulse; visible arterial bounding pulse with quick upstroke in
de Musset's sign	the carotids
Quincke's sign	Head bobbing
Muller's sign	Visible capillary pulsations of the base of the nail beds
Traube's sign	Pulsations of the uvula
Duroziez's sign	Loud systolic sounds ("pistol shot") over the femoral arteries
	Systolic murmur heard over the femorals with proximal compression of the artery by a stethoscope, diastolic murmur when compressed distally

ventricular diastolic pressure. The inability to augment stroke volume due to normal ventricular size causes a profound and life-threatening decrease in forward flow. The only possible compensatory mechanism in the setting of acute, severe aortic regurgitation is tachycardia.

Patients with acute aortic regurgitation are critically ill with respiratory failure from pulmonary edema, hypotension, and shock from diminished cardiac output and a compensatory tachycardia. Interestingly, despite a dramatic clinical presentation, the diagnosis of acute aortic regurgitation may be difficult because the diastolic murmur is typically early and soft in acute aortic insufficiency and may be obscured by extensive pulmonary rales from the associated pulmonary edema. The absence of the compensatory mechanisms described previously prevents the development of the classic peripheral signs of chronic, severe aortic regurgitation (i.e., wide pulse pressure, Duroziez's sign). For these reasons, prompt diagnosis depends upon heightened clinical suspicion for the condition; acute aortic regurgitation should always be considered by the clinician faced with an acutely ill patient with pulmonary edema and hypotension of unclear etiology.

Hemodynamic Findings

In chronic, well-compensated aortic regurgitation, the hemodynamic findings typically reflect the associated marked increases in left ventricular volume and stroke volume. The central aortic pressure waveform is characterized by high systolic pressure, low diastolic pressure, and, consequently, a wide pulse pressure (Figure 5-1). The marked increase in stroke volume forms the basis of several hemodynamic findings. Increased systolic flow across an abnormal valve leads to turbulence and a prominent anacrotic notch during systole on

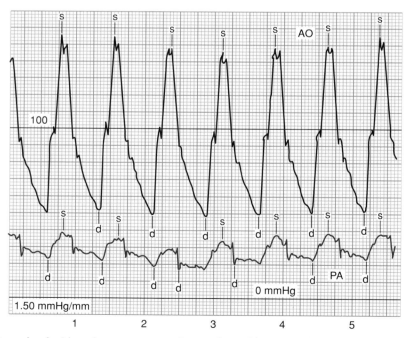

FIGURE 5-1. Example of wide pulse pressure seen in a patient with severe, chronic aortic regurgitation. Note the systolic hypertension, a common feature of chronic aortic regurgitation.

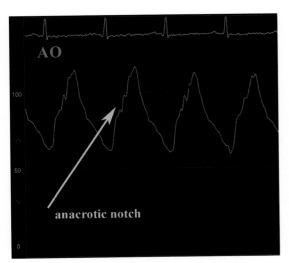

FIGURE 5-2. The anacrotic notch, or shoulder *(arrow)*, may appear prominently in cases of severe aortic regurgitation due to turbulence associated with the abnormal valve. Mild stenosis of this bicuspid valve was also present.

the central aortic waveform (Figure 5-2). The normal physiologic phenomenon of peripheral amplification is even further exaggerated, yielding systolic pressures in the femoral artery greatly exceeding central aortic pressures (Figure 5-3). This phenomenon accounts for many of the peripheral signs of aortic regurgitation described earlier.

Additional hemodynamic findings reflect left ventricular function and the state of compensation. Asymptomatic patients with chronic severe aortic regurgitation whose ventricular function remains normal and who have achieved excellent compensation often exhibit fairly normal, resting hemodynamics, with the exception of the wide aortic pulse pressure and marked peripheral amplification noted. Left ventricular end-diastolic pressure remains low with right-sided pressures unaffected. With the development of symptoms or left ventricular dysfunction, the left ventricular diastolic pressure rises. Typically, early diastolic pressure is normal then rapidly rises by end diastole. The aortic and ventricular diastolic pressures may

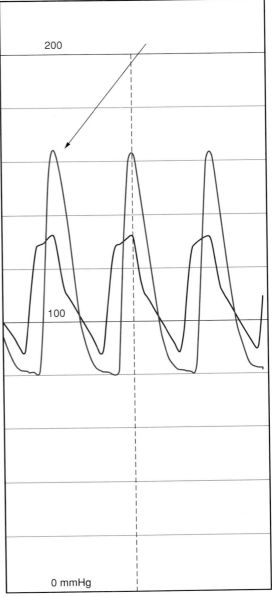

FIGURE 5-3. Marked peripheral amplification in the femoral artery pressure *(arrow)* compared to the central aortic pressure in a patient with severe, chronic aortic regurgitation.

become equal in late diastole, a phenomenon known as *diastasis* (Figure 5-4). The point at which diastasis occurs defines the end of the diastolic murmur; at this time, flow no longer occurs between the aorta and the left ventricle. This fact accounts for the shortening of the

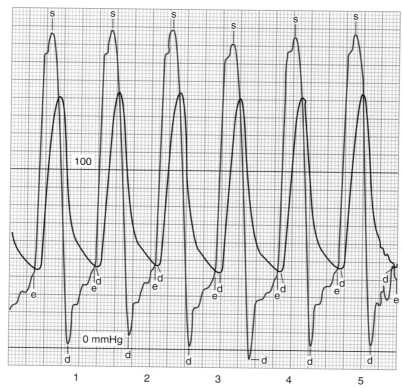

FIGURE 5-4. Simultaneous left ventricular and femoral artery sheath pressure in a patient with severe aortic regurgitation from an old porcine aortic valve prosthesis. Note the rapid rise in left ventricular diastolic pressure and equalization of the left ventricular end-diastolic and arterial diastolic pressure *(diastasis)*. A systolic pressure gradient also occurs across this failing prosthetic valve.

murmur with decompensation and the associated rise in left ventricular diastolic pressure. The degree of elevation of the left ventricular end-diastolic pressure with decompensation varies widely; values in excess of 50 mmHg are not unheard of (Figure 5-5). With the development of decompensation, chronic aortic regurgitation may lead to elevations in right-sided pressures typically associated with heart failure.

Chronic severe aortic regurgitation may elevate right ventricular end-diastolic pressure in the absence of elevation of the pulmonary capillary wedge pressure or pulmonary artery systolic pressure. This has been explained on the basis of a *Bernheim* effect, in which the increased left ventricular volume and the elevations

in left ventricular diastolic pressures are transmitted to the right ventricle, thus elevating right ventricular pressures.

With chronic aortic regurgitation, the low aortic diastolic pressure may adversely affect coronary perfusion. The combination of decreased coronary perfusion coupled with increased demand from increased myocardial mass may lead to ischemia from supply-versus-demand mismatch. Importantly, other causes of a wide pulse pressure exist besides chronic, severe aortic regurgitation (Figure 5-6). They include marked bradycardia, severe systolic hypertension, the presence of a rigid and inelastic aorta as often seen in the elderly or in patients with vascular disease, and the presence of a high output state as observed in patients with severe

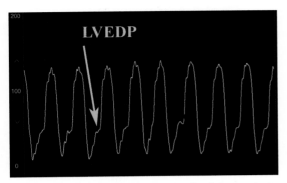

FIGURE 5-5. Marked elevation in the left ventricular end-diastolic pressure *(arrow)* in a patient with severe, chronic aortic regurgitation with recent decompensation.

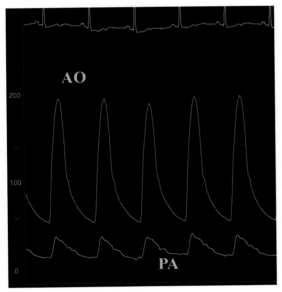

FIGURE 5-6. A wide pulse pressure may be present on the aortic pressure tracing in conditions other than aortic insufficiency. This tracing shows a wide pulse pressure in an elderly woman with hypertensive heart disease and no aortic regurgitation.

anemia, hyperthyroidism, anxiety, significant arteriovenous fistulas, or a large patent ductus.

Hemodynamic findings of acute aortic regurgitation reflect the physiologic effects of acute volume overload and diminished forward flow. Left ventricular diastolic pressure increases with a rapidly rising slope, obscuring the *a* wave and culminating in marked elevation of the left

ventricular end-diastolic pressure. Diastasis is commonly seen. By mid or late diastole, left ventricular diastolic pressure may exceed left atrial pressure, resulting in preclosure of the mitral valve (Figure 5-7). Pulmonary edema and subsequent elevations in right-sided pressures ensue with associated hypotension and low cardiac output from diminished forward flow, despite a compensatory tachycardia.

An unusual but interesting finding may be present on the aortic pressure trace in acute aortic regurgitation. In the setting of acute, severe aortic regurgitation, premature diastolic opening of the aortic valve may occur from marked elevations in left ventricular diastolic pressure. With a prematurely opened aortic valve, the additional increase in left ventricular pressure from atrial systole may transmit to the aortic pressure wave, inscribing an *a* wave on the aortic waveform (Figure 5-8). This rare finding is highly sensitive for acute aortic regurgitation.[3]

Angiography in Aortic Regurgitation

Grading the severity of aortic regurgitation in the cardiac catheterization laboratory is based on angiography and not hemodynamics. The hemodynamic abnormalities described provide information regarding the physiologic consequences of aortic regurgitation and the extent of compensation. Nevertheless, when performing cardiac catheterization on patients with aortic regurgitation, both angiography and hemodynamics are important and provide valuable complementary information to the clinician regarding this valvular lesion. Echocardiographic methods of grading aortic regurgitation have been extensively discussed elsewhere.[4]

Grading the severity of aortic regurgitation is based on contrast aortography

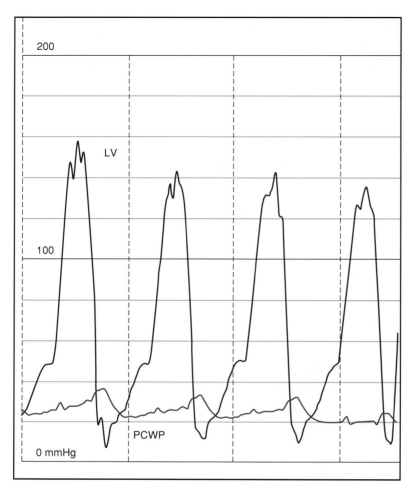

FIGURE 5-7. Patient with severe, acute aortic regurgitation and marked elevation in the left ventricular diastolic pressure exceeding the pulmonary capillary wedge pressure.

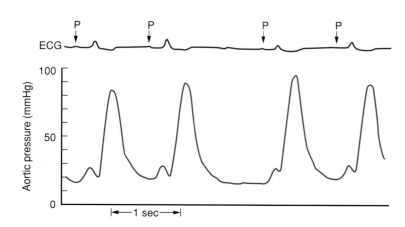

FIGURE 5-8. Premature opening of the aortic valve in severe, acute aortic regurgitation may result in transmission of a pressure wave from atrial contraction to the aorta and appears as an *a* wave on the aortic pressure trace, as shown here. (Reproduced with permission from Alexopoulos D, Sherman W. Unusual hemodynamic presentation of acute aortic regurgitation following percutaneous balloon valvuloplasty. *Am Heart J* 1988;116: 1622–1623.)

of the ascending aorta, using a pigtail catheter positioned carefully above the aortic valve. Optimal opacification usually requires about 60 mL of iodinated contrast delivered rapidly (flow rate of 30 mL/sec). A commonly used, semiquantitative scale for grading aortic regurgitation is shown in Table 5-3.

The degree of regurgitation can also be calculated by determining the regurgitant volume, which is simply a comparison of the angiographically determined stroke volume and the forward stroke volume determined by the Fick or thermodilution method, as shown by the formula

$$\text{Regurgitant Fraction} = \frac{(\text{Stroke Volume}_{angiography}) - (\text{Stroke Volume}_{forward})}{(\text{Stroke Volume}_{angiography})}$$

The angiographic stroke volume is estimated from the ventricular volumes obtained by angiography and is equal to the difference between end-diastolic volume and end-systolic volume. The forward stroke volume is calculated by dividing the cardiac output (determined by either the Fick or thermodilution method) by the heart rate. Regurgitant fraction of 0%–20% represents mild aortic regurgitation, 20%–40% represents moderate aortic regurgitation, and >40% indicates severe aortic regurgitation.

TABLE 5-3.	Angiographic Grading of the Severity of Aortic Regurgitation
1+	Small amount of contrast in the left ventricle during diastole that clears with each beat and never completely fills the left ventricular chamber
2+	Faint opacification of the entire left ventricle
3+	Dense opacification of the left ventricle (as dense as the aorta)
4+	Complete and dense opacification of the left ventricle during the first cardiac cycle and the left ventricle is more densely opacified than the aorta

Aortic Stenosis

Aortic valve stenosis is one of the most commonly observed valvular lesions in clinical practice. Adult patients who present with aortic stenosis at relatively younger ages (i.e., less than age 65) typically have a congenitally bicuspid valve, whereas patients who present greater than this age have calcific, tricuspid aortic valves (termed *calcific aortic stenosis* or *senile aortic stenosis*). Other disease processes rarely cause aortic valvular stenosis and include rheumatic heart disease, radiation-induced valvulitis, Paget's disease of bone, and renal failure. Note the importance of distinguishing aortic valvular stenosis from related conditions causing obstruction to left ventricular outflow, such as hypertrophic obstructive cardiomyopathy, subvalvular membranes, supravalvular aortic stenosis, or coarctation of the aorta.

Physiology of Aortic Valve Stenosis

The presence of a pressure gradient across the aortic valve defines aortic valvular stenosis. Normally, a small pressure gradient is present very early in systole when simultaneous left ventricular and aortic pressures are measured with sensitive, high-fidelity catheter-tipped micromanometers that represent an *impulse gradient* during the rapid phase of ventricular ejection.[5] The pathological gradient of aortic stenosis persists through systole.

Obstruction leads to pressure overload of the left ventricle and compensatory left ventricular hypertrophy. Aortic stenosis is progressive. The rate of progression is variable for any individual, but the annual increase in pressure gradient averages 7 mmHg, and the annual decrease in aortic valve area averages 0.1 cm^2.[6] Patients with aortic stenosis remain asymptomatic for prolonged periods until valve stenosis is severe. Symptoms include anginal chest pain, caused primarily by subendocardial ischemia from coronary blood flow supply-demand mismatch, syncope from a diminished and fixed cardiac output, and heart failure. Sudden cardiac death occurs primarily in symptomatic patients with severe aortic stenosis; it is rarely observed in adult patients without symptoms.

Several complex factors impact the pressure gradient that exists between the left ventricle and the ascending aorta in patients with valvular aortic stenosis. Note the importance of understanding these components when evaluating the various techniques used to measure the degree of valve obstruction. The first set of factors relates to the complex nature of fluid mechanics and flow through a stenotic orifice (Figure 5-9). Theoretical considerations of flow through a stenotic orifice predict the presence of intraventricular pressure gradients due to a drop in pressure from the body of the left ventricle to the outflow tract from a tapering of the flow field, with subsequent acceleration of blood flow as it approaches the stenotic orifice. This observation has been confirmed in patients with valvular

aortic stenosis. Elegant investigations using micromanometer catheters to precisely measure chamber pressure in patients with severe valvular aortic stenosis reveal that subvalvular gradients comprise nearly half of the total pressure gradient.[7] This observation is critically important to clinicians using cardiac catheterization to estimate the severity of aortic stenosis because failure to properly position the catheter deep within the left ventricle may incompletely estimate the true transvalvular gradient. Fluid dynamic theory also predicts the phenomenon of *pressure recovery*. The maximum pressure drop and the zone of minimal pressure and maximum velocity exist at the site of obstruction (vena contracta) with the development of turbulent flow and loss of energy. Distal to the obstruction, some of this energy is recovered with the reestablishment of laminar flow, and, consequently, an increase in pressure occurs from *recovery* of some of the pressure dropped across the stenotic valve. This phenomenon has been observed in patients with significant aortic stenosis, using micromanometer catheters to carefully measure pressure

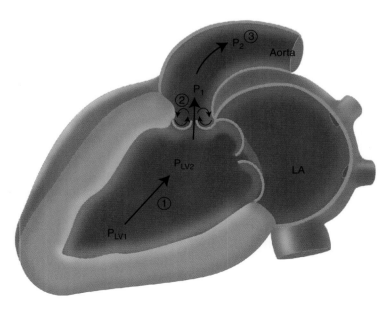

FIGURE 5-9. Schematic diagram of the important factors involved in generation and interpretation of a pressure gradient. Intracavitary tapering of the flow field causes an intraventricular pressure gradient *(1)* where pressure at the apex *(P_{LV1})* exceeds pressure below the aortic valve *(P_{LV2})*. Just after the site of obstruction, where maximum velocity (vena contracta) occurs *(2)*, is the site of minimal pressure. Turbulence in this area leads to pressure recovery *(3)*. Thus, aortic pressure at P_1 is lower than aortic pressure at P_2.

from the left ventricle to the ascending aorta.[7] The zone of minimal pressure occurred just above the aortic valve and the zone of pressure recovery occurred higher in the ascending aorta. The magnitude of pressure recovery averaged 10 mmHg. Although the fluid-filled catheters with multiple side-holes used for clinical estimation of valve area are unlikely to detect pressure recovery, clinicians should be aware of this phenomenon and position the aortic catheter in the most proximal location. Neglecting the concept of pressure recovery and improper positioning of the aortic catheter when measuring a transvalvular gradient will lead to underestimation of the gradient and overestimation of the aortic valve area with greater disparity observed with more severely narrowed aortic valves.[8]

The second set of factors that affect the pressure gradient relates to the pressure gradient being proportional not only to orifice area, but also to flow across the valve. Flow will vary with heart rate, contractile state of the heart, and the degree of preload and afterload. Thus, flow may vary from beat to beat and with the respiratory cycle. Common arrhythmias, including marked sinus arrhythmia, atrial fibrillation with variations in the R–R interval, and frequent premature atrial or ventricular beats or intermittent pacing, will impact greatly on the transvalvular pressure gradient (Figure 5-10). For this reason, the use of invasive techniques to estimate the severity of aortic valve stenosis mandate simultaneous left ventricular and aortic pressure measurements and relative stability of these factors during data collection.

Determination of the Severity of Aortic Valve Stenosis

Estimating the severity of aortic stenosis often begins with noninvasive

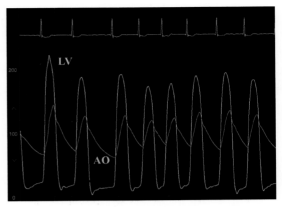

FIGURE 5-10. Simultaneous left ventricular and aortic pressure tracings obtained in a patient with severe aortic stenosis and atrial fibrillation, demonstrating the varying systolic pressure gradients associated with varying R–R intervals.

methods using echocardiographic techniques, using Doppler methodology.[4] These well-established methods provide accurate estimations of the extent of valve narrowing by estimating the transvalvular gradients and aortic valve orifice area. Many clinical decisions are based on these measurements alone. In some cases, noninvasive techniques may be inconclusive, of inadequate quality, or provide data that are discordant with the clinical exam or a patient's symptoms. In such cases, clinicians turn to an invasive assessment.

Invasive methodology applies an adaptation of the Gorlin formula to calculate the area of the stenotic aortic valve. This technique has been in clinical use for many years, is fairly simple to calculate from variables obtained during catheterization, and provides clinicians and patients an easy-to-visualize number (i.e., aortic valve area in cm^2).

Gorlin's Formula for Estimation of Aortic Valve Area

The mathematical derivation of Gorlin's formula to estimate orifice area is based on the idealized physics of hydraulic systems and has been explained during the discussion of mitral valve stenosis (see Chapter 4). Gorlin solved the equation using the valve area of a stenotic mitral valve measured at autopsy from a single patient to determine the value of the coefficient C to be 0.7 and then compared the calculated valve area to the area measured at either autopsy (six patients) or operation (five patients) for validation.[9] Gorlin noted that the formula could be adapted to the aortic valve by using the systolic ejection period (SEP) to account for the time that flow occurs across the aortic valve, but he did not know the value of the coefficient. This has subsequently never been determined. Nevertheless, the Gorlin formula applied to the aortic valve is generally used as follows:

$$\text{Aortic Valve Area} = \frac{\text{Cardiac Output}}{\text{Heart Rate (SEP)(44.5)C}(\sqrt{P_1 - P_2})}$$

The coefficient C has traditionally been set at 1.0 (based on the assumption that the effective and anatomic orifice areas are identical for the aortic valve), with P_1-P_2 representing the mean transvalvular pressure gradient.

Although Gorlin's formula for the aortic valve is generally well established by the cardiology community and has been the basis of clinical decision making in valvular heart disease for over a generation, several important criticisms are known of the equation, potentially limiting its use. Although the formula calculates a *valve area* in cm², the formula actually provides the *effective* orifice area rather than a determination of a true anatomic area. The formula is based on an idealized view of a stenotic valve and assumes that the stenotic orifice is round and the degree of narrowing is rigid and fixed. In fact, the usual stenotic aortic valve is a highly distorted orifice and there often remains some degree of mobility that may vary in the

orifice area, depending on the flow across the valve. The coefficients used by the formula are not constant and may vary with both the size of the gradient and the cardiac output. In addition, the formula is not valid in the setting of significant regurgitation because flow across the valve represents the summation of both forward flow and the difficulty to quantify regurgitant flow. Finally, Gorlin's formula depends on precise measurement of the transvalvular gradient, systolic ejection period, and cardiac output, each of which may represent considerable challenges.

In the majority of patients with aortic stenosis, the portion of Gorlin's formula described in the denominator as *heart rate × systolic ejection period × 44.5* calculates to around 1000. Thus, Gorlin's formula can be simplified by the formula described by Hakki et al.[10]:

$$\text{AVA} = \frac{\text{Cardiac Output in L/min}}{\sqrt{\text{Pressure Gradient}}}$$

In a study of 60 patients with varying degrees of aortic stenosis, the calculated aortic valve area using Hakki's[10] formula correlated extremely well to valve area determined by the more complex Gorlin formula even when peak was substituted for mean gradient. The observed difference between the two calculations rarely exceeded 0.2 cm², especially in patients with valve areas less than 0.7 cm², providing confidence that a designation of *severe* aortic stenosis would not change depending on the formula used. Although valve areas in most patients with moderate degrees of aortic stenosis were within 0.2 cm², the observed difference in valve areas between the two formulas was as high as 0.42 cm², suggesting that the more detailed Gorlin formula may be more appropriate to correctly classify the stenosis severity in patients with borderline degrees of stenosis.

An alternative to the gravity-based Gorlin formula for describing the severity of valve stenosis is the estimation of valve resistance.[11,12] Resistance simply relates flow and pressure using Ohm's law and is easily calculated as the mean pressure gradient across the valve divided by the mean flow rate during systolic ejection. This measurement does not require an empiric constant like the Gorlin formula and is unlikely to change under different flow conditions. Unfortunately, this method has not been embraced by the cardiology community, likely because the relatively abstract resistance units (dynes $\times$ sec $\times$ cm^{-5}) are more difficult to conceptualize than an orifice area.

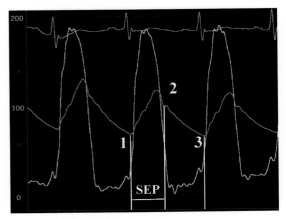

FIGURE 5-11. Determination of the SEP for calculation of the aortic valve area using Gorlin's formula. Systole begins when left ventricular and aortic pressures first cross *(point 1)* and end at the dicrotic notch *(point 2)*. The systolic ejection period represents the time from *point 1* to *point 2* in seconds. The cardiac cycle ends at *point 3*.

Application of Gorlin's Formula for Estimation of Aortic Valve Area

Gorlin's formula for calculation of aortic valve area requires measurement of cardiac output, systolic ejection period, heart rate, and mean transvalvular pressure gradient. Cardiac output is easily and routinely measured in the cardiac catheterization laboratory, using either thermodilution or Fick methods; however, it should be emphasized that great care must be taken in making this determination because small differences in cardiac output translate to potentially important changes in the calculated valve area. Similarly, variations in measurement of the systolic ejection period may result in differences in valve areas. The systolic ejection period begins when intraventricular pressure rises above aortic pressure. The end of the systolic ejection period has been variably defined as either the second left ventricular aortic pressure crossover point or at the aortic incisura (Figure 5-11). Carefully performed hemodynamic studies have shown that the aortic incisura more accurately reflects the end of aortic ejection rather than the second LV–AO pressure crossover point.[13]

Modern-day catheterization laboratories outfitted with computerized physiologic recording systems provide automated calculations of aortic valve area, obviating the need for physicians to recall the formula, to manually measure specific variables, or to perform the calculations. The required elements for the Gorlin formula are either directly entered into the computer (e.g., cardiac output) or obtained from computerized analysis of the waveforms (Figure 5-12). These automated systems are usually highly accurate; however, the careful physician should always review the computerized analysis for errors in measurement of the gradient, heart rate, or systolic ejection period, particularly if the waveforms or surface electrocardiogram contains artifact or are of poor quality. Patients with conditions that result in varying heart rate or changing pressure gradients, as observed in atrial fibrillation or marked respiratory variation, require an analysis of at least ten consecutive beats for the most accurate estimation of valve area.

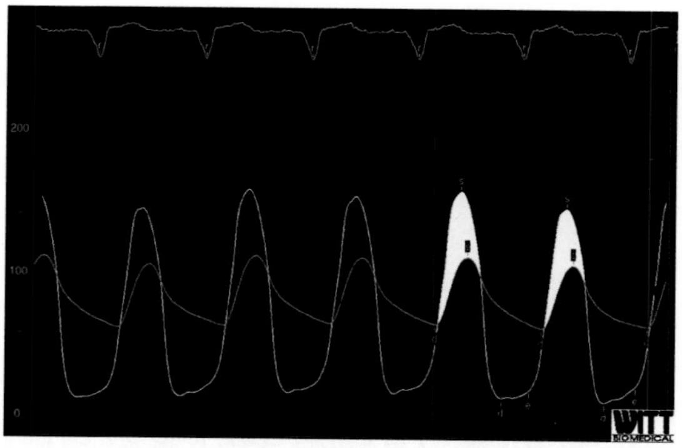

FIGURE 5-12. Example of an automated computerized analysis for determination of several of the variables required to calculate aortic valve area with the Gorlin formula. In this case, the computer determined a mean systolic gradient (*white shaded area*) of 32.4 mmHg, a heart rate of 86 beats per minute, and a systolic ejection period of 0.394 seconds. The cardiac output measured 4.3 L/min or 4300 mL/min. Thus, the calculated aortic valve area is 0.5 cm².

Measurement of the Transvalvular Pressure Gradient

Confusion often occurs regarding the various terms used to describe the pressure gradient. The *peak-to-peak* gradient is the difference between the peak left ventricular and aortic systolic pressure and is often used to quickly report the transvalvular gradient in the cardiac catheterization laboratory, but it has no physiologic relevance because these peaks occur at different times. The *peak instantaneous* gradient describes the Doppler-derived gradient and represents the largest gradient that exists between the left ventricle and the aorta. Finally, the *mean* gradient, used in the Gorlin formula, represents the average of each instantaneous gradient that exists during systole.

Accurate invasive measurement of the transvalvular pressure gradient represents the most significant challenge in determining the severity of aortic valve narrowing. Clinicians use various methods to obtain this measurement (Table 5-4),[14] and many are fraught with the potential for significant error.

The ideal method takes into account the presence of intraventricular pressure

TABLE 5-4. Methods of Measuring a Transvalvular Gradient in Aortic Stenosis

LV via transseptal; AO catheter retrograde above AO valve
LV retrograde with pressure wire; AO catheter retrograde above AO valve
LV retrograde with pigtail; AO catheter retrograde above AO valve
LV and AO retrograde with dual lumen pigtail
LV retrograde with pigtail; AO pressure from side arm of long sheath
LV retrograde with pigtail; AO pressure from side is of femoral sheath
LV retrograde with pigtail and "pullback" pressure from LV to AO

gradients and the phenomenon of pressure recovery in the ascending aorta described earlier and avoids positioning a catheter across the aortic valve to record left ventricular pressure, thereby preventing additional orifice obstruction by the profile of the catheter itself.[15] This ideal catheter configuration can be achieved by simultaneously recording pressure from two catheters: one positioned directly above the aortic valve from a retrograde approach via the femoral or brachial artery and one placed by a transseptal approach from the femoral vein, across the atrial septum and mitral valve into the body of the left ventricle toward the apex (Figure 5-13). This technique may also alleviate the concern regarding the risk of cerebral embolic events from retrograde crossing of a stenotic aortic valve.[16,17] However, many physicians who perform routine diagnostic catheterization lack transseptal catheterization skills, and thus this catheter arrangement is not commonly used unless the aortic valve cannot be crossed by a retrograde approach.

An elegant method uses a pressure wire (designed to assess intracoronary pressure) positioned across the aortic valve, using a retrograde approach to measure left ventricular pressure while simultaneously measuring aortic pressure from a

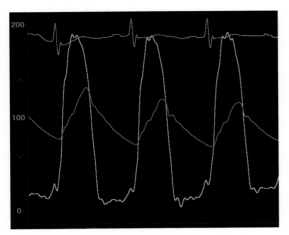

FIGURE 5-13. Simultaneous left ventricular and central aortic pressures in a patient with severe aortic stenosis. To avoid the presence of a catheter across the aortic valve, which may contribute additional obstruction to flow, the left ventricular pressure was recorded from a catheter placed into the left ventricle by a transseptal approach. Central aortic pressure was recorded from a catheter positioned just above the aortic valve from a retrograde approach via the femoral artery. Note the marked delay in upstroke, presence of a crisp dicrotic notch, and lack of time delay on the central aortic pressure. This method represents the ideal technique for recording the transvalvular pressure gradient.

catheter placed just above the aortic valve. Advantages of this method include the extremely low profile of the 0.014-inch pressure wire across the valve, preventing the potential for additional obstruction, the generation of high-fidelity waveforms from the micromanometer near the wire tip, and the requirement of only a single arterial site to obtain this data (Figure 5-14). A major disadvantage relates to the significant additional cost of the pressure wire compared to the relatively inexpensive table-mounted transducers. A detailed description of this method has been described.[14]

Simultaneous left ventricular and aortic pressures can be very accurately measured from a retrograde catheter placed across the aortic valve into the left ventricle and a second catheter positioned from another arterial site in the ascending aorta just above the valve. This arrangement provides high-quality hemodynamic data but is not very

popular because it requires two arterial punctures, thereby potentially increasing the risk of a vascular complication. In addition, the presence of a catheter across the aortic valve may contribute additional obstruction, although this effect is usually small.

The dual lumen pigtail catheter (or Langston catheter) allows simultaneous pressure measurements above and below the valve from a single arterial access site, thereby avoiding the need for two arterial punctures. Criticism of earlier versions of this catheter centered on the relatively small size of the aortic pressure lumen, resulting in dampened waveforms and loss of fidelity. Current versions (Vascular Solutions; Minneapolis) of this catheter perform well (Figure 5-15). Available in several French sizes (6–8) and shapes (pigtail, multipurpose A2, and straight), the aortic side-holes lie about 8 cm from the end of the catheter, allowing positioning well within the ventricle and just above the aortic valve, in most cases.

Many physicians favor the use of a retrograde catheter placed across the aortic valve to measure left ventricular pressure while simultaneously recording the femoral artery sheath side arm pressure as a surrogate for central aortic pressure. This technique requires using a sheath at least one French size greater than the pigtail catheter. Importantly, the operator must first demonstrate that the femoral artery is nearly the same as central aortic pressure before the aortic valve is crossed. Although this method may prove adequate in the presence of a large transvalvular pressure gradient and good correlation between central aortic and femoral arterial sheath pressures, this arrangement is fraught with potential error and may easily mislead the unwary physician regarding the severity of aortic valve narrowing. The error is most likely to have a clinical

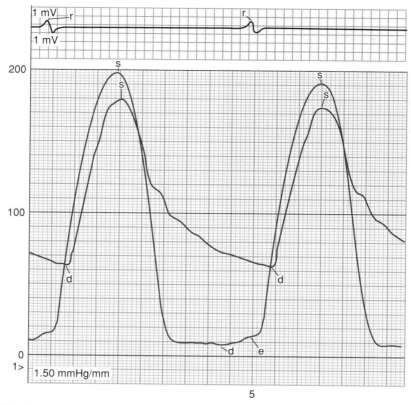

FIGURE 5-14. Simultaneous left ventricular and central aortic pressures in a patient with mild aortic stenosis. Left ventricular pressure was obtained with a 0.014-inch pressure wire, and central aortic pressure was obtained from a catheter positioned above the aortic valve using a retrograde approach via the femoral artery.

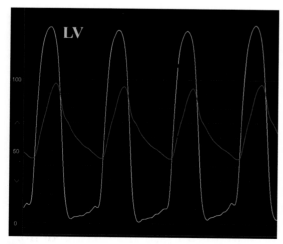

FIGURE 5-15. Simultaneous left ventricular and central aortic pressures collected from a dual lumen (Langston) catheter in a patient with severe aortic stenosis.

impact when stenosis of moderate severity is present or if a marked discrepancy occurs between the femoral artery sheath and central aortic pressure. One important source of error relates to the temporal lag between central aortic and peripheral artery pressure; this time delay in femoral artery sheath relative to left ventricular pressure falsely raises the mean transvalvular pressure gradient. An additional source of error is due to peripheral amplification, resulting in a higher systolic pressure in the femoral artery compared to the central aorta. This will falsely lower the mean transvalvular pressure gradient.

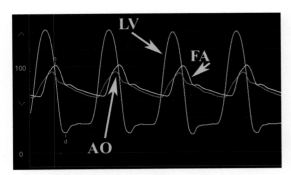

FIGURE 5-16. Simultaneous recordings from the side arm of a 7 French femoral arterial *(FA)* sheath and a dual lumen pigtail recording central aortic *(AO)* and left ventricular *(LV)* pressures in a patient with severe aortic stenosis. Note the significant time delay and systolic pressure amplification apparent on the femoral artery sheath pressure. An overestimation of the gradient occurs because of the time delay as well as an underestimation due to peripheral amplification. The effect of these two opposing errors may, in fact, come close to canceling each other out and would not likely change the valve area calculation in most cases of severe aortic stenosis. However, this error would have more potential impact in borderline cases. Although phase shifting can correct the time delay, it will not correct the effect of peripheral amplification and would only exacerbate the error, leaving the effect of peripheral amplification unopposed.

Figure 5-16 depicts the effect of temporal delay and systolic pressure amplification typically observed in cases of aortic stenosis. These two errors have opposing effects and, in many cases, actually negate each other, impacting little on the valve area calculation. The temptation to correct for the time delay by phase shifting the femoral artery sheath tracing to the left should be resisted because this will leave the effect of peripheral amplification unopposed and will actually exacerbate the error.

A major source of error in this technique occurs when femoral artery sheath pressure records lower than central aortic pressure. This can be observed in the presence of an iliac stenosis from peripheral vascular disease, vessel tortuosity, or when a clot or kink occurs in the sheath. These common situations falsely raise the gradient, overestimating

the severity of aortic stenosis. A long (55 cm) sheath positioned distal to the origin of the subclavian artery minimizes these effects.[18]

The final technique for measuring transvalvular gradient relies on a recording of pressure during *pullback* from the left ventricle to the aorta. This method is simply not a valid means for measurement of the pressure gradient in patients with aortic stenosis and should be used only as a method of screening for the presence of a gradient in patients who undergo cardiac catheterization for definition of coronary anatomy. The effects of the respiratory cycle, ventricular ectopy, and rhythm irregularity greatly impact the pressure gradient; thus, accurate estimation of the gradient mandates simultaneous pressure recordings (Figure 5-17).

The various techniques used to measure the transvalvular gradient have been evaluated.[19,20] Compared to simultaneous left ventricular and central aortic pressure, the left ventricle to aorta pullback method underestimates the degree of stenosis.[19] One study compared the pressure gradient in 15 patients with aortic stenosis from 8 different catheter configurations.[20] All eight catheter configurations measured left ventricular pressure by a retrograde approach from two positions within the left ventricle: the body of the left ventricle near the apex and the outflow tract just below the aortic valve. For aortic pressure, the study compared four different methods: ascending aorta at the level of the coronary arteries, ascending aorta 5 cm distal to the valve, femoral artery sheath pressure unadjusted for the time delay, and femoral artery sheath pressure adjusted (i.e., realigned) for the time delay. Compared to the gradients measured from catheters in the body of the left ventricle and the aorta at the level of the coronary

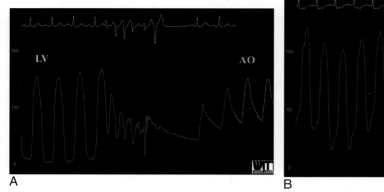

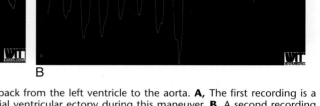

FIGURE 5-17. Recording of pressure during a pullback from the left ventricle to the aorta. **A,** The first recording is a patient with mild aortic stenosis and shows substantial ventricular ectopy during this maneuver. **B,** A second recording shows marked respiratory variation. Determination of the presence or extent of a pressure gradient without simultaneous pressure recordings in these cases is not possible.

arteries, all other positions underestimated the gradient. Most of the difference was attributable to the presence of an intraventricular gradient rather than pressure recovery stressing the importance of positioning the catheter in the body of the left ventricle instead of in the left ventricular outflow tract. Furthermore, use of an aligned femoral artery sheath pressure was associated with substantial underestimation of valve area. Importantly, patients with moderate aortic stenosis exhibited the maximum variation (0.3 cm^2)—a group in whom this degree of difference in valve area may change management decision.

Hemodynamic Findings in Aortic Stenosis

The calculated valve area is often used to assign the severity of aortic stenosis. The designations are somewhat arbitrary; nevertheless, a valve area >1.2 cm^2 is considered *mild* because symptoms are rare without other heart disease; a valve area calculation of 0.9–1.1 cm^2 is often classified as *moderate,* with symptoms seen only during stress, such as fever, extreme exertion, or tachyarrhythmia.

A calculated valve area <0.8 cm^2 represents *severe* aortic stenosis, with symptoms associated with rest or minimal exertion. The term *critical* aortic stenosis is somewhat of an emotional term to describe very severe aortic stenosis with a calculated valve area <0.5–0.7 cm^2. Clinicians must remain mindful of the limitations in valve area calculation and not base decisions solely on a number but to take into account the patient's symptoms, ventricular function, compensatory processes, physical exam, and results of noninvasive tests, in addition to calculated valve area.[4]

Mild aortic stenosis results in small transvalvular gradients, normal aortic upstroke, and normal right-sided pressures. With severe aortic stenosis, a variety of interesting hemodynamic findings are possible. The left ventricular, central aortic peak-to-peak systolic pressure gradient generally exceeds 50 mmHg and may top 100 mmHg. In cases of severe aortic stenosis, when a retrograde approach is used to obtain left ventricular pressure, the profile of the catheter may contribute to obstruction, adding to the transvalvular gradient. This may be observed as a rise in the aortic pressure of at least 5 mmHg when the catheter is withdrawn from the left ventricle and is known as *Carabello's sign* after the original observer of this phenomenon who noted this occurrence in patients with valve area <0.6 cm^2 (Figure 5-18).[21]

One of the cardinal features of severe aortic stenosis is the marked delay in upstroke on the aortic pressure waveform. Additionally, a prominent anacrotic notch or shoulder may appear within the upstroke from turbulent flow across the valve (Figure 5-19). Pulsus

alternans is a rare finding in patients with severe aortic stenosis and is usually associated with heart failure and poor left ventricular function (Figure 5-20).[22]

Although right-sided pressures are usually normal unless there is heart failure, pulmonary hypertension may be seen in up to a third of patients with severe aortic stenosis and portends a poor prognosis, although it generally improves after aortic valve replacement.[23,24]

Low Gradient–Low Output Aortic Stenosis

Aortic stenosis observed in the setting of severe ventricular dysfunction and a low cardiac output represents a unique challenge, especially when associated with a relatively low (<30 mmHg) transvalvular gradient. The low gradient may indicate one of two conditions, each managed quite differently. The patient may truly have severe aortic stenosis with a low gradient from diminished cardiac output. If flow is augmented,

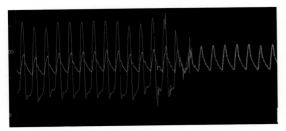

FIGURE 5-18. Example of Carabello's sign in severe aortic stenosis. During pullback of a pigtail catheter from the left ventricle to the aorta, the systolic pressure in the aortic waveform increases with relief of additional obstruction caused by the profile of the catheter.

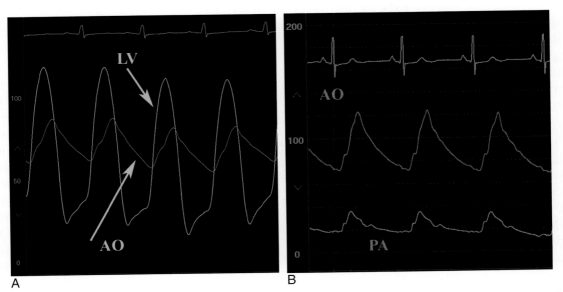

A   B

FIGURE 5-19. Example of the marked delay in upstroke on the aortic pressure tracing in a patient with severe aortic stenosis. **A** depicts simultaneous left ventricular and aortic pressure; **B** shows aortic and pulmonary artery pressure. Note the anacrotic notch on the upstroke of the aortic pressure tracing.

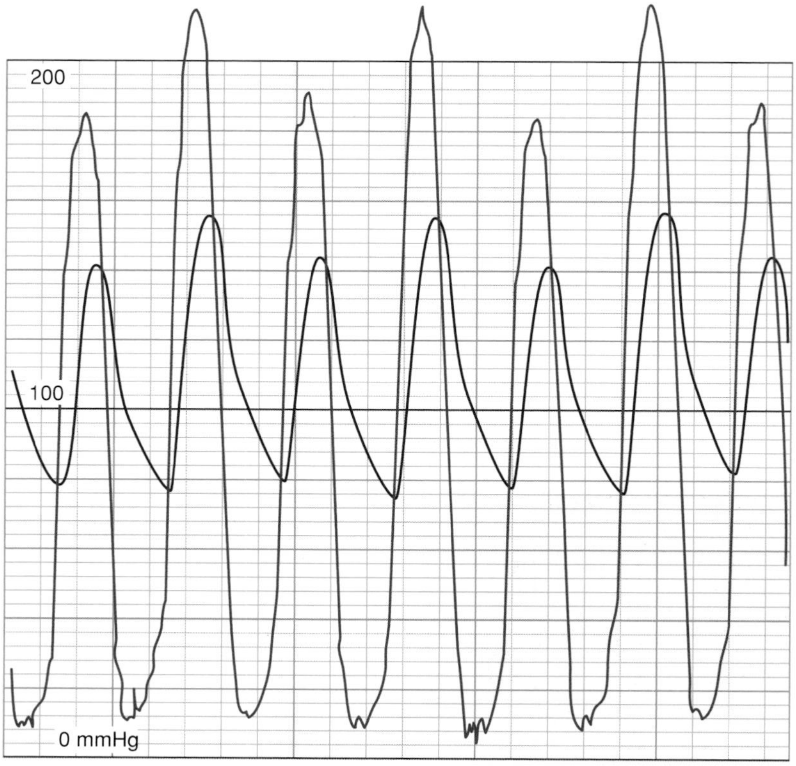

FIGURE 5-20. Pulsus alternans in a patient with severe aortic stenosis.

the gradient will rise accordingly. Such a patient will benefit greatly from aortic valve replacement. On the other hand, the presence of marked left ventricular dysfunction and weak forward flow may not allow a mildly stenotic aortic valve to open adequately, giving a false impression of severe aortic stenosis (*pseudo* severe aortic stenosis); valve replacement will not improve symptoms or ventricular function in this individual, and prognosis is generally poor with valve surgery.[25] In this circumstance, the valve area is not fixed but is dependent on flow; increasing flow will result in no change (or even a decrease) in the pressure gradient with a larger calculated aortic valve area. An additional complicating issue in these situations relates to the Gorlin formula being inaccurate in low flow states.[26]

To sort out these two clinical entities and determine who will benefit most from aortic valve replacement is difficult. Dobutamine infusion has been proposed as a method to increase flow and can be applied to both the cardiac catheterization and echocardiographic evaluations.[27,28] However, it is not entirely clear how dobutamine can best be used to discriminate patients likely to benefit from valve replacement. The Mayo Clinic first described its use in the cardiac catheterization laboratory to determine the need for surgery and found severe aortic stenosis present at surgery in those whose gradient increased to >30 mmHg and had a valve area <1.2 cm^2.[27] Another study using echocardiography observed an operative mortality of only 5% for patients who exhibited contractile reserve (defined as >20% increase in stroke volume) compared to 32% for those without contractile reserve.[28] Whether it is the presence of an increased pressure gradient, cardiac output or ejection fraction that best selects patients remains to be determined.

Coexisting Aortic Regurgitation

Significant aortic regurgitation complicates the invasive assessment of aortic stenosis severity, primarily because Gorlin's formula requires knowledge of transvalvular flow during systole. The Fick and thermodilution methods assess only the effective forward flow, whereas transvalvular flow in mixed aortic regurgitation and stenosis includes regurgitant and forward flow. Using the Fick or thermodilution methods will *underestimate* total flow, providing an *overestimation* of the severity of the stenosis. There is no consensus on how to correct for this or how to report the results. Many clinicians report that the true valve area is *no less than* that calculated by Gorlin's formula. This may reassure the clinician in cases of moderate or mild aortic stenosis but is not helpful if the calculation suggests severe aortic stenosis.

Prosthetic Aortic Valves

The normally functioning prosthetic valve often results in some degree of obstruction. The degree of obstruction depends on the type and size of prosthesis; expected gradients are often provided by the manufacturers. Expected gradients average 0–15 mmHg for bioprosthetic valves and for St. Jude mechanical valves in the aortic position, whereas the gradients seen with the higher profile Starr–Edward valve range from 0–30 mmHg. To calculate a *valve area* is meaningless when hemodynamically assessing an aortic prosthesis and most clinicians simply

report a pressure gradient. One study of 135 patients with normally functioning prosthetic aortic valves compared Gorlin-derived valve area with the actual orifice area of the prosthesis and, in many cases, found poor correlation with both overestimation and underestimation by >0.25 cm^2.[29]

Measurement of left ventricular pressure in patients with prosthetic valves requires special attention. Bioprosthetic valves can be crossed retrograde using similar methods as for native valves; mechanical valves cannot be crossed with conventional catheters in a retrograde fashion because of potential catheter entrapment or propping open of a leaflet, causing acute severe regurgitation, which may not be tolerated. Traditionally, transseptal puncture has been used to measure left ventricular pressure in this setting. Recently, however, Parnham et al.[30] demonstrated the safety and success of using a 0.014-inch pressure wire to measure left ventricular pressure by a retrograde approach in patients with St. Jude aortic valve prostheses; an example is shown in Figure 5-21.

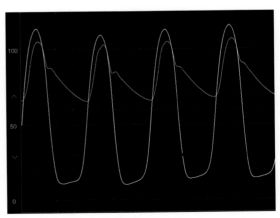

FIGURE 5-21. Simultaneous left ventricular and central aortic pressures in a patient with a St. Jude aortic valve prosthesis. The left ventricular pressure was measured with a 0.014-inch pressure wire with micromanometer positioned into the left ventricle, using a retrograde approach.

Aortic Balloon Valvuloplasty

Aortic balloon valvuloplasty for calcific aortic stenosis improves the hemodynamics of severe aortic stenosis to a modest degree. The average valve area increases from 0.5–0.8 cm^2, peak-to-peak systolic pressure gradients decrease from 55–29 mmHg, and small improvements in left ventricular end-diastolic pressure, pulmonary artery pressure, and cardiac output are noted.[31,32] The high procedural complication rates coupled with unacceptably high restenosis rates within 6 months of the procedure led to the abandonment of this procedure for calcific aortic stenosis in adults, except as a form of palliation in those with debilitating symptoms who are not operative candidates. Figure 5-22 is an example of the effect of balloon valvuloplasty on the transvalvular gradient in an elderly woman with severe aortic stenosis and refractory heart failure who was not a candidate for aortic valve replacement.

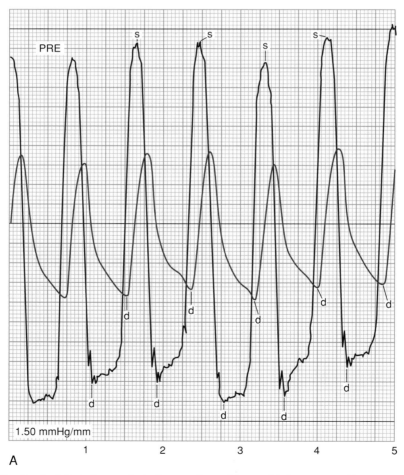

FIGURE 5-22. Results of aortic balloon valvuloplasty performed in an elderly woman with severe aortic stenosis and heart failure who was not an operative candidate as a palliative procedure. **A,** The transvalvular gradient that exceeded 60 mmHg prevalvuloplasty was reduced to 20 mmHg with this procedure **(B).**

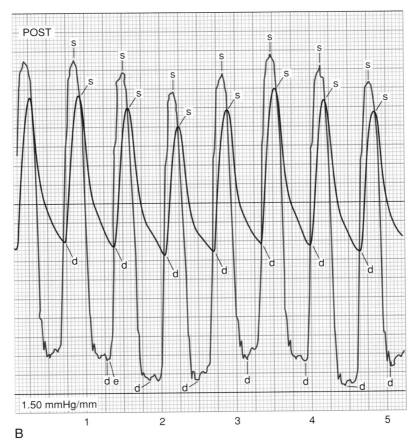

B

FIGURE 5-22—cont'd.

References

1. Bekeredjian R, Grayburn PA. Valvular heart disease: Aortic regurgitation. *Circulation* 2005;112: 125–134.
2. Carabello BA. Progress in mitral and aortic regurgitation. *Prog Cardiovasc Dis* 2001;43:457–475.
3. Alexopoulos D, Sherman W. Unusual hemodynamic presentation of acute aortic regurgitation following percutaneous balloon valvuloplasty. *Am Heart J* 1988;116:1622–1623.
4. Otto CM. Valvular aortic stenosis. Disease severity and timing of intervention. *J Am Coll Cardiol* 2006; 47:2141–2151.
5. Murgo JP. Systolic ejection murmurs in the era of modern cardiology. What do we really know? *J Am Coll Cardiol* 1998;32:1596–1602.
6. Freeman RV, Otto CM. Spectrum of calcific aortic valve disease. Pathogenesis, disease progression, and treatment strategies. *Circulation* 2005;111: 3316–3326.
7. Laskey WK, Kussmaul WG. Subvalvular gradients in patients with valvular aortic stenosis. Prevalence, magnitude and physiologic importance. *Circulation* 2001;104:1019–1022.
8. Laskey WK, Kussmaul WG. Pressure recovery in aortic valve stenosis. *Circulation* 1994;89:116–121.
9. Gorlin R, Gorlin SG. Hydraulic formula for calculation of the area of the stenotic mitral valve, other cardiac valves and central circulatory shunts. *Am Heart J* 1951;41:1–29.
10. Hakki AH, Iskandrian AS, Bemis CE, et al. A simplified valve formula for the calculation of stenotic cardiac valve areas. *Circulation* 1981;63:1050–1055.
11. Ford LE, Feldman T, Chiu YC, Carroll JD. Hemodynamic resistance as a measure of functional impairment in aortic valvular stenosis. *Circ Res* 1990;66:1–7.
12. Ford LE, Feldman T, Carroll JD. Valve resistance. *Circulation* 1994;89:893–895.
13. Bermejo J, Rojo-Alvarez JL, Antoranz JC, et al. Estimation of the end of ejection in aortic stenosis. An unreported source of error in the invasive assessment of severity. *Circulation* 2004;110:1114–1120.
14. Fusman B, Faxon D, Feldman T. Hemodynamic rounds: Transvalvular pressure gradient measurement. *Catheter Cardiovasc Interv* 2001;53:553–561.
15. Adele C, Vaitkus PT, Tischler MD. Evaluation of the significance of a transvalvular catheter on aortic valve gradient in aortic stenosis: A direct hemodynamic and Doppler echocardiographic study. *Am J Cardiol* 1997;79:513–516.
16. Omran H, Schmidt H, Hackenbroch M, et al. Silent and apparent cerebral embolism after retrograde catheterisation of the aortic valve in valvular

stenosis: A prospective randomised study. *Lancet* 1994;361:1241–1246.

17. Meine TJ, Harrison JK. Should we cross the valve: The risk of retrograde catheterization of the left ventricle in patients with aortic stenosis. *Am Heart J* 2004;148:41–42.

18. Hays J, Lujan M, Chilton R. Aortic stenosis catheterization revisited: A long sheath single puncture technique. *J Invasive Cardiol* 2006;18:262–267.

19. Brogan WC, Lange RA, Hillis LD. Accuracy of various methods of measuring the transvalvular pressure gradient in aortic stenosis. *Am Heart J* 1992; 123:948–953.

20. Assey ME, Zile MR, Usher BW, et al. Effect of catheter positioning on the variability of measured gradient in aortic stenosis. *Cathet Cardiovasc Diagn* 1993;30:287–292.

21. Carabello BA, Barry WH, Grossman W. Changes in arterial pressure during left heart pullback in patients with aortic stenosis: A sign of severe aortic stenosis. *Am J Cardiol* 1979;44:424–427.

22. Schaefer S, Malloy CR, Schmitz JM, Dehmer GJ. Clinical and hemodynamic characteristics of patients with inducible pulsus alternans. *Am Heart J* 1988;115:1251–1257.

23. Silver K, Aurigemma G, Krendel S, et al. Pulmonary artery hypertension in severe aortic stenosis: Incidence and mechanism. *Am Heart J* 1993;125: 146–150.

24. Malouf JF, Enriquez-Sarano M, Pellika PA, et al. Severe pulmonary hypertension in patients with severe aortic stenosis: Clinical profile and prognostic implications. *J Am Coll Cardiol* 2002;40:789–795.

25. Carabello BA, Green LH, Grossman W, et al. Hemodynamic determinants of prognosis of aortic valve replacement in critical aortic stenosis and advanced congestive heart failure. *Circulation* 1980;62:42–48.

26. Cannon JD Jr, Zile MR, Crawford FA Jr, Carabello BA. Aortic valve resistance as an adjunct to the Gorlin formula in assessing the severity of aortic stenosis in symptomatic patients. *J Am Coll Cardiol* 1992;20:1517–1523.

27. Nishimura RA, Grantham JA, Connolly HM, et al. Low-output, low-gradient aortic stenosis in patients with depressed left ventricular systolic function: The clinical utility of the dobutamine challenge in the catheterization laboratory. *Circulation* 2002; 106:809–813.

28. Monin JL, Quere JP, Monchi M, et al. Low-gradient aortic stenosis: Operative risk stratification and predictors for long-term outcome: A multicenter study using dobutamine stress hemodynamics. *Circulation* 2003;108:319–324.

29. Cannon SR, Richards KL, Crawford MH, et al. Inadequacy of the Gorlin formula for predicting prosthetic valve area. *Am J Cardiol* 1988;62: 113–116.

30. Parnham W, Shafei AE, Rajjoub H, et al. Retrograde left ventricular hemodynamic assessment across bileaflet prosthetic aortic valves: The use of a high-fidelity pressure sensor angioplasty guidewire. *Catheter Cardiovasc Interv* 2003;59:509–513.

31. NHLBI Balloon Valvuloplasty Registry Participants. Percutaneous balloon aortic valvuloplasty. Acute and 30 day follow-up results in 674 patients from the NHLBI Balloon Valvuloplasty Registry. *Circulation* 1991;84:2383–2397.

32. Otto CM, Mickel MC, Kennedy JW, et al. Three-year outcome after balloon aortic valvuloplasty. Insights into prognosis of valvular aortic stenosis. *Circulation* 1994;89:642–650.

CHAPTER 6

Hypertrophic Cardiomyopathy and Related Conditions

Michael Ragosta, MD

Hypertrophic cardiomyopathy is a myocardial disorder characterized by the presence of excessive ventricular hypertrophy in the absence of conditions causing physiologic hypertrophy such as hypertension, aortic stenosis, or the athletic heart. Hypertrophy is severe and often asymmetric; the ventricular septum is disproportionately involved with septal thickening in excess of 20 mm. Viewed microscopically, the myocardium demonstrates a characteristic pattern of myocyte fiber disarray and fibrosis. Hypertrophic cardiomyopathy is a genetic disorder, usually autosomal dominant, and is the most common form of inherited heart disease affecting 1 of 500 persons. Multiple genetic mutations that involve the cardiac muscle contractile proteins have been described with the most common genetic mutation involving the beta-myosin heavy chain gene. The clinical presentation and natural history of hypertrophic cardiomyopathy vary widely from a relative benign and asymptomatic condition to one characterized by disabling symptoms or sudden cardiac death.[1-4]

Impressive and interesting hemodynamic consequences arise in patients with hypertrophic cardiomyopathy, depending on whether or not ventricular outflow tract obstruction develops and manifest as a pressure gradient between the left ventricle (LV) and the aorta. Hypertrophic cardiomyopathy is often classified as *obstructive* or *nonobstructive*, based on the presence of this finding. When present, the dynamic nature of obstruction causes marked variability in pressure gradients, depending on the loading conditions and contractile state of the heart. Obstructive forms may exhibit gradients at rest with pronounced lability in the degree of obstruction, or obstruction may be *latent*, indicating that it is absent at rest and present after provocation only. The nonobstructive forms of hypertrophic cardiomyopathy lack resting or provocable gradients.

Pathophysiology

Excessive and inappropriate hypertrophy leads to several important consequences (Table 6-1). Hypertrophy impairs left ventricular compliance and diastolic dysfunction is common, resulting in elevations in the left atrial and pulmonary artery pressures. This causes symptoms of dyspnea and exercise intolerance. Arrhythmias frequently complicate the course, particularly atrial fibrillation and nonsustained ventricular tachycardia. Atrial fibrillation may be poorly tolerated because of the presence of associated diastolic dysfunction and a greater importance of the atrial contribution to cardiac output. Importantly, arrhythmias (particularly ventricular) represent the primary mechanism of sudden cardiac death, the most dreaded consequence of hypertrophic cardiomyopathy. An increase in myocardial oxygen consumption from excessive hypertrophy outstrips myocardial blood supply, potentially causing myocardial ischemia. This may occur despite normal coronary arteries. In addition, ischemia may originate from reduced coronary flow reserve from abnormalities of the small, resistance vessels. Finally, systolic compression of the coronaries (due

TABLE 6-1.	Pathophysiologic and Clinical Consequences of Hypertrophic Cardiomyopathy

PATHOPHYSIOLOGIC ABNORMALITY	CLINICAL SYNDROME
Diastolic dysfunction	Dyspnea
	Exercise intolerance, fatigue
	Arrhythmia
Myocardial ischemia	Angina
	Dyspnea
	Arrhythmia
Obstruction	Dyspnea
	Exercise intolerance, fatigue
	Chest pain
	Syncope
	Endocarditis
	Arrhythmia

to intramyocardial bridging) has been observed and may cause ischemia.

One of the most important physiologic abnormalities in hypertrophic cardiomyopathy is the presence of left ventricular outflow tract obstruction. A resting or provocable gradient is observed in about 25%–50% of cases.[5] The mechanism of obstruction had previously been a focus of considerable debate. However, extensive investigations over the years have established the role of systolic anterior motion of the mitral valve leaflet as the cause of outflow tract obstruction.[5-7] Extreme hypertrophy distorts the normal relationship between the mitral apparatus and the muscular outflow tract. The asymmetrically hypertrophied proximal intraventricular septum narrows the orifice of the outflow tract. Distortion of the ventricle causes redundancy of the mitral leaflets, leading to systolic anterior motion (SAM) of the leaflets, causing obstruction (Figure 6-1). It was thought that turbulence within the outflow tract led to a Venturi effect, drawing the anterior mitral leaflet into the outflow tract; however, SAM begins prior to the onset of ejection, suggesting that the Venturi effect contributes little to the outflow tract obstruction. Systolic anterior motion of the mitral valve also results in mitral regurgitation, explaining the association of significant mitral regurgitation in the presence of outflow tract obstruction. Obstruction causes

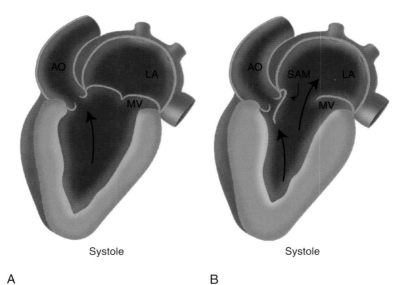

FIGURE 6-1. **A,** In normal patients, the mitral valve closes during systole, leaving the outflow tract unobstructed. **B,** In patients with hypertrophic obstructive cardiomyopathy, distortion of ventricular geometry and severe septal hypertrophy causes systolic anterior motion of the mitral valve, the mechanism of outflow tract obstruction in hypertrophic obstructive cardiomyopathy, and is associated with significant mitral regurgitation.

symptoms of dyspnea, fatigue, exercise intolerance, anginal chest pain, and syncope.

Hemodynamic Abnormalities

A wide spectrum of hemodynamic findings may be observed in patients with hypertrophic cardiomyopathy and depends on the consequences of severe hypertrophy on diastolic function and on the presence and extent of left ventricular outflow tract obstruction.

Diastolic Dysfunction

Impaired relaxation of the LV represents the predominant diastolic abnormality associated with the severe hypertrophy of hypertrophic cardiomyopathy. The associated increase in chamber stiffness from increased myocardial mass and lower chamber volumes also impairs diastolic function.[5]

Impaired relaxation limits rapid, passive left ventricular filling occurring in early diastole. To compensate for reduced rapid filling, atrial systolic filling is exaggerated. This phenomenon is clinically observed by a prominent fourth heart sound on physical examination and by the often dramatic clinical deterioration seen when patients with hypertrophic cardiomyopathy develop atrial fibrillation or other loss in atrial synchrony.

Abnormal diastolic function correlates with the degree of hypertrophy. Patients with severe resting gradients have the highest elevations of left ventricular end-diastolic pressure compared to those with latent gradients or no obstruction.[5] In addition, there may be abnormalities in early diastolic pressure. Normally, left ventricular diastolic pressure is low in early diastole; patients with hypertrophic cardiomyopathy may have marked elevations in pressure at the beginning of

diastole, reflecting abnormal ventricular relaxation (Figure 6-2). Reduced compliance of the LV is readily apparent by a prominent *a* wave on the left ventricular waveform (Figure 6-3). Left ventricular diastolic abnormalities elevate the pulmonary capillary wedge and pulmonary artery systolic pressures, and, in some cases, pulmonary pressures may be markedly elevated, ultimately causing structural changes and increased pulmonary vascular resistance with fixed pulmonary hypertension similar to chronic heart failure.

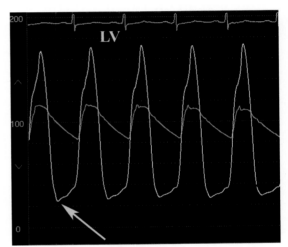

FIGURE 6-2. Diastolic dysfunction is common in hypertrophic cardiomyopathy. Abnormal relaxation is manifest by elevation of the early diastolic pressure (arrow).

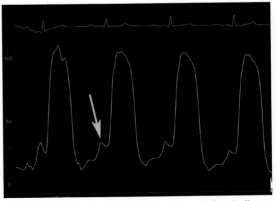

FIGURE 6-3. A prominent *a* wave (arrow) that indicates noncompliance of the LV in a patient with severe, nonobstructive hypertrophic cardiomyopathy.

Left Ventricular Outflow Tract Obstruction

The dynamic nature of the obstruction characterizing hypertrophic obstructive cardiomyopathy possesses important hemodynamic distinctions from the fixed obstruction observed in valvular aortic stenosis. In valvular aortic stenosis, fixed obstruction impedes ventricular ejection fairly uniformly throughout systole. This leads to the characteristic delayed upstroke in the aortic pressure waveform and the presence of a large systolic gradient beginning early in systole and peaking at maximum left ventricular pressure (Figure 6-4). In the case of hypertrophic obstructive cardiomyopathy, no obstruction exists at the onset of ventricular ejection. Instead, obstruction progressively develops during systole as the contractile force of the LV builds. Early in systole, left ventricular ejection is relatively unimpeded, resulting in a brisk, initial upstroke of the aortic waveform culminating in a peak systolic pressure. As systole continues and obstruction reaches a maximum, aortic pressure drops and the aortic pressure waveform transforms to appear similar to valvular stenosis with a delayed upstroke. This pattern of initial unimpeded ejection followed by progressive obstruction leads to the characteristic

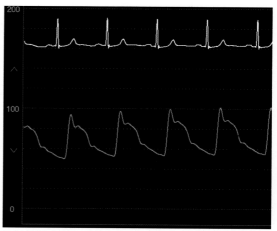

FIGURE 6-5. In patients with hypertrophic obstructive cardiomyopathy, the initial upstroke of the aortic pressure wave is normal, because early ejection is unimpeded. As obstruction to outflow develops, a fall in pressure occurs, with a spike-and-dome configuration, as shown.

"spike and dome" configuration of the aortic waveform in hypertrophic obstructive cardiomyopathy and is also responsible for the *bifid* pulse described in this condition (Figure 6-5).

Another hallmark of dynamic obstruction, and a clinically useful feature distinguishing hypertrophic obstructive cardiomyopathy from valvular aortic stenosis, is the drop in the aortic pulse pressure in the first normally conducted beat after the compensatory pause from a premature ventricular contraction (PVC). This finding, known as *Brockenbrough's sign*, was first described over 40 years ago.[8] This phenomenon is due to augmentation of the contractile force of the post-PVC beat. In valvular aortic stenosis with *fixed obstruction*, the increased contractile force of the post-PVC beat increases both left ventricular and aortic pressures. The systolic gradient increases from an associated increase in cardiac output across the valve. Importantly, the pulse width on the aortic pressure waveform also increases (Figure 6-6). In patients with *dynamic obstruction* exemplified by hypertrophic obstructive cardiomyopathy, the increased contractile force of the

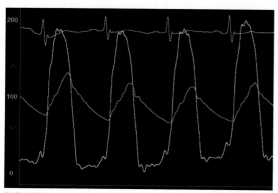

FIGURE 6-4. Fixed obstruction due to valvular aortic stenosis causes a marked delay in the upstroke of the aortic pressure wave.

FIGURE 6-6. The LV and aortic pressures (shown here as the femoral artery *[FA]* pressure) both increase in the post-PVC beat in a patient with valvular aortic stenosis, resulting in an increase in the transvalvular gradient and an increase in the aortic pulse pressure.

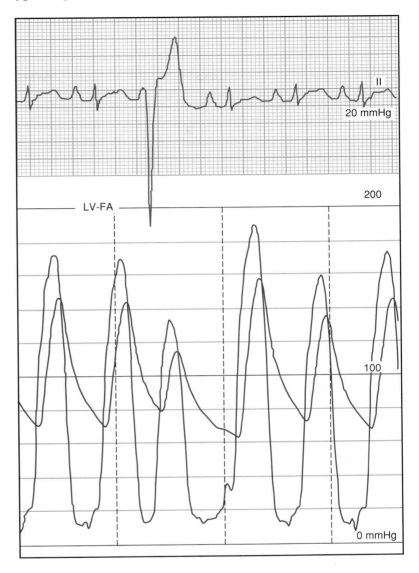

post-PVC beat worsens the degree of obstruction. This increases the left ventricular systolic pressure and the systolic gradient but decreases aortic systolic pressure, narrowing the pulse pressure (Figure 6-7). The Brockenbrough's sign requires an analysis of the aortic waveform post-PVC only, because the crucial feature is simply the narrowing of the aortic pulse pressure on the post-PVC beat. The Brockenbrough's sign distinguishes fixed from dynamic obstruction but also helps distinguish true outflow tract obstruction from an intraventricular

gradient due to severe hypertrophy and midcavity obliteration or catheter entrapment; the Brockenbrough's sign is observed only in the presence of true outflow tract obstruction. The absence of the Brockenbrough's sign, however, does not entirely exclude outflow tract obstruction. Analysis of the left ventricular ejection time on the post-PVC beat is another simple hemodynamic finding that distinguishes fixed from dynamic obstruction. The left ventricular ejection time (LVET) is defined as the time from the initial upstroke of the aortic pressure

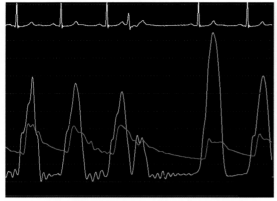

FIGURE 6-7. Patients with hypertrophic obstructive cardiomyopathy develop worsening obstruction in the post-PVC beat because of augmented contractility. This results in the classic Brockenbrough's sign demonstrated here as a drop in aortic pulse pressure in the post-PVC beat.

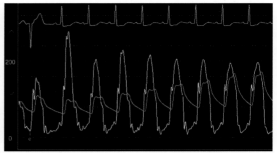

FIGURE 6-8. Obstruction is dynamic in patients with hypertrophic cardiomyopathy. The left ventricular-aortic (LV-AO) pressure gradient often varies spontaneously, as shown. Note the augmentation of the gradient on the post-PVC beat.

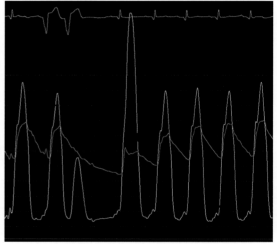

FIGURE 6-9. Provocation of the pressure gradient by introduction of a premature ventricular beat. The resting, peak-to-peak systolic gradient in this patient was approximately 40–50 mmHg and increased to over 140 mmHg on the post-PVC beat. Note both the Brockenbrough's sign and the classic spike-and-dome configuration on the aortic pressure wave of the post-PVC beat.

tracing to the dicrotic notch. An increase of the LVET on the post-PVC beat >20 msec was noted in 11 of 12 patients with hypertrophic obstructive cardiomyopathy and not in normal patients or those with valvular aortic stenosis.[9]

The dynamic nature of the gradient between the LV and the aorta in hypertrophic obstructive cardiomyopathy reflects the loading conditions of the heart as well as the inotropic state of the myocardium. Significant variations in the gradient are observed at rest.[10] Inspiration causes a decrease in the gradient. Beat-to-beat fluctuations in the gradient can be seen without changes in catheter position or in respiratory status (Figure 6-8).

Patients with latent obstruction lack a gradient at rest. Provocative maneuvers should be considered in those without a resting gradient in whom obstruction is suspected. A variety of techniques have been used; any condition reducing preload or afterload or increasing contractile force augments dynamic obstruction, unmasking a systolic gradient. Physiologic-based methods are best. The simplest method is to induce premature ventricular contractions with a catheter in the right or left ventricle (Figure 6-9).

Exercise may be used and is more likely to accurately reproduce the hemodynamic condition experienced by the patient's clinical syndrome. This is often difficult to perform in the catheterization laboratory, however, and may be best suited with noninvasive assessment by echocardiography. The Valsalva maneuver increases intrathoracic pressure lowering preload and thus augments obstruction.[11] The Valsalva is an effective method but may be difficult for some patients to comply correctly. During the strain phase, left ventricular diastolic and systolic pressures rise and aortic systolic pressures fall. The provoked gradient appears maximal during and at the end of the strain phase (Figure 6-10).

Pharmacologic techniques for provocation of a gradient include nitrates to reduce preload and afterload,[11] and inotropic stimulation to increase contractility. These techniques are problematic and may not accurately reflect the patient's true physiologic status. In one study, a poor correlation existed between the gradient provoked by nitrates and the gradient provoked by exercise; older patients with narrower outflow tracts had a larger gradient provoked by nitrates than exercise, whereas patients who exercised to higher workloads showed higher gradients with exercise than nitrates.[12] Greater concern relates to the use of direct inotropic stimulation with agents such as dobutamine. Expert panels do not recommend the use of these agents to decide treatment strategies,[1] because it has been well recognized that excessive inotropic stimulation may provoke gradients in normal hearts or in conditions other than hypertrophic cardiomyopathy such as, for example, in the setting of severe hypertrophy.[13,14] In addition, administering inotropic agents in patients with underlying severe hypertrophic obstructive cardiomyopathy may be harmful.

Potential Pitfalls in Hemodynamic Assessment

An important point to emphasize is that sloppy cardiac catheterization technique, improper catheter position, or inattention to several essential details may confuse the operator or lead to an erroneous diagnosis. Patients with hypertrophic cardiomyopathy who undergo hemodynamic assessment in the cardiac catheterization should be approached in a fashion similar to patients with valvular aortic stenosis in whom catheterization is performed to assess the transvalvular gradient and to calculate orifice area (see Chapter 5). Therefore, the gradient between the LV and the ascending aorta is ideally assessed by recording simultaneous LV and ascending aortic pressures. Although a femoral artery sheath pressure is often used as a surrogate for aortic pressure after first confirming that the sheath and aortic pressures are similar, this introduces potential inaccuracies (see Chapter 5). A dual lumen catheter can obviate many of these concerns. The optimal catheter to record LV pressure and characterize the outflow tract gradient is one with an end-hole and two side-holes near its tip. A pigtail catheter should specifically be avoided. A pigtail catheter often underestimates or even fails to identify the gradient because several of its side-holes may lie above the obstruction (Figure 6-11).

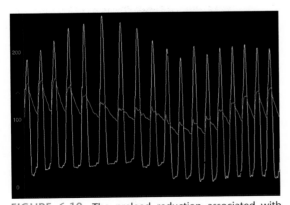

FIGURE 6-10. The preload reduction associated with the strain phase of the Valsalva maneuver worsens obstruction and augments the pressure gradient in hypertrophic obstructive cardiomyopathy. On the left side of the panel, the resting gradient is seen and measured about 40 mmHg. The strain phase of the Valsalva maneuver causes a rise in the LV diastolic pressure and a marked increase in the gradient.

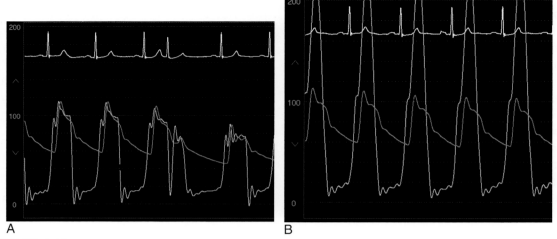

A   B

FIGURE 6-11. The pigtail catheter is not optimal for measurement of a gradient in hypertrophic obstructive cardio-myopathy. **A,** Example of the hemodynamics obtained using a pigtail catheter in the LV in a patient with hypertrophic cardiomyopathy. No gradient is present despite the observation of a spike-and-dome configuration of the simultaneously obtained femoral artery pressure trace. **B,** The pigtail catheter was exchanged for an end-hole catheter, and a large outflow tract gradient became readily apparent.

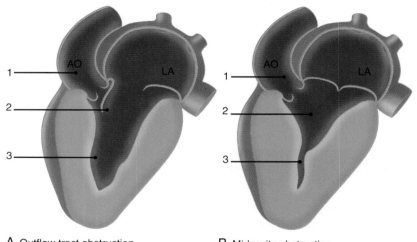

A Outflow tract obstruction   B Midcavity obstruction

FIGURE 6-12. Of importance is to distinguish true outflow tract obstruction from midcavity obstruction, both of which may demonstrate pressure gradients between the LV and the aorta. **A,** True outflow tract obstruction is present due to systolic anterior motion of the mitral valve. Pressure in the ventricular apex (point 3) will be higher than the aorta (point 1), but a gradient will also exist between the aorta (point 1) and the left ventricle at the level of the mitral valve (point 2). **B,** In contrast, when midcavity obstruction occurs, a gradient will be present between the left ventricular apex (point 3) and the aorta (point 1) but not between the aorta (point 1) and the left ventricle at the level of the mitral valve (point 2).

A gradient between the LV and aorta may not always represent true outflow tract obstruction. Another cause of a gradient between the LV and the aorta is due to midcavity or apical obstruction.

Severe hypertrophy coupled with hyperdynamic ventricular function and/or reduced ventricular volumes may obliterate the LV cavity from the midportion of the ventricle to the apex (Figure 6-12).

A catheter tip in that portion of the ventricle will record high ventricular systolic pressures and a systolic gradient. In such cases, other features typical to hypertrophic obstructive cardiomyopathy, such as the Brockenbrough's sign or a spike-and-dome configuration to the aortic waveform, will be absent (Figure 6-13). Systolic anterior motion of the mitral valve will specifically be absent, as well as associated mitral regurgitation. Careful positioning of the catheter in the outflow tract will fail to record a systolic pressure gradient.

A related pitfall occurs when entrapment of the LV catheter tip occurs within the excessively hypertrophied myocardium. This artifact may provide the appearance of an intraventricular pressure gradient often confused with the dynamic obstruction seen in hypertrophic cardiomyopathy. However, several features suggest artifact rather than true obstruction.[15] First, this finding is usually seen when the tip of an end-hole catheter is buried into the hypertrophied myocardium. The operator will be unable to draw blood back from the catheter with absence of pulsatile flow during systole from the disconnected catheter. The peak LV systolic pressure is seen later in systole, usually at

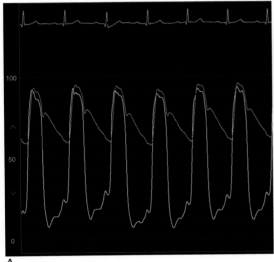

A

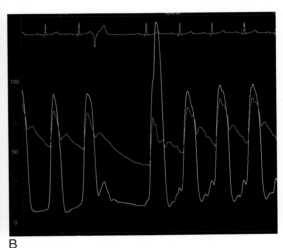

B

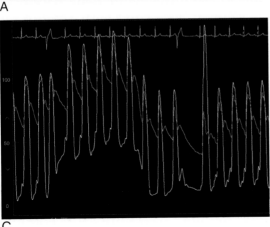

C

FIGURE 6-13. This set of waveforms was obtained in a patient with severe hypertrophy to determine if there was outflow tract obstruction. **A,** With a dual lumen, end-hole catheter positioned near the left ventricular apex, no gradient is present between the left ventricle and the aorta, and the aortic waveform has a normal morphology. However, a marked elevation of the left ventricular diastolic pressure occurs with a prominent *a* wave. **B,** Post-PVC, there appeared to be provocation of a gradient; however, the aortic pressure wave remained normal in morphology and the pulse pressure was unchanged. **C,** A Valsalva maneuver did not change the gradient. Again, note the PVC and augmentation of the gradient with the post-PVC beat, but no change in aortic waveform morphology or drop in the aortic pulse pressure occurred. These hemodynamics are most consistent with obstruction in the midcavity location and not true outflow tract obstruction due to systolic anterior motion of the mitral valve.

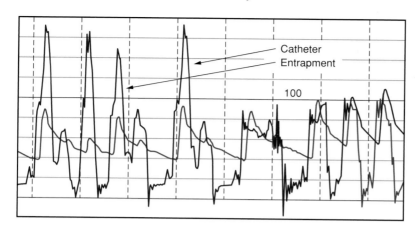

Catheter
Entrapment

100

FIGURE 6-14. These tracings were obtained using an end-hole catheter in a patient with severe hypertrophy. The left ventricular pressure tracings of the post-PVC beats have a bizarre and spiked appearance with a peak pressure that occurs late in systole. The aortic pressure wave forms do not show a spike-and-dome morphology or evidence of the Brockenbrough's sign post-PVC. The ventricular pressure tracings likely represent catheter entrapment artifact.

the dicrotic notch of the aortic pressure wave. Repositioning the catheter tip in the outflow tract at the level of the mitral valve will confirm the absence of a true outflow tract gradient. Often, the contour of the ventricular waveform appears bizarre with a narrow, spiked appearance and an initially normal appearance with no gradient early in systole (Figure 6-14). The Brockenbrough's sign and spike-and-dome appearance to the aortic pressure waveform are absent. The LV ejection time is prolonged in true obstruction and decreased with entrapment.[16]

Effects of Treatment

The majority of symptomatic patients with obstruction are treated with medical therapy consisting of beta blockers, calcium channel blockers, or disopyramide. Although beta blockers improve symptoms, they have shown inconsistent effects on reducing the degree of obstruction or improving diastolic function.[17] Verapamil has been more extensively studied than other calcium channel blockers in this condition and is associated with both modest reductions in the outflow tract gradient and improved diastolic function. Disopyramide is effective at acutely reducing resting or provoked gradients with a 50% reduction in

gradient sustained over 3 years and no apparent proarrhythmia.[18]

Patients with continued severe symptoms on medical therapy (New York Heart Association Class 3 or 4) with gradients in excess of 30–50 mmHg at rest or greater than 50–60 mmHg following physiologic provocation are candidates for either surgical myectomy or catheter-based alcohol septal ablation. The advantages and disadvantages of these two approaches continue to supply bountiful and passionate discussion in the literature.[19,20] Although no randomized data are available to compare the two techniques, both methods reduce outflow tract gradients and improve symptoms with a higher rate of heart block, requiring permanent pacemaker placement associated with alcohol septal ablation.[21] Surgical myectomy is a well-established technique with more than 4 decades of experience. In the hands of experienced, dedicated surgical centers, surgical myectomy is highly effective at eliminating the outflow tract gradient in more than 98% of patients and is associated with excellent long-term survival similar to the general population.[22,23]

The technique for alcohol septal ablation has improved since its inception in the early 1990s. The technique uses conventional angioplasty equipment but requires a sophisticated understanding of septal anatomy and myocardial perfusion. A detailed description of currently used techniques and issues has been described.[24] Appropriate candidates for this technique include patients with greater than 1.8 cm septal thickness, Class 3 or 4 symptoms despite medical therapy, and at least a 30-mmHg resting systolic gradient or more than a 60-mmHg provocable gradient. The technique depends on the presence of suitable septal anatomy. Identification of discrete septal perforators is necessary. Ideally, the septal perforators should supply only the proximal intraventricular septum at the point of contact between the septum and the mitral leaflet during systolic anterior motion. This can be confirmed with myocardial contrast echocardiography and selective injection of a myocardial contrast agent into a candidate septal perforator. Also of importance is to demonstrate that the septal perforator does not also supply other areas of myocardium such as the inferior wall. If the septal anatomy is appropriate, a small diameter, over-the-wire balloon is positioned and inflated to occlude the septal perforator. Angiographic contrast is injected into both the lumen of the balloon, to ensure no spillage into the left anterior descending artery, and into the left coronary artery, to show that no anterograde flow occurs around the balloon. The procedure requires placement of a temporary pacemaker because of the high incidence of transient heart block. Denatured alcohol (1–5 mL) is slowly injected through the lumen of the inflated balloon into the septal perforator and allowed to dwell for 5–10 minutes, causing a dense septal infarction and, when successful, elimination of obstruction. The typical hemodynamic effects obtained from alcohol septal ablation are provided in Figure 6-15. The effects on hemodynamics have been described in large series of patients who

undergo alcohol septal ablation.[25] An immediate improvement occurs in the outflow tract gradient, which continues to improve over time (Figure 6-16).

Related Conditions

Apical Variant

A rare variant of hypertrophic cardiomyopathy, first described by the Japanese, consists of marked hypertrophy that involves only the apex of the LV. Giant negative T waves on the precordial leads of the electrocardiogram and a characteristic "spade-shape" appearance of the left ventriculogram confirm the diagnosis. No specific hemodynamic feature is characteristic of apical hypertrophic cardiomyopathy. Similar to other patients with severe hypertrophy, diastolic abnormalities may be observed (Figure 6-17). Because this condition is not associated with LV outflow tract obstruction, no outflow tract gradient, spike-and-dome configuration, or Brockenbrough's sign is present. Symptoms such as dyspnea are due to diastolic abnormalities. This condition is not associated with sudden cardiac death and carries a relatively benign prognosis with the major morbidity due to atrial arrhythmias.[26]

Acquired Obstruction

Dynamic LV outflow tract obstruction can be seen in conditions other than hypertrophic obstructive cardiomyopathy. The mechanism of obstruction is similar and is due to systolic anterior motion of the mitral valve. It has been reported in the setting of severe, concentric LV hypertrophy from hypertension or aortic stenosis, particularly under excessive inotropic stimulation or severe volume depletion. In addition, dynamic outflow tract obstruction due

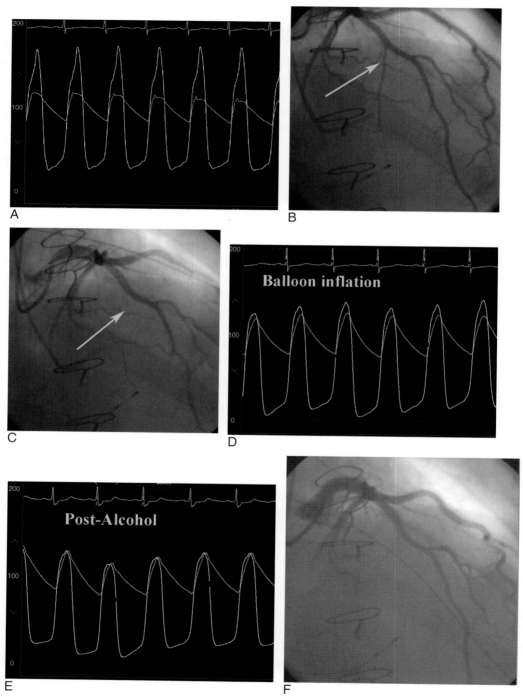

FIGURE 6-15. Alcohol septal ablation results in immediate improvement in the hemodynamics of hypertropic cardiomyopathy. **A,** At rest, a gradient of nearly 60 mmHg is present. **B,** Coronary angiography confirmed the presence of a suitable first septal perforator. **C,** A small, 2.0-mm over-the-wire balloon was positioned in this branch and inflated to temporarily obstruct flow. **D,** The pressure gradient during balloon inflation immediately decreased to 10–15 mmHg. **E,** Alcohol was injected through the balloon lumen while the balloon was inflated, and the hemodynamics obtained immediately after alcohol delivery showed resolution of the pressure gradient. **F,** The septal perforator typically occludes on the post-procedure angiography in successful cases.

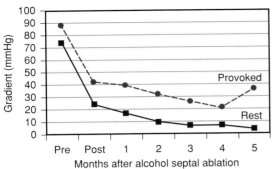

FIGURE 6-16. Time course of pressure gradient changes after alcohol septal ablation. Continued improvement occurs in the pressure gradient after the initial procedure. (From Fernandes VL, Nagueh SF, Franklin J, et al. A prospective follow-up of alcohol septal ablation for symptomatic hypertrophic obstructive cardiomyopathy—The Baylor experience (1996–2002). *Clin Cardiol* 2005;28:124–130, with permission.)

to systolic anterior motion of the mitral valve has been described as a rare occurrence in the setting of an acute anterior myocardial infarction or with myocardial "stunning" in the setting of an acute coronary syndrome when excessive basal

left ventricular hypercontractility is present.[27–32] In fact, it should be considered in the differential diagnosis of cardiogenic shock in patients with acute infarction.

A very unusual but interesting example of a patient with acquired obstruction is shown in Figure 6-18. This patient presented to the emergency room with acute onset of unresponsiveness and profound hypotension, with an electrocardiogram that demonstrated a left bundle branch block and an emergent, quickly performed bedside echocardiogram that showed hypokinesis of the anterior wall. The patient was thought to be in cardiogenic shock and therefore underwent emergent catheterization, revealing normal coronary arteriography. The hemodynamics suggested outflow tract obstruction. Left ventriculogram confirmed an anterior wall motion abnormality, and repeat echocardiography

FIGURE 6-17. Abnormal diastolic function in a patient with apical variant of hypertrophic cardiomyopathy. Diastolic pressure is highest early in diastole, representing abnormal relaxation. *LVEDP,* Left ventricular end-diastolic pressure; *PCWP,* pulmonary capillary wedge pressure.

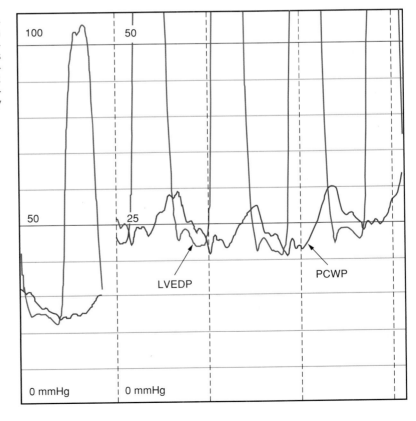

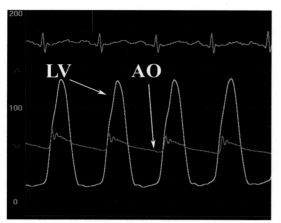

FIGURE 6-18. Left ventricular outflow tract obstruction may be due to causes other than hypertrophic cardiomyopathy, as shown. This tracing was obtained in a profoundly hypotensive, unresponsive patient taken emergently to the cardiac catheterization laboratory. The coronary arteries were normal. A large gradient is present on simultaneous LV-AO pressure tracings, and echocardiography confirmed a large anterior wall motion abnormality and systolic anterior motion of the mitral valve. The patient was found to have a subarachnoid hemorrhage with neurogenic stunning of the left ventricle and acquired outflow tract obstruction.

revealed systolic anterior motion of the mitral valve as the mechanism of obstruction without evidence of ventricular hypertrophy. The patient was found to have a subarachnoid hemorrhage with neurogenic stunning of the anterior wall and acquired obstruction.

Subaortic Membrane

In contrast to hypertrophic obstructive cardiomyopathy, in which LV obstruction is due to systolic anterior motion of the mitral valve, the outflow tract obstruction seen in association with a subaortic membrane is caused by the anatomic presence of a discrete membrane, a fibromuscular ridge, or a fibromuscular tunnel that narrows the outflow tract. In addition to the usual symptoms attributed to obstruction, the high velocity jet may cause progressive and severe aortic regurgitation.

The hemodynamic effects of a subaortic membrane appear similar to those of

valvular aortic stenosis. Distinguishing the two conditions requires careful catheterization technique. The membrane lies only about 1 cm below the aortic valve. If a pigtail catheter is used to assess LV pressure, it will not discriminate the precise location of the obstruction because of the numerous side-holes on the catheter. An end-hole catheter is better suited to determine the exact level of obstruction within the outflow tract. Simultaneous aortic and LV pressure waveforms (using an end-hole catheter) document a large systolic pressure gradient. As the ventricular catheter is withdrawn, a pressure gradient within the ventricle will appear to exist just below the aortic valve. No pressure gradient is present across the aortic valve.

Although both hypertrophic obstructive cardiomyopathy and subaortic membranes exhibit LV outflow tract obstruction, obstruction from a subaortic membrane is *fixed* and thus will behave more like valvular aortic stenosis than hypertrophic obstructive cardiomyopathy. Similar to valvular stenosis, early ejection will be impaired and no spike-and-dome configuration is present to the aortic waveform, as seen with dynamic obstruction. The Brockenbrough's sign is usually absent, although it may rarely be seen when a predominantly muscular component exists to the membrane.

Supravalvular Aortic Stenosis

Supravalvular aortic stenosis is a rare condition in which the level of obstruction is above the aortic valve in the ascending aorta. It has classically been described in association with William's syndrome (elfin facies, peripheral pulmonary artery stenosis, coarctation of the aorta, and supravalvular aortic stenosis) but is actually more commonly observed as an isolated, sporadic form. Rarely, it may appear as a familial autosomal dominant form associated with peripheral pulmonary artery stenosis.

The hemodynamic findings of supravalvular aortic stenosis are shown in Figure 6-19. A gradient is present between the LV and the femoral artery sheath pressure. As the LV catheter is withdrawn across the aortic valve, the absence of systolic pressure gradient between the

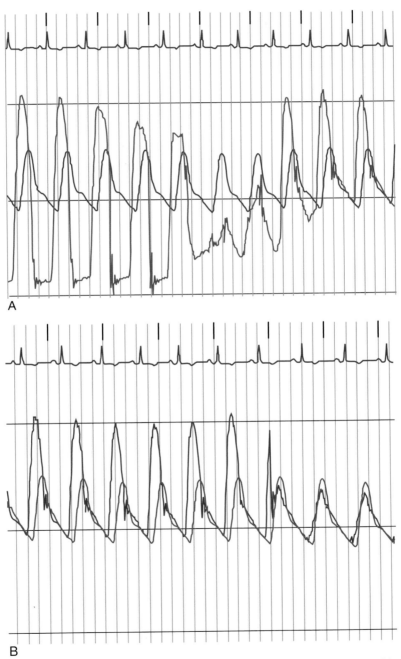

FIGURE 6-19. Simultaneous left ventricular and femoral artery pressure tracings in a patient with supravalvular aortic stenosis. **A,** A pressure gradient exists between the left ventricle and the femoral artery *(left of panel)* and the aorta just above the aortic valve and the femoral artery on pullback from the ventricle *(right of panel).* **B,** Continued catheter withdrawal above the aortic valve in the ascending aorta discerns the precise location of obstruction.

LV and the proximal few centimeters of the aorta is apparent. This finding excludes the presence of valvular or subvalvular stenosis. As the catheter is withdrawn further, the precise location of the pressure gradient is identified in the ascending aorta. Coarctation of the aorta exhibits similar hemodynamics with the systolic pressure gradient localized in the descending aorta at the ligamentum arteriosum.

References

1. Maron BJ, McKenna WJ (Co-Chair). American College of Cardiology/European Society of Cardiology clinical expert consensus document on hypertrophic cardiomyopathy. *J Am Coll Cardiol* 2003;42:1687–1713.
2. Roberts R, Sigwart U. New concepts in hypertrophic cardiomyopathies, part I. *Circulation* 2001;104:2113–2116.
3. Roberts R, Sigwart U. New concepts in hypertrophic cardiomyopathies, part II. *Circulation* 2001;104:2249–2252.
4. Cannan CR, Reeder GS, Bailey KR, et al. Natural history of hypertrophic cardiomyopathy. A population-based study, 1976 through 1990. *Circulation* 1995;92:2488–2495.
5. Wigle ED, Sasson Z, Henderson MA, et al. Hypertrophic cardiomyopathy: The importance of the site and the extent of hypertrophy. A review. *Prog Cardiovasc Dis* 1985;28:1–83.
6. Pollick C, Rakowski H, Wigle ED. Muscular subaortic stenosis: The quantitative relationship between systolic anterior motion and the pressure gradient. *Circulation* 1984;69:43–49.
7. Jiang L, Levine RA, King ME, Weyman AE. An integrated mechanism for systolic anterior motion of the mitral valve in hypertrophic cardiomyopathy based on echocardiographic observations. *Am Heart J* 1987;113:633–644.
8. Brockenbrough EC, Braunwald E, Morrow AG. A hemodynamic technic for the detection of hypertrophic subaortic stenosis. *Circulation* 1961;23:189–194.
9. White CW, Zimmerman TJ. Prolonged left ventricular ejection time in the post-premature beat. A sensitive sign of idiopathic hypertrophic subaortic stenosis. *Circulation* 1975;52:306–312.
10. Kizilbash AM, Heinle SK, Grayburn PA. Spontaneous variability of left ventricular outflow tract gradient in hypertrophic obstructive cardiomyopathy. *Circulation* 1998;97:461–466.
11. Braunwald E, Oldham HN, Ross J, et al. The circulatory response of patients with idiopathic hypertrophic subaortic stenosis to nitroglycerin and to the Valsalva maneuver. *Circulation* 1964;29:422–431.
12. Marwick TH, Nakatani S, Haluska B, et al. Provocation of latent left ventricular outflow tract gradients with amyl nitrate and exercise in hypertrophic cardiomyopathy. *Am J Cardiol* 1995;75: 805–809.
13. Luria D, Klutstein MW, Rosenmann D, et al. Prevalence and significance of left ventricular outflow gradient during dobutamine echocardiography. *Eur Heart J* 1999;20:386–392.
14. Pellikka PA, Oh JK, Bailey KR, et al. Dynamic intraventricular obstruction during dobutamine stress echocardiography. A new observation. *Circulation* 1992;86:1429–1432.
15. Wigle DE, Marquis Y, Auger P. Muscular subaortic stenosis: Initial left ventricular inflow tract pressure in the assessment of intraventricular pressure differences in man. *Circulation* 1967;35:1100–1117.
16. Wigle DE, Marquis Y, Auger P. Muscular subaortic stenosis: The direct relation between the intraventricular pressure difference and the left ventricular ejection time. *Circulation* 1967;36:36–44.
17. Yoerger DM, Weyman AE. Hypertrophic obstructive cardiomyopathy: Mechanism of obstruction and response to therapy. *Rev Cardiovasc Med* 2003; 4:199–215.
18. Sherrid MV, Barac I, McKenna WJ, et al. Multicenter study of the efficacy and safety of disopyramide in obstructive hypertrophic cardiomyopathy. *J Am Coll Cardiol* 2005;45:1251–1258.
19. Maron BJ, Dearani JA, Ommen SR, et al. The case for surgery in obstructive hypertrophic cardiomyopathy. *J Am Coll Cardiol* 2004;44:2044–2053.
20. Hess OM, Sigwart U. New treatment strategies for hypertrophic obstructive cardiomyopathy. Alcohol ablation of the septum: The new gold standard? *J Am Coll Cardiol* 2004;44:2054–2055.
21. Nagueh SF, Ommen SR, Lakkis NM, et al. Comparison of ethanol septal reduction therapy with surgical myectomy for the treatment of hypertrophic obstructive cardiomyopathy. *J Am Coll Cardiol* 2001;38:1701–1706.
22. Woo A, Williams WG, Choi R, et al. Clinical and echocardiographic determinants of long-term survival after surgical myectomy in obstructive hypertrophic cardiomyopathy. *Circulation* 2005;111:2033–2041.
23. Ommen SR, Maron BJ, Olivotto I, et al. Long-term effects of surgical septal myectomy on survival in patients with obstructive hypertrophic cardiomyopathy. *J Am Coll Cardiol* 2005;46:470–476.
24. Holmes DR, Valeti US, Nishimura RA. Alcohol septal ablation for hypertrophic cardiomyopathy: Indications and technique. *Catheter Cardiovasc Interv* 2005;66:375–389.
25. Fernandes VL, Nagueh SF, Franklin J, et al. A prospective follow-up of alcohol septal ablation for symptomatic hypertrophic obstructive cardiomyopathy— The Baylor experience (1996–2002). *Clin Cardiol* 2005;28:124–130.
26. Eriksson MJ, Sonnenberg B, Woo A, et al. Long-term outcome in patients with apical hypertrophic cardiomyopathy. *J Am Coll Cardiol* 2002;39: 638–645.
27. San Roman Sanchez D, Medina O, Jimenez F, et al. Dynamic intraventricular obstruction in acute myocardial infarction. *Echocardiography* 2001;18: 515–518.
28. Haley JH, Sinak LJ, Tajik JA, et al. Dynamic left ventricular outflow tract obstruction in acute coronary syndromes: An important cause of new systolic murmur and cardiogenic shock. *Mayo Clin Proc* 1999;74:901–906.

29. Armstrong WF, Marcovitz PA. Dynamic left ventricular outflow tract obstruction as a complication of acute myocardial infarction. *Am Heart J* 1996;131:827–830.
30. Villareal RP, Achari A, Wilansky S, Wilson JM. Anteroapical stunning and left ventricular outflow tract obstruction. *Mayo Clin Proc* 2001;76:79–83.
31. Landesman KA, Sadaniantz A. Left ventricular outflow tract obstruction after myocardial infarction due to a hyperdynamic basal septum. *Echocardiography* 2001;18:291–294.
32. Joffe II, Riley MF, Katz SE, et al. Acquired dynamic left ventricular outflow tract obstruction complicating acute anterior myocardial infarction: Serial echocardiographic and clinical evaluation. *J Am Soc Echo* 1997;10:717–721.

CHAPTER 7

Right-Sided Heart Disorders: Hemodynamics of the Tricuspid and Pulmonic Valves and Pulmonary Hypertension

MICHAEL RAGOSTA, MD

After Werner Forssmann boldly inserted a urological catheter into his own right atrium, the right heart became accessible to clinical investigation, allowing the study of right-heart physiology in both normal and diseased states.[1] Many cardiac diseases influence right-heart hemodynamics. The primary cause of right-heart failure is left-heart failure; therefore, the myriad cardiac disorders associated with left-heart failure often impact right-heart hemodynamics. In addition, right ventricular infarction, congenital heart diseases, and disorders of the pericardium affect right-heart hemodynamics. These aspects are extensively covered in the corresponding chapters. This chapter will focus on disorders unique to the right heart, including tricuspid and pulmonic valvular diseases and the effect of pulmonary hypertension.

Tricuspid Valve Stenosis

This rare valvular lesion is most often due to rheumatic heart disease and is almost always associated with mitral stenosis; isolated rheumatic tricuspid stenosis is rare.[2] Very rarely, tricuspid stenosis is caused by other conditions, including

carcinoid syndrome, endomyocardial fibrosis, congenital tricuspid valve stenosis, pacemaker lead–related leaflet fibrosis, atrial myxoma, or prosthetic valve dysfunction (both bioprosthetic and mechanical).

Tricuspid stenosis impairs right atrial emptying and elevates right atrial pressure. Diminished filling of the right ventricle reduces cardiac output. The combination of tricuspid and mitral stenosis reduces the cardiac output to levels lower than expected on the basis of either valvular lesion alone. Clinical consequences of severe tricuspid stenosis include fatigue, elevated jugular veins, peripheral edema, hepatic congestion, and ascites. If unsuspected, the diagnosis may prove challenging because symptoms mimic other conditions such as pericardial disease, cirrhosis of the liver, or pulmonary hypertension, which may, in fact, be present from associated mitral stenosis.

The hemodynamic abnormalities observed in tricuspid stenosis have been well described.[3–6] Right atrial pressure is elevated. The *a* wave reaches giant proportions in patients in normal sinus rhythm and may exceed 20 mmHg. However, an enlarged *a* wave is not specific for tricuspid stenosis because it may be seen in the presence of pulmonary hypertension and right ventricular hypertrophy; although, in the absence of pulmonary hypertension, a prominent *a* wave supports a diagnosis of tricuspid stenosis.

Similar to mitral stenosis, the presence of a pressure gradient observed while simultaneously measuring pressure in the right atrium and right ventricle during diastole characterizes tricuspid valve stenosis (Figure 7-1). Because of the lower right-sided pressures, the relatively lower cardiac output and greater size of the tricuspid orifice as compared to the mitral valve, the observed gradients are

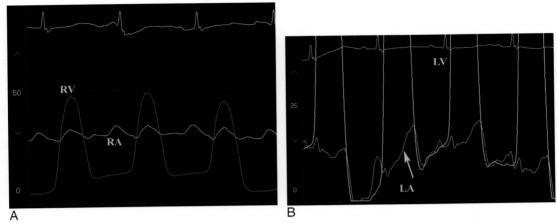

FIGURE 7-1. These hemodynamics were obtained from a 19-year-old patient with a mechanical (tilting disc) tricuspid valve presenting with severe right-sided heart failure and thrombosis of the mechanical valve. The right ventricular pressure waveform was obtained via right ventricular puncture. **A,** The right atrial pressure is markedly elevated with a prominent *a* wave and a large diastolic pressure gradient. This case differs from the more commonly seen **(B)** rheumatic tricuspid stenosis, which typically also has associated mitral stenosis, absent in this case (simultaneous left ventricular and left atrial pressure).

correspondingly relatively small, ranging from 2–12 mmHg with 90% of gradients less than 7 mmHg.[6] A *mean* diastolic gradient >2 mmHg is diagnostic of tricuspid stenosis. Small gradients (2–3 mmHg) that exist only in early diastole may be observed in patients with predominantly tricuspid regurgitation without significant stenosis.[3,6] In patients with tricuspid stenosis and normal sinus rhythm, a small pressure gradient early in diastole increases at end-diastole because of the rise in atrial pressure from atrial contraction. For patients with atrial fibrillation, right atrial pressure remains uniformly elevated throughout the cardiac cycle, and the pressure gradient is greatest in early diastole when the right ventricular diastolic pressure is lowest. The transtricuspid valve pressure gradient increases with inspiration, predominantly due to a fall in the diastolic pressure with inspiration. The gradient increases with exercise due to an increase in the right atrial pressure. An increase in volume will also increase the gradient.

Calculation of the tricuspid valve orifice area has been estimated, using Gorlin's formula (see Chapter 4). Similar to mitral stenosis, the mean pressure gradient across the valve, the diastolic filling period, the heart rate, and the cardiac output are the important measured variables entered into the formula; however, unlike the mitral valve, the coefficient has not been determined and has been arbitrarily set at 1.0 (similar to the aortic valve area). The formula has not been well validated in tricuspid stenosis, although small series have correlated the calculated valve area with the area determined at surgery.[6] Similar to mitral stenosis with associated mitral regurgitation, if there is associated tricuspid regurgitation, Gorlin's formula will underestimate the valve area because the true transvalvular flow is not known.

Tricuspid Valve Regurgitation

This represents the most commonly encountered right-sided valvular heart lesion. Mild-to-moderate degrees of tricuspid regurgitation are very commonly detected on 2D echocardiography and are of little to no significance. Severe tricuspid regurgitation, however, is an important valvular lesion that causes progressive right-heart failure and increased mortality.[7] Among the numerous possible etiologies (Table 7-1), functional tricuspid regurgitation from right ventricular pressure or volume overload accounts for most cases; primary regurgitation due to organic tricuspid valve pathology is much less prevalent.[8] Common in patients with rheumatic heart disease (with a prevalence of nearly 40% in patients with mitral stenosis), tricuspid regurgitation is due to several potential mechanisms, including rheumatic tricuspid valve involvement (primary tricuspid regurgitation) or functional regurgitation as a consequence of pressure or volume overload of the right ventricle.[9] Elucidation of the mechanism of tricuspid regurgitation seen in association with rheumatic mitral stenosis is important for proper treatment. Observation of normal pulmonary pressures suggests

TABLE 7-1.	Causes of Tricuspid Regurgitation

STRUCTURALLY NORMAL TRICUSPID VALVE (FUNCTIONAL TRICUSPID REGURGITATION)

Annular dilatation from volume or pressure
  overload
  Atrial septal defect
  Right ventricular infarction
  Congestive heart failure
  Pulmonary hypertension
  Post-heart transplantation

STRUCTURALLY ABNORMAL TRICUSPID VALVE

  Rheumatic heart disease
  Carcinoid
  Radiation-induced valvular regurgitation
  Endocarditis
  Trauma
  Right ventricular biopsy induced
  Pacemaker-lead induced
  Myxomatous degeneration

primary valve disease. In patients with pulmonary hypertension, echocardiography can help distinguish functional regurgitation from organic tricuspid valve disease.

Tricuspid regurgitation causes volume overload of the right ventricle and atrium. Over time, the right ventricle dilates further, worsening the degree of regurgitation. In the presence of pulmonary hypertension, severe tricuspid regurgitation causes both volume and pressure overload and is less well tolerated, leading to earlier onset of symptoms. Symptoms of severe tricuspid regurgitation reflect right-heart failure and include edema, ascites, distended neck veins, and profound fatigue from decreased cardiac output.

The hemodynamic abnormalities of severe tricuspid regurgitation include elevation of right atrial pressure, decreased cardiac output, and abnormalities of the right atrial pressure waveform. Because the jugular veins mirror the abnormalities present in the right atrium, it is no surprise that the characteristic atrial waveform abnormalities attributed to tricuspid regurgitation were first observed on analysis of jugular venous pressure waveforms[10] (Figure 7-2). Normally, an x descent exists on the right atrial waveform, reflecting descent of the base of the heart during systole. Classically, in tricuspid regurgitation, the x descent is attenuated (Figure 7-3). The x descent ultimately disappears and is replaced by a systolic wave with a *peak-dome* contour often termed the *c-v* wave.[1,11-13] The v wave is classically prominent, and the y descent is very rapid (Figure 7-4). Ventricularization of the right atrial pressure waveform may occur (Figure 7-5). In some cases, the right atrial pressure wave is nearly indistinguishable from the right ventricular pressure contour (Figure 7-6). The v wave may increase further during exercise.

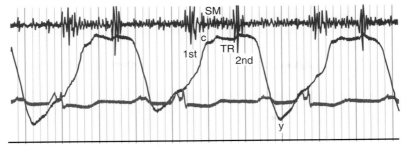

FIGURE 7-2. Venous pressure waveform in severe tricuspid regurgitation demonstrating a large *c-v* wave. (From Messer AL, Hurst JW, Rappaport MB, Sprague HB. A study of the venous pulse in tricuspid valve disease. *Circulation* 1950;1:388–393, with permission.)

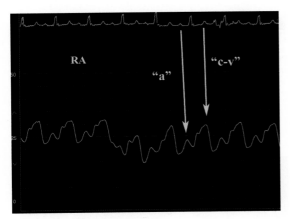

FIGURE 7-3. Right atrial waveform from a patient with secondary tricuspid regurgitation from associated severe left-sided heart failure and right-sided heart failure. Attenuation of the *x* descent is present, leading to a prominent *c-v* wave.

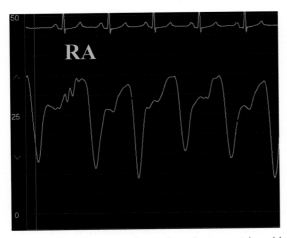

FIGURE 7-4. Right atrial waveform in severe tricuspid regurgitation demonstrating absence of the *x* descent and a large *c-v* wave with a prominent *y* descent.

Unfortunately, these hemodynamic findings are not always helpful to diagnose tricuspid regurgitation. Atrial fibrillation without tricuspid regurgitation may distort the atrial waveform in a similar fashion with absence of the *x* descent (because no atrial contraction is present), causing the *c-v* wave to appear prominent and similar to that of tricuspid regurgitation.[13,14] Similarly, finding a normal right atrial pressure, normal *x* descent and absence of prominent *v* waves do not exclude significant tricuspid regurgitation.[14–16] Ventricularization of right atrial pressure is very specific for severe tricuspid regurgitation but is seen in only 40% of patients.[16] Similar to mitral regurgitation, the size of the *v* wave in tricuspid regurgitation depends upon the volume status and compliance of the right atrium and does not necessarily correlate with the presence or severity of tricuspid regurgitation.[17] A subtle hemodynamic finding is perhaps more sensitive for tricuspid regurgitation. Instead of the normal fall in right atrial pressure with inspiration, one study found that all patients with tricuspid regurgitation demonstrated either a rise or no change in right atrial pressure during deep inspiration.[16] This finding was very sensitive for tricuspid regurgitation but was also apparent in several patients with severe (>90 mmHg) pulmonary hypertension; thus, in the

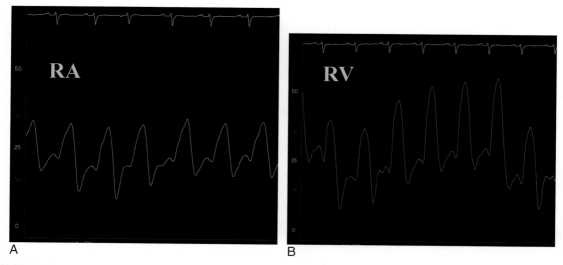

FIGURE 7-5. These tracings were obtained from a patient with severe tricuspid regurgitation due to profound biventricular heart failure. **A,** The right atrial waveform shows *ventricularization.* Compare this to **(B),** the right ventricular waveform from this patient.

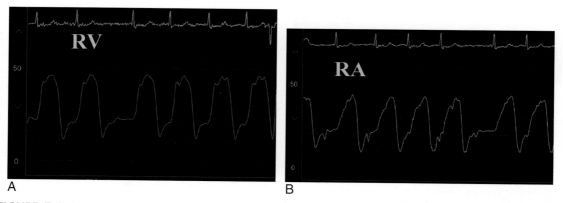

FIGURE 7-6. Severe tricuspid regurgitation may result in complete ventricularization of the right atrial waveform. **A,** The right ventricular pressure wave; note the **(B)** nearly indistinguishable appearance of the right atrial waveform.

absence of severe pulmonary hypertension, this sign may help diagnose tricuspid regurgitation. In contrast to mitral regurgitation, angiographic assessment of tricuspid regurgitation is problematic and rarely used, because the presence of a catheter across the tricuspid valve to perform right ventriculography may interfere with tricuspid valve function and cause regurgitation; however, this method

is useful for proving the absence of tricuspid regurgitation.

Some of the clinical and hemodynamic aspects of severe tricuspid regurgitation may be confused with constrictive pericarditis.[18] The predominant symptoms of both conditions (edema, ascites, prominent neck veins, and fatigue) are very similar. In addition, the right atrial pressure waveform may appear similar with a prominent y descent, particularly if the patient's rhythm is atrial fibrillation. The finding of ventricular interdependence is an important clue that may distinguish these two conditions[19] (see Chapter 8).

Cardiac output determination using the thermodilution method may be problematic in patients with tricuspid regurgitation because severe degrees of regurgitation underestimate the cardiac output.[20] The Fick methodology is more accurate in this setting.

Pulmonic Valve stenosis

Pulmonic stenosis is the most common abnormality of the pulmonary valve and is nearly always due to congenital causes. It may be seen in association with other congenital heart defects or exist in isolation. Often detected in childhood, pulmonic stenosis rarely presents in adults. In the majority of cases, the valve

leaflets are fused and amenable to balloon or surgical valvotomy. The 10%–15% of pulmonic valves stenosed from dysplastic conditions (as seen in association with Noonan's syndrome) are often not treatable by valvotomy.

Obstruction causes a pressure gradient across the pulmonic valve, with right ventricle systolic pressure exceeding pulmonary artery systolic pressure (Figure 7-7).[21] Pressure overload and subsequent hypertrophy of the right ventricle ensues. The hemodynamic abnormalities depend upon the severity of stenosis and the cardiac output. In mild cases, the pressure gradient across the pulmonic valve is less than 20 mmHg, and the cardiac output increases normally with exercise.[21,22] With severe pulmonic stenosis, the pressure gradient exceeds 40 mmHg and may reach very high levels (>100 mmHg), causing the right ventricular pressure to equal systemic arterial

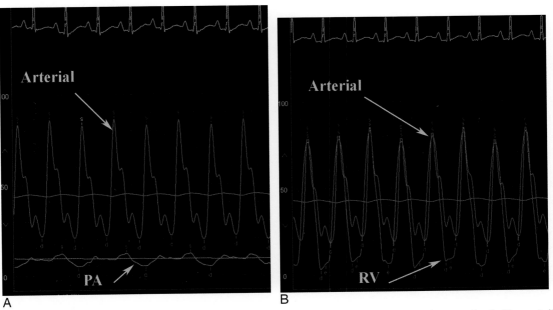

FIGURE 7-7. Right-heart pressures obtained in an infant with severe, congenital pulmonic stenosis. **A,** The systolic pulmonary artery pressure measured 15 mmHg with **(B),** a right ventricular pressure reaching systemic levels at nearly 80 mmHg.

pressures. The right ventricular stroke volume is fixed and unable to augment with exercise.[22] In addition, because of diminished right ventricular compliance from concentric hypertrophy of the right ventricle, severe pulmonic stenosis elevates right ventricular end-diastolic pressure, both at rest and with exercise. An elevated right ventricular end-diastolic pressure may raise right atrial pressure and cause right-to-left shunting if there is a patent foramen ovale leading to cyanosis or paradoxical embolism. Furthermore, right ventricular diastolic pressure rises have been associated with elevations in left ventricular end-diastolic pressures likely from interactions via the septum.[23] Interestingly, many individuals are asymptomatic even with severe stenosis. Symptoms of severe stenosis include dyspnea, fatigue, syncope, and exercise intolerance.

Valve area can be calculated using Gorlin's formula, as described in Chapter 4, and adapted to the pulmonic valve.[24] However, most clinicians classify the severity of pulmonic stenosis and base treatment decisions upon the extent of the transvalvular gradient alone. Current guidelines recommend either surgical or balloon valvuloplasty for symptomatic patients with a peak systolic gradient >30 mmHg by catheterization or for asymptomatic patients with a peak systolic gradient >40 mmHg.[25] Outcomes with balloon valvuloplasty are excellent with little chance of recurrence (Figure 7-8).

Related conditions that cause similar physiologic and hemodynamic effects on the right heart include peripheral pulmonary artery stenosis (discussed in Chapter 11) and right ventricular infundibular stenosis. Infundibular stenosis is commonly associated with severe pulmonic stenosis because compensatory right ventricular hypertrophy narrows and obstructs the outflow tract.

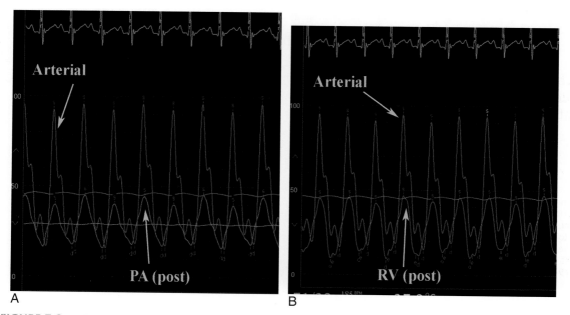

FIGURE 7-8. Balloon valvuloplasty performed in the patient mentioned in Figure 7-7 resulted in elimination of the pressure gradient between the pulmonary artery **(A)** and the right ventricle **(B)**.

With relief of valvular obstruction, hypertrophy regresses and the extent of infundibular stenosis regresses.[26]

Pulmonic Valve Regurgitation

Pulmonary insufficiency is uncommon and most often seen in association with congenital heart disease, typically as a consequence of either surgical or balloon valvulotomy for pulmonic stenosis or from repair of tetralogy of Fallot (see Chapter 11). Other causes include rheumatic heart disease, endocarditis, dilatation of the pulmonary artery (either idiopathic or from pulmonary hypertension), traumatic disruption of the pulmonic valve, syphilis, or an isolated congenital defect.[27,28] The low pressure circuit of the right heart causes pulmonary regurgitation to behave differently than aortic regurgitation.[29] Right atrial contraction can maintain forward pulmonary blood flow despite severe regurgitation, and the pulmonary resistance is typically very low, allowing blood to easily pass through the lungs and preventing significant backward flow during diastole. Thus, the volume overload on the right ventricle is substantially less than that seen in severe aortic regurgitation and allows this lesion to be tolerated for longer periods. Conditions that increase pulmonary vascular resistance, however, will increase the regurgitant volume and may lead to detrimental effects. Eventually, the right ventricle dilates and becomes dysfunctional, leading to reduced exercise capacity and right-heart failure.

The hemodynamic abnormalities reflect the severity of pulmonic regurgitation. Patients with severe pulmonary regurgitation demonstrate an increased pulse pressure, a rapid dicrotic collapse, and early equilibration of the diastolic pressures between the pulmonary artery and right ventricle[27,28,30] (Figures 7-9 and 7-10). Milder forms of pulmonary regurgitation affect the pulse pressure to a lesser degree and equilibration of the pressure between the right ventricle and pulmonary artery occurs only at end-diastole.

Pulmonary Hypertension

The normal pulmonary artery systolic pressure is <25 mmHg. Pulmonary hypertension has been variably defined using several criteria. Recent expert consensus defines pulmonary hypertension as a mean pulmonary artery pressure >25 mmHg, in the setting of a pulmonary capillary wedge pressure <15 mmHg, and normal or reduced cardiac output or by a pulmonary vascular

FIGURE 7-9. Diastasis of pressure between the right ventricle and pulmonary artery pressure is a hemodynamic finding of severe pulmonic insufficiency. (From Nemickas R, Roberts J, Gunnar RM, Tobin JR. Isolated congenital pulmonic insufficiency. Differentiation of mild from severe regurgitation. *Am J Cardiol* 1964;14:456–463, with permission.)

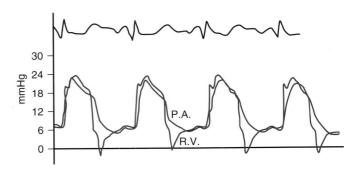

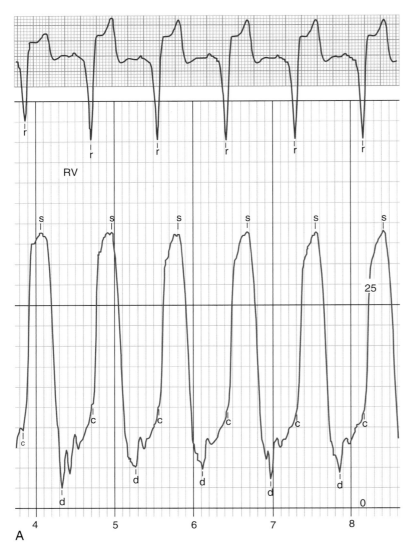

FIGURE 7-10. These tracings were obtained from a patient with severe pulmonic insufficiency after surgical correction of tetralogy of Fallot. **A,** The right ventricular pressure.

resistance in excess of 3 Wood units.[31] Pulmonary vascular resistance (PVR) is easily calculated using Ohm's Law in Wood units, as follows:

$$PVR = \frac{\text{(Mean pulmonary artery pressure)} - \text{(Mean wedge pressure)}}{\text{Cardiac output}}$$

Multiplying the resistance calculated in Wood units by 80 converts to the resistance units of dynes-sec-cm[5]; a normal pulmonary vascular resistance is roughly 70 dynes-sec-cm[5].

Pulmonary hypertension is often classified as *primary,* if cause is not known, or *secondary,* if hypertension is due to an identifiable, underlying cause. Primary pulmonary hypertension is a rare disorder of unknown cause characterized by increased pulmonary vascular resistance due to structural changes in the pulmonary vasculature.[31,32] Secondary pulmonary hypertension is more common and can be seen in association with multiple, diverse conditions that either raise pulmonary venous pressure and,

FIGURE 7-10—cont'd. **B,** The pulmonary artery pressure. Note the wide pulse pressure on the pulmonary artery tracing with equilibration of diastolic pressures.

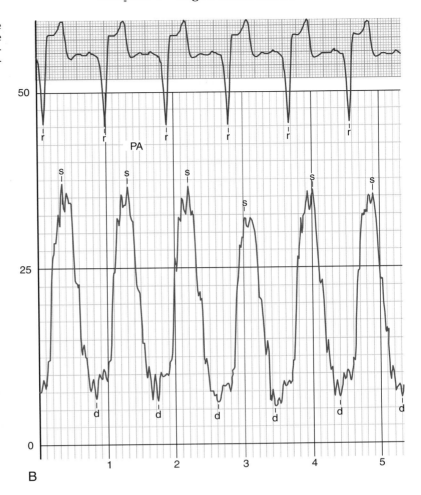

consequently, the pulmonary arterial pressure or increase the pulmonary vascular resistance. The World Health Organization classifies the causes of pulmonary hypertension based on the underlying pathophysiology leading to elevated pulmonary pressures. This classification scheme and the more commonly observed causes of secondary pulmonary hypertension are presented in Table 7-2.

In most cases of secondary pulmonary hypertension, the underlying cause is obvious and dominates the clinical presentation. For example, the most common cause of pulmonary hypertension seen by most adult cardiologists in the United States is from pulmonary venous hypertension due to the multiple left-sided heart diseases that raise left atrial pressure, such as congestive heart failure and left-sided valvular disorders. In addition, many of the pulmonary diseases that cause pulmonary hypertension are clinically apparent when pulmonary hypertension is diagnosed.

On occasion, physicians are surprised to discover pulmonary hypertension, either by echocardiography or during performance of right-heart catheterization, and there is no readily apparent cause.

TABLE 7-2.	World Health Organization Classification of Pulmonary Hypertension (partial list)

I. PRIMARY ARTERIAL HYPERTENSION

Primary pulmonary hypertension (idiopathic)
Related to:
   Collagen vascular diseases (scleroderma, lupus, etc.)
   Congenital heart disease with left-to-right shunt
      Ventricular septal defect
      Patent ductus arteriosus
      Atrial septal defect
   Cirrhosis of the liver and portal hypertension
   Human immunodeficiency virus infection
   Drugs and toxins

II. PULMONARY VENOUS HYPERTENSION

Left-sided heart disease
Left heart failure
Left-sided valvular lesions
Extrinsic compression (tumors, adenopathy)
Pulmonary veno-occlusive disease

III. PULMONARY ARTERIAL HYPERTENSION CAUSED BY LUNG DISEASE

Chronic obstructive pulmonary disease
Interstitial lung disease
Obstructive sleep apnea
Hypoventilation disorders
Chronic high-altitude exposure

IV. PULMONARY ARTERIAL HYPERTENSION CAUSED BY CHRONIC THROMBOTIC OR EMBOLIC DISEASE

Thromboembolic obstruction of proximal pulmonary arteries
Obstruction of distal pulmonary arteries
   Pulmonary embolism
   Parasitic diseases
   In situ thrombosis
   Sickle cell disease

V. PULMONARY ARTERIAL HYPERTENSION CAUSED BY DISEASES OF THE PULMONARY VASCULATURE

Inflammatory diseases
   Sarcoidosis
   Schistosomiasis
Pulmonary capillary hemangiomatosis

Several common conditions should be carefully considered and require additional diagnostic testing. Demonstrating a normal wedge pressure on right-heart catheterization eliminates pulmonary venous hypertension and the left-sided heart disorders such as mitral valve disease, heart failure, or restrictive cardiomyopathy as the inciting causes. Other diagnostic tests search for the presence of occult lung disease and include chest X-ray, chest computed tomographic scan, arterial blood gas for chronic hypoxemia, and pulmonary function tests. A sleep study is important to rule out obstructive sleep apnea. Finally, all patients with pulmonary hypertension of unclear cause deserve an evaluation for chronic pulmonary embolism.

The hemodynamic abnormalities observed in pulmonary hypertension depend on the underlying condition, the magnitude of pressure elevation, and its effect on the right ventricle. Pulmonary pressures may be only modestly elevated with systolic pressure in the 40- to 50-mmHg range, or they may reach very high at systemic levels of greater than 100 mmHg. The pulmonary capillary wedge pressure will be normal in cases of primary pulmonary hypertension or when due to causes other than pulmonary venous hypertension (Figure 7-11). It may prove very difficult to obtain an accurate wedge pressure when there is severe pulmonary hypertension. Hybrid tracings are very common and will overestimate the wedge pressure. In addition, the operator should exhibit great care when attempting to wedge the pulmonary artery catheter in severe pulmonary hypertension, because these patients are at increased risk for pulmonary artery rupture, a highly morbid and potentially fatal event.

The right atrial waveform may show a prominent *a* wave when contracting against higher right ventricular diastolic pressures (Figure 7-12). The right atrial waveform may also demonstrate a finding consistent with tricuspid regurgitation (described earlier) because this condition is very commonly associated with pulmonary hypertension. Pulmonary hypertension leads to right ventricular hypertrophy and reduced compliance. A prominent *a* wave on the right ventricular waveform is a hemodynamic manifestation of this abnormality (Figure 7-13). Pulsus alternans that affects only the right-sided chamber pressures (i.e., right ventricular and pulmonary arterial waveforms) is an unusual and rare finding in severe pulmonary hypertension (Figure 7-14).

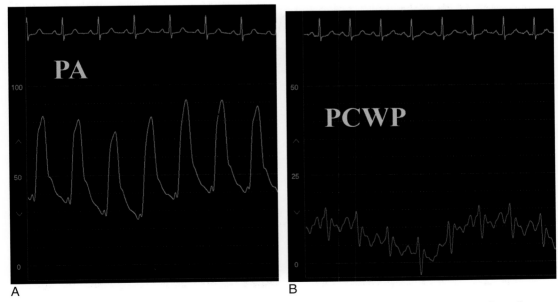

FIGURE 7-11. Right-heart catheterization findings in severe pulmonary hypertension due to end-stage liver disease and portal hypertension. **A,** The pulmonary artery pressures are markedly elevated, reaching systemic levels (mean pressure = 56 mmHg). **B,** The mean pulmonary capillary wedge pressure is normal (10 mmHg), eliminating left-heart failure and left-side valve lesions as a cause of secondary pulmonary hypertension. With a cardiac output of 6 L/min, the pulmonary vascular resistance is markedly elevated at 7.7 Wood units.

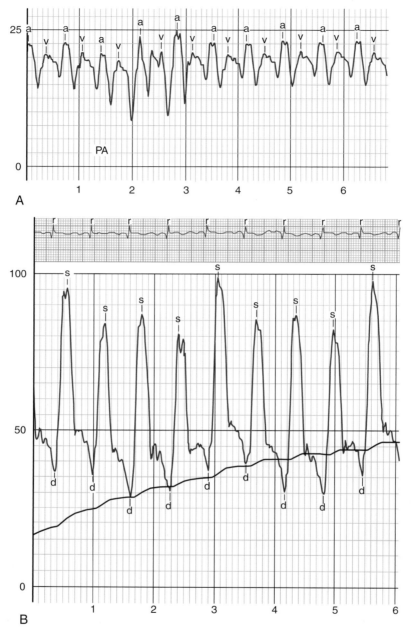

FIGURE 7-12. **A,** Example of a prominent *a* wave on the right atrial waveform in a patient with pulmonary hypertension from sarcoidosis. **B,** Pulmonary arterial pressures are markedly elevated.

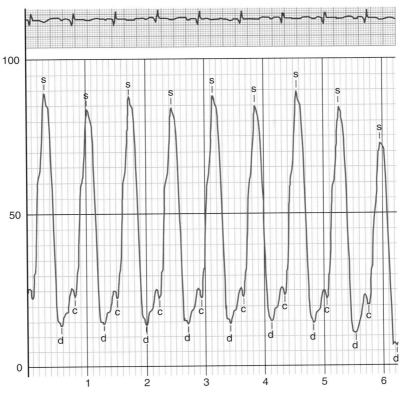

FIGURE 7-13. Right ventricular pressure waveform from the same patient depicted in Figure 7-12, demonstrating non-compliance of the right ventricle manifest as a prominent *a* wave on the right ventricular pressure tracing.

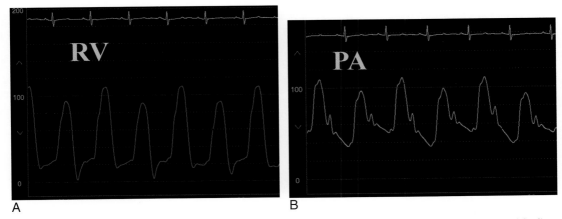

FIGURE 7-14. These tracings from a patient with primary pulmonary hypertension demonstrate the unusual finding of **(A)** pulsus alternans on the right ventricular and **(B)** pulmonary arterial waveforms.

References

1. Bloomfield RA, Lauson HD, Cournand A, et al. Recording of right heart pressures in normal subjects and in patients with chronic pulmonary disease and various types of cardio-circulatory disease. *J Clin Invest* 1946;25:639–664.
2. Roguin A, Rinkevich D, Milo S, et al. Long-term follow-up of patients with severe rheumatic tricuspid stenosis. *Am Heart J* 1998;136:103–108.
3. McCord MC, Swan H, Blount SG. Tricuspid stenosis: Clinical and physiologic evaluation. *Am Heart J* 1954;48:405–415.
4. Whitaker W. The diagnosis of tricuspid stenosis. *Am Heart J* 1955;50:237–241.

5. Yu PN, Harken DW, Lovejoy FW, et al. Clinical and hemodynamic studies of tricuspid stenosis. *Circulation* 1956;13:680–691.
6. Killip T, Lukas DS. Tricuspid stenosis: Physiologic criteria for diagnosis and hemodynamic abnormalities. *Circulation* 1957;16:3–13.
7. Nath J, Foster E, Heidenreich PA. Impact of tricuspid regurgitation on long-term survival. *J Am Coll Cardiol* 2004;43:405–409.
8. Behm CZ, Nath J, Foster E. Clinical correlates and mortality of hemodynamically significant tricuspid regurgitation. *J Heart Valve Dis* 2004;13:784–789.
9. Raman SV, Sparks EA, Boudoulas H, Wooley CF. Tricuspid valve disease: Tricuspid valve complex perspective. *Curr Probl Cardiol* 2002;27:103–142.
10. Messer AL, Hurst JW, Rappaport MB, Sprague HB. A study of the venous pulse in tricuspid valve disease. *Circulation* 1950;1:388–393.
11. McCord MC, Blount SG. The hemodynamic pattern in tricuspid valve disease. *Am Heart J* 1952;44:671–680.
12. Sepulveda G, Lukas DS. The diagnosis of tricuspid insufficiency. Clinical features in 60 cases with associated mitral valve disease. *Circulation* 1955;11:552–563.
13. Hansing CE, Rowe GG. Tricuspid insufficiency: A study of hemodynamics and pathogenesis. *Circulation* 1972;45:793–799.
14. Cairns KB, Kloster FE, Bristow JD, et al. Problems in the hemodynamic diagnosis of tricuspid insufficiency. *Am Heart J* 1968;75:173–197.
15. Rubeiz GA, Nassar ME, Dagher IK. Study of the right atrial pressure pulse in functional tricuspid regurgitation and normal sinus rhythm. *Circulation* 1964;30:190–193.
16. Lingamnemi R, Cha SD, Maranhao V, et al. Tricuspid regurgitation: Clinical and angiographic assessment. *Cathet Cardiovasc Diagn* 1979;5:7–17.
17. Pitts WR, Lange RA, Cigarroa JE, Hillis LD. Predictive value of prominent right atrial V waves in assessing the presence and severity of tricuspid regurgitation. *Am J Cardiol* 1999;83:617–618.
18. Studley J, Tighe DA, Joelson JM, Flack JE 3rd. The hemodynamic signs of constrictive pericarditis can be mimicked by tricuspid regurgitation. *Cardiol Rev* 2003;11:320–326.
19. Hurrell DG, Nishimura RA, Higano ST, et al. Value of dynamic respiratory changes in left and right ventricular pressures for the diagnosis of constrictive pericarditis. *Circulation* 1996;93:2007–2013.
20. Balik M, Pachl J, Hendl J. Effect of the degree of tricuspid regurgitation on cardiac output measurements by thermodilution. *Intensive Care Med* 2002;28:1117–1121.
21. Dow JW, Levine HD, Elkin M, et al. Studies of congenital heart disease: IV. Uncomplicated pulmonic stenosis. *Circulation* 1950;1:267–287.
22. Moller JH, Rao S, Lucas RV. Exercise hemodynamics of pulmonary valvular stenosis: Study of 64 children. *Circulation* 1972;46:1018–1026.
23. Herbert WH, Yellin E. Left ventricular diastolic pressure elevation consequent to pulmonary stenosis. *Circulation* 1969;40:887–892.
24. Moller JH, Adams P Jr. A simplified method for calculating the pulmonary valve area. *Am Heart J* 1966;72:463–465.
25. Bonow RO, Carabello BA, Chatterjee K, et al. ACC/AHA 2006 guidelines for the management of patients with valvular heart disease. A report of the American College of Cardiology/American Heart Association Task Force on Practice Guidelines (Writing committee to revise the 1998 guidelines for the management of patients with valvular heart disease). *J Am Coll Cardiol* 2006;48:e1.
26. Fawzy ME, Galal O, Dunn B, et al. Regression of infundibular pulmonary stenosis after successful balloon pulmonary valvuloplasty in adults. *Cathet Cardiovasc Diagn* 1990;21:77–81.
27. Morton RF, Stern TN. Isolated pulmonic valvular regurgitation. *Circulation* 1956;14:1069–1072.
28. Kohout FW, Katz LN. Pulmonic valvular regurgitation. Report of a case with catheterization data. *Am Heart J* 1955;49:637–642.
29. Bouzas B, Kilner PJ, Gatzoulis MA. Pulmonary regurgitation: Not a benign lesion. *Eur Heart J* 2005;26:433–439.
30. Nemickas R, Roberts J, Gunnar RM, Tobin JR. Isolated congenital pulmonic insufficiency. Differentiation of mild from severe regurgitation. *Am J Cardiol* 1964;14:456–463.
31. McLaughlin VV, McGoon MD. Pulmonary arterial hypertension. *Circulation* 2006;114:1417–1431.
32. Archer S, Rich S. Primary pulmonary hypertension. A vascular biology and translational research "work in progress." *Circulation* 2000;102:2781–2791.

CHAPTER 8

Pericardial Disease and Restrictive Cardiomyopathy

Michael Ragosta, MD

Pericardial diseases represent an interesting and diverse group of disorders with complex and fascinating hemodynamics. A list of etiologies of pericardial pathology appears similar to the table of contents of an internal medicine textbook because nearly all major disease processes potentially affect the pericardium (Table 8-1). Despite this wide array of inciting processes, pericardial disease presents as one or more of four distinct syndromes: acute pericarditis, effusion and tamponade, pericardial constriction, and effusive-constrictive pericarditis. Syndromes may overlap, for example, as when a large effusion complicates acute pericarditis or when acute inflammation smolders chronically, causing pericardial scarring and constriction. Often observed is that any given etiology causes a predominant syndrome more frequently than others; for instance, viral infections more commonly cause acute pericarditis, whereas malignancy usually results in effusion and tamponade. Although generally true, any of the conditions listed in Table 8-1 is capable of producing any of these syndromes.

This chapter will emphasize the pericardial syndromes associated with hemodynamic consequences, namely, pericardial effusions, pericardial constriction, and effusive-constrictive pericarditis. In addition, because the clinical presentation and hemodynamic abnormalities of restrictive cardiomyopathy behave similarly to constrictive pericarditis, the rare entity of restrictive cardiomyopathy will also be discussed.

Normal Pericardial Anatomy and Related Physiology

The normal pericardium consists of an inner, single layer of serous membrane known as the *visceral pericardium* and a fibrous, outer structure called the *parietal pericardium,* normally about 1-mm thick. The serous pericardium attaches to the surface of the heart and the inner surface of the parietal pericardium, defining the limits of the pericardial space; this space normally contains less than 50 mL of serous fluid.

Although a human can live without a pericardium without ill effects, the normal pericardium does serve specific functions.[1] The major function relates to the relatively rigid and noncompliant nature of the parietal pericardium, limiting cardiac chamber distension with changes in volume and contributing to ventricular stiffness in diastole. These properties facilitate interaction and coupling of the cardiac chambers via the interventricular septum, an important role in cardiac physiology both inhealth and disease. The noncompliant nature of the pericardium results in a rapid rise in pericardial pressure with acute accumulation of fluid in the pericardial space. The volume that can be accommodated without increasing pressure in the pericardial space is known as the *pericardial reserve volume* and is normally only about 50–75 mL. Slow and gradual accumulation of fluid stretches the pericardium, allowing a greater pericardial reserve volume. For this reason, relatively large volumes of fluid can collect over time without increasing pressure. Once the pericardial reserve volume is reached, the relatively steep pressure-volume curve for the pericardium

TABLE 8-1. Causes of Pericardial Disease

Infectious
Bacterial
   Streptococcus, Staphylococcus, gram (–) rods
Mycobacterial
   Tuberculosis
Viral
   Coxsackie, echovirus, adenovirus, Epstein-Barr virus
   Human immunodeficiency virus
Fungal
   Aspergillosis, Candida, histoplasmosis
Protozoal
   Amoebic

Neoplastic
Primary mesothelioma
Metastatic
   Breast, lung, skin, lymphoma, leukemia

Metabolic
Uremia, myxedema, amyloidosis

Immune/inflammatory
Connective tissue disorders (lupus, scleroderma,
   polyarteritis nodosa, rheumatoid arthritis)
Sarcoidosis
Post-MI (myocardial infarction), post-pericardiotomy
   syndrome

Iatrogenic
Radiation induced
Cardiac perforation from interventional procedures
Drugs (warfarin, minoxidil, procainamide)

Trauma
Direct trauma
Aortic dissection

Congenital
Pericardial cyst

Idiopathic

mandates rapid pressure increases in the pericardial space with small additional increments of fluid (Figure 8-1). This explains the *last-drop* effect, in which a small increase in fluid causes a patient to deteriorate dramatically but also explains why removal of just a small amount of fluid leads to rapid improvement.[2]

Complex interactions exist between the pericardium, the pericardial space, the cardiac chambers, and the thoracic cavity during cardiac and respiratory cycles. The spectrum of hemodynamic abnormalities observed in pericardial diseases can best be interpreted by first understanding these important physiologic relationships.

The relationships between the cardiac chambers, the great vessels of the heart, the thoracic cavity, and the pericardial space are summarized in Figure 8-2. Importantly, the pericardial space sits within the thoracic cavity, reflecting intrathoracic pressure (roughly −6–0 mmHg). While the cardiac chambers lie within the confines of the pericardial space, the pulmonary venous system does not. The pulmonary veins exist outside of the pericardial space but within the thoracic cavity, thereby directly influenced by changes in intrathoracic pressure. Both the inferior and superior vena cava lie outside the pericardial space and only partially within the thoracic cavity. Therefore, the systemic venous circulation is mostly independent of changes in intrathoracic pressures.

In the presence of a normal pericardium, a variety of changes in cardiac physiology occurs with inspiration and expiration (Figure 8-3). During inspiration, intrathoracic pressure decreases, resulting in decreased pressure in the cardiac chambers. With little or no corresponding reduction in systemic venous pressure with inspiration, the pressure drop in the right heart chambers augments right heart filling. The pulmonary venous bed lies within the thoracic cavity; therefore, the inspiratory reduction in intrathoracic pressure also decreases pressure within the pulmonary veins. With pressure falling uniformly in the left atrium, the left ventricle, and the pulmonary veins, no major change occurs in left ventricular (LV) filling with inspiration. Opposite changes occur with expiration with the net effect being a decrease in right-sided filling. Inspiratory augmentation of right ventricular (RV) filling with no change in LV filling causes bowing of the septum from the right to the left, impairing left-sided output (Figure 8-4). This results in a small, inspiratory drop

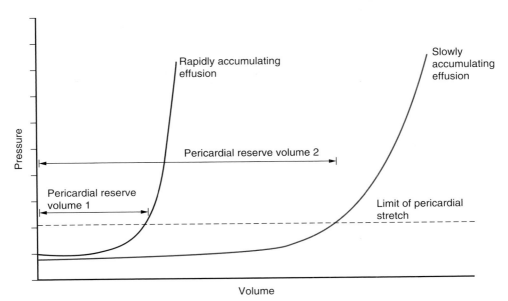

FIGURE 8-1. Schematic representation of the pressure-volume relationship for the pericardium. The pericardial reserve volume represents the amount of fluid that the pericardial space can accommodate before a rise occurs in pericardial pressure. A rapidly accumulating effusion reaches the limit of pericardial stretch at a lower volume than a slowly accumulating effusion. Chronic and slow fluid accumulation allows the pericardium to stretch, creating a larger pericardial reserve volume. (Adapted from Spodick DH. Acute tamponade. *N Engl J Med* 2003;349:684–690.)

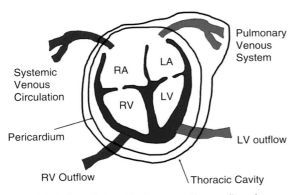

FIGURE 8-2. Relationship between the cardiac chambers, the pericardial space, and the thoracic cavity. The cardiac chambers lie within the pericardial space as well as the thoracic cavity while the pulmonary venous system sits within the thoracic cavity but outside of the pericardial space.

in systolic pressure known as a *pulsus paradox*, normally measuring less than 12 mmHg (Figure 8-5).

In the presence of a normal pericardium and vacant pericardial space, the diastolic pressures of the right and left ventricles vary during the respiratory cycle independent of each other (Figure 8-6). In contrast, the systolic pressures of the right

and left ventricles change during the respiratory cycle in parallel fashion. In the presence of a normal, compliant pericardium, augmented filling of the right ventricle with inspiration is easily accommodated by the compliant right ventricle and does not lead to an increase in pressure in the right ventricle with inspiration. Instead, the changing forces with respiration cause the pressure in both chambers to decrease with inspiration and increase with expiration. Thus, the right and left ventricular systolic pressures normally parallel each other during the respiratory cycle (Figure 8-7).

Pericardial Effusions and Tamponade

Pericardial effusions occur commonly in clinical practice from any of the multiple causes listed in Table 8-1. Although easily diagnosed with echocardiography, the nonspecific presenting symptoms

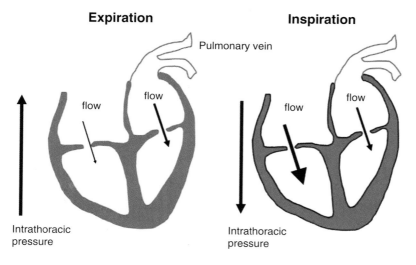

Expiration **Inspiration**

FIGURE 8-3. Effects of the respiratory cycle on normal cardiac chamber filling. See text for details.

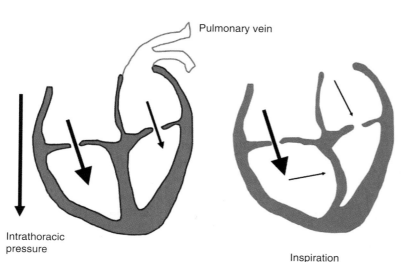

FIGURE 8-4. Proposed mechanism of a pulsus paradoxus. Inspiration lowers intrathoracic pressure, resulting in no change in left ventricular filling as both pulmonary venous pressure and left ventricular pressure drop in parallel. However, right ventricular filling increases with inspiration, resulting in bowing of septum to the left, impairing left-sided output.

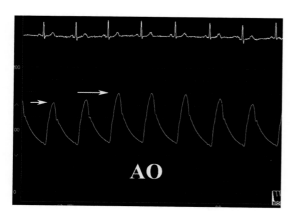

FIGURE 8-5. Example of the normally observed or *physiologic* pulsus paradoxus on an aortic pressure waveform. The inspiratory drop in systolic pressure, or *pulsus paradoxus,* normally does not exceed 12 mmHg.

are often attributed to other conditions, failing to trigger early clinical suspicion and recognition. The lack of suspicion during the early phases of an effusion prevents appropriate therapy. The unrecognized effusion frequently progresses followed by cardiovascular collapse. At this point, the diagnosis becomes obvious. Unfortunately, the naive physician is now faced with management of crisis instead of basking in the joy of a clever diagnosis auspiciously treated.

Dyspnea, fatigue, and chest pain constitute the most common symptoms of an effusion. Manifestations associated

FIGURE 8-6. The diastolic pressures of the right and left ventricles normally separate during the respiratory cycle.

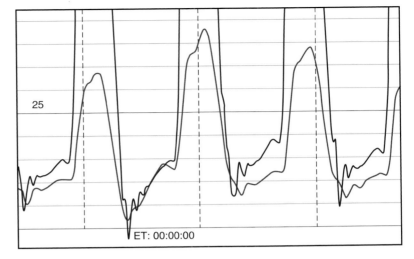

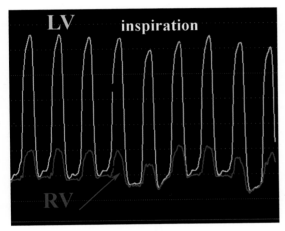

FIGURE 8-7. Normally, concordance of the left and right ventricular systolic pressure is present during inspiration. See text for details.

with more profound hemodynamic sequelas include syncope, confusion, renal failure, and shock. Patients with subacute or chronic effusions may exhibit peripheral edema due to increased right atrial (RA) pressure; similarly, patients may present with abdominal pain from hepatic distension. Physical examination nearly always reveals distended and tense neck veins. Tachycardia, arterial hypotension, and a pulsus paradox >12 mmHg provide further evidence of a hemodynamically significant pericardial effusion. Two other physical examination findings are noteworthy.

Beck's triad describes the constellation of elevated neck veins, hypotension, and a quiet precordium, named after the American surgeon Claude Schaffer Beck, who first described these findings in tamponade from acute, traumatic effusions. Ewart's sign describes the finding of dullness to percussion with bronchial breath sounds and evidence of lung consolidation below the left scapula seen with large, chronic pericardial effusions.[3] An echocardiogram easily identifies pericardial effusions even in the presence of poor acoustic windows. Pericardial effusions are sometimes diagnosed surreptitiously by chest X-ray (appearing as an enlarged cardiac silhouette), chest computerized tomography (CT), or magnetic resonance imaging (MRI). The electrocardiogram (ECG) is nonspecific; it may show low voltage, electrical alternans, and diffuse ST elevation consistent with pericarditis.

Once an effusion is identified, it is important to determine its hemodynamic effect. The hemodynamic sequelas of an effusion depend on the rate and volume of fluid accumulation, compliance of the cardiac chambers and the pericardium, and the filling pressures in the heart. The commonly asked question *Is there tamponade?*, usually following an echocardiographic diagnosis of an effusion, is best addressed by describing its hemodynamic impact instead of deciding whether a patient is "in tamponade." This concept has been elegantly elucidated by Reddy and Curtiss,[4,5] who emphasize that tamponade is not an "all or none" phenomenon but rather, represents a spectrum of hemodynamic abnormalities, beginning with isolated elevation of pericardial pressure and ending with the profound abnormalities classically attributed to tamponade.

Figure 8-8 depicts the progressive hemodynamic derangements that occur with incremental accumulation of pericardial fluid. Initially, just pericardial pressure rises. Elevated pericardial pressure triggers compensatory mechanisms (venoconstriction and fluid retention), raising systemic venous pressure to adequately fill the right heart. This causes both RA and RV diastolic pressures to increase. During this early phase of tamponade, cardiac output is maintained and a normal inspiratory fall in systolic pressure of less than 10–12 mmHg occurs. With additional accumulation of fluid, further elevation and equilibration of pericardial, RA, and RV diastolic pressures occur. Left ventricular diastolic pressure then increases, ultimately equilibrating with the right-sided diastolic pressures. This results in *equalization* of diastolic pressures across the cardiac chambers. Additional fluid accumulation drops stroke volume; cardiac output falls despite a compensatory tachycardia. The inspiratory fall in systolic pressure (pulsus paradoxus) becomes more prominent but may remain below the upper limits of normal. The final phase of tamponade, more classically recognized as *tamponade*, exhibits elevated and equalized diastolic pressures, a prominent inspiratory fall in systolic pressure, and a precipitous drop in cardiac output and blood pressure.

Hemodynamics of Pericardial Effusion and Tamponade

Tamponade causes continuous compression of the heart throughout the cardiac cycle, preventing rapid atrial emptying when the tricuspid valve opens. This correlates with the echocardiographic finding of RV diastolic collapse and absence of the *y* descent on the RA waveform. This abnormality occurs relatively early in tamponade (Figure 8-9, *A*). Right atrial pressure is typically seen to equilibrate with pericardial pressure (Figure 8-9, *B*). In advanced stages of tamponade, the RA pressure waveform

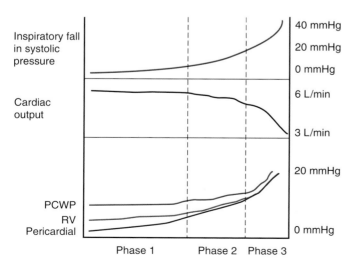

FIGURE 8-8. Depiction of the various hemodynamic phases of tamponade, demonstrating the concept of the spectrum of tamponade and the effects of progressive accumulation of pericardial fluid. In phase 1, the pericardial pressure is the first to rise and leads to elevation of the right ventricular diastolic pressure. The pulmonary capillary wedge pressure, cardiac output, and the inspiratory fall in systolic pressure are not yet affected. In phase 2, equalization of the diastolic pressures occurs, and cardiac output begins to fall with a greater fall in systolic pressure with inspiration evident. Phase 3 tamponade represents *classic* tamponade with a dramatic drop in cardiac output and marked pulsus paradoxus. (From Reddy PS, Curtiss EI, Uretsky BF. Spectrum of hemodynamic changes in cardiac tamponade. *Am J Cardiol* 1990;66:1487–1491.)

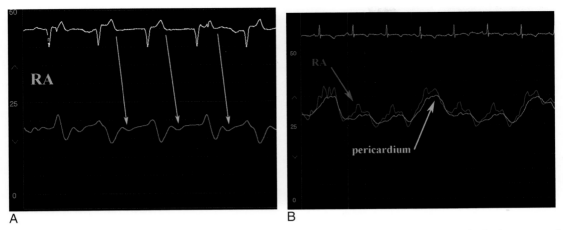

FIGURE 8-9. **A,** Loss of the *y* descent *(arrows)* usually on the right atrial waveform in tamponade. **B,** As tamponade becomes more significant, the right atrial pressure waveform usually appears as an undulating line with no discernible *a* or *v* waves or *x* and *y* descents, and equilibration with the pericardial pressure is present.

appears as an undulating line without discernible *a* and *v* waves or *x* and *y* descents. Typically, patients with tamponade present with elevated and equalized right-sided diastolic pressures that measure 20 mmHg; this appears to a common level associated with presentation of a low cardiac output and hypotension (Figure 8-10). Right ventricular and pulmonary artery pressure waveforms often appear abnormally thin and asthenic because of reduced right-sided output from compression. Marked elevation of the pulmonary artery systolic pressure is not usually present. In severe tamponade, pulmonary artery systolic pressure may be only slightly higher than diastolic pressure. Pulmonary edema is generally not a feature of tamponade for poorly understood reasons but likely because patients first present with hypotension and shock when diastolic pressures reach about 20 mmHg, before achieving an LA pressure associated with pulmonary edema. Accordingly, arterial hypoxemia should not be attributed to tamponade physiology. Its presence should prompt a search for other etiologies.

As described earlier, an inspiratory drop in systolic pressure (pulsus paradox) of up to 10–12 mmHg is part of normal cardiac physiology. Advanced phases of tamponade exaggerate this finding with the inspiratory fall in systolic pressure that exceeds 12 mmHg because the presence of pericardial fluid within the inelastic confines of the pericardium allows only a certain volume to fill the cardiac chambers and prevents one cardiac chamber from accommodating any additional volume without a corresponding impairment in filling of the adjacent chamber.[6] Therefore, the augmentation in right-heart filling with inspiration competes with filling of the left heart, reducing stroke volume and systolic pressure to a greater degree than seen normally.

Kussmaul[5] first described this phenomenon over a century ago:

The pulse of all arteries—with the heart movement continuing steadily—becomes very small in certain intervals that regularly occur with each inspiration, or it disappears completely, only to immediately return with expiration. I suggest to term this pulse the paradox pulse, in part, because of the obvious disparity between the heart action and arterial pulse, and, in part, because the pulse—though seemingly irregular—is in fact a pulse stopping or decreasing with regular repetition.

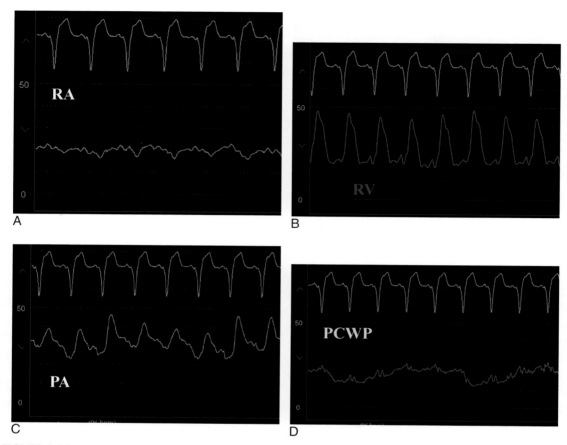

FIGURE 8-10. This set of tracings was obtained in a patient with tamponade and demonstrates many of the characteristic findings. The right atrial pressure is **(A)** elevated with loss of *y* descent and is **(B)** equal to the right ventricular diastolic pressure and **(C)** close to the pulmonary artery diastolic pressure and **(D)** equal to the pulmonary capillary wedge pressure.

Not specific for tamponade, other conditions may exhibit a prominent pulsus paradox (Table 8-2).[6,7] Circumstances that prevent a pulsus paradox despite a large and significant effusion include a coexisting atrial septal defect (because the inspiratory increase in venous return is shared between the atria), aortic regurgitation (because filling of the left ventricle is independent of respiration), or if there is marked elevation of the LV end-diastolic pressure.

Accurate measurement of a pulsus paradox helps define the hemodynamic significance of an effusion. On physical examination, measurement of a pulsus paradox involves inflation of the blood pressure cuff above systolic pressure followed by careful auscultation during very slow deflation until any Korotkoff sound is heard with any cardiac cycle. This marks the upper limit of systolic pressure. With continued slow deflation

TABLE 8-2.	Causes of an Inspiratory Drop in Systolic Pressure >12 mmHg (Pulsus Paradoxus)

Pericardial tamponade
Effusive-constrictive pericarditis
Right ventricular infarction
Asthma
Chronic obstructive pulmonary disease
Congestive heart failure
Obesity
Ascites
Pregnancy
Pulmonary embolism
Tension pneumothorax

of the cuff, the pressure at which Korotkoff sounds are heard with each cardiac cycle is noted and defines the lower limit of systolic pressure. The difference between these two recordings is the pulsus paradox. This procedure should be carried out while the patient is breathing normally. Arterial pressure recordings identify a pulsus paradox with greater sensitivity than physical examination (see Figure 8-5). In tamponade, the pulsus paradox may be dramatic, completely obliterating the pulse, as described by Kussmaul (Figure 8-11).

The classic hemodynamic findings of tamponade may be obscured or absent in several conditions. Right ventricular hypertrophy and pulmonary hypertension prevent an effusion from fully compressing the right ventricle during diastole. Accordingly, early diastolic filling may not be impaired; the y descent on the RA waveform may appear normal despite tamponade (Figure 8-12). Patients with preexisting elevation of

LV diastolic pressure may not have equalization of LV diastolic or pulmonary capillary wedge pressure with right-sided chamber diastolic pressures. Diastolic pressures may not equalize across all chambers, if there is marked pulmonary hypertension, despite advanced tamponade, or, if there is a loculated effusion that selectively compresses just the right heart. This latter scenario is most common in a postoperative effusion.[8] As noted earlier, a pulsus paradox may be absent in the presence of an atrial septal defect, significant aortic regurgitation, elevated LV end-diastolic pressure, or localized tamponade.

Elevated and equalized right-sided diastolic pressures characterize classic tamponade. However, a pericardial effusion may cause serious hemodynamic compromise, despite low (6–12 mmHg) diastolic pressures. This so-called *low-pressure tamponade* was initially described predominantly in the setting of hypovolemia.[2,9] It may be seen with acute

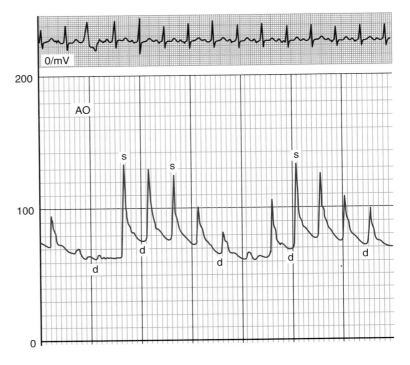

FIGURE 8-11. The arterial pressure waveform in this tracing obtained in a patient with tamponade demonstrates total pulsus paradoxus with complete obliteration of the arterial pressure with inspiration.

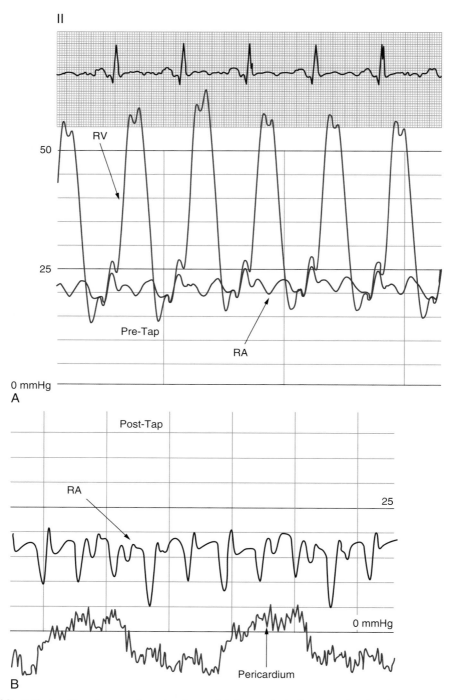

FIGURE 8-12. Patients with pulmonary hypertension and right ventricular hypertrophy often have preservation of the *y* descent on the right atrial pressure waveform, despite tamponade as shown in this example of a patient with tamponade from post-pericardiotomy syndrome after mitral valve replacement for chronic mitral regurgitation. The patient had known pulmonary hypertension prior to surgery, with pulmonary pressure in the 70-mmHg systolic range. **A,** Pressures obtained prior to pericardiocentesis. **B,** Pressures obtained after successful pericardiocentesis show that the average pericardial pressure was reduced to less than 0 mmHg; the right atrial pressure waveform remains abnormal with a more prominent *y* descent.

FIGURE 8-12—cont'd. **C,** Pressures also obtained post-pericardiocentesis; compare this to *(A)* and note the greater prominence of the *y* descent.

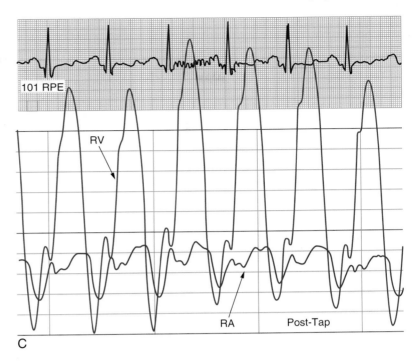

101 RPE

RV

RA   Post-Tap

C

tamponade, particularly from hemorrhage into the pericardium, as may occur from iatrogenic perforation during a coronary intervention or electrophysiologic procedure (Figure 8-13). The fall in intravascular volume associated with hemorrhage into the pericardium prevents the aforementioned compensatory increase in venous pressure further exacerbating the consequences of cardiac compression, manifest by cardiovascular collapse, despite *low* right-sided pressures.

The syndrome of low pressure tamponade has not been properly defined or systematically studied. A recently published study that involved 143 patients with an effusion who underwent careful hemodynamic studies at the time of pericardiocentesis provides important information regarding this syndrome.[10] The authors' proposed criteria first define the presence of tamponade as equalization of intrapericardial and RA pressure with right transmural pressure <2 mmHg. Low-pressure tamponade is

then defined as the presence of an intrapericardial pressure <7 mmHg before pericardiocentesis and RA pressure <4 mmHg after intrapericardial pressure had been lowered to near 0 mmHg by pericardiocentesis. Using this definition, low-pressure tamponade was present in 20% of patients who underwent pericardiocentesis. These patients were less likely to exhibit clinical signs of classic tamponade; the presence of pulsus paradox was present in only 7% of patients. The frequency of symptoms, effusion size by echocardiography, and preexisting use of diuretics were not different than patients with classic tamponade.[10]

Treatment of Tamponade

Small-to-moderate sized effusions without significant hemodynamic sequelae often do not require any specific treatment. It is important to prevent dehydration and avoid vasodilator drugs in these patients due to their

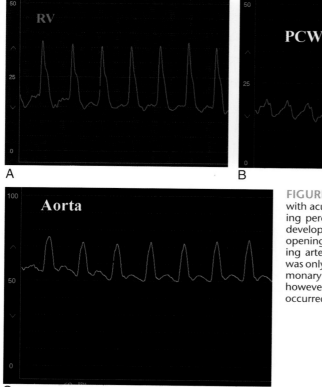

A

B

C

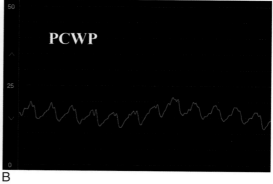

FIGURE 8-13. Low-pressure tamponade in a patient with acute tamponade from coronary perforation during percutaneous coronary intervention. The patient developed acute hypotension during an attempt at opening a chronically occluded left anterior descending artery. **A,** The right ventricular diastolic pressure was only mildly elevated at 13 mmHg, and **(B)** the pulmonary capillary wedge pressure was only 16 mmHg; however, profound **(C)** hemodynamic collapse occurred with marked hypotension and tachycardia.

dependence on preload. In the presence of significant hemodynamic consequences or symptoms, the effusion requires removal. Hypotension can be improved with a rapid infusion of normal saline and intravenous pressor agents while preparing for pericardiocentesis. Removal of the pericardial fluid should proceed without delay in clinically unstable patients. The treatment of choice in most patients is percutaneous pericardiocentesis.[1,2] Compromised patients with loculated effusions or in whom pericardiocentesis is not successful need surgical drainage, often accomplished by the creation of a pericardial window. Finally, percutaneous balloon pericardiotomy has a role in reducing recurrent effusions in patients with malignant pericardial effusion.[11]

Pericardiocentesis is often performed in the catheterization laboratory but can be accomplished at the bedside in a critically ill patient who is rapidly deteriorating from the effusion or cannot be transported to the catheterization laboratory because of clinical instability. Echo guidance identifies the ideal site for percutaneous access to the effusion and determines whether loculation is present. A right-heart catheterization procedure performed in conjunction with pericardiocentesis allows an assessment of hemodynamics before and after fluid removal. The goal of pericardiocentesis is to remove all fluid and achieve a pericardial pressure of zero (or less). Inability to obtain a pericardial pressure of zero indicates loculation (Figure 8-14). Right-heart pressure measurements obtained after successful pericardiocentesis show reduction in right-sided diastolic pressures and return of the *y* descent on RA pressure waveforms. Fluid analysis may

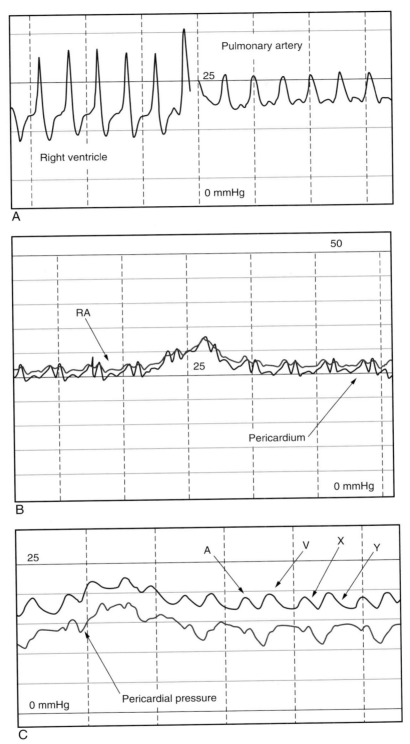

FIGURE 8-14. Loculation of fluid is suggested by the inability to reduce the pericardial pressure to zero or less with peri-cardiocentesis. In this example, **(A)** typical tamponade is present with equalization and elevation of the right ventricular end-diastolic and pulmonary artery pressure and **(B)** the right atrial and pericardial pressures. **C,** After pericardiocentesis, elevation of the pericardial pressure is still present. Note that evidence exists for some hemodynamic improvement with a return of the *x* and *y* descents post-pericardiocentesis.

provide valuable insight regarding the etiology of the effusion.

Pericardial Constriction

Constrictive pericarditis can be caused by any of the disorders that affect the pericardium shown in Table 8-1 with idiopathic causes, prior radiation exposure, postoperative state, connective tissue disorders, and viral and/or other infectious causes of pericarditis representing the most likely etiologies in the modern era.[12–14] Often noted as one of the classic causes of pericardial constriction, tuberculosis is rare in developed countries.

Constrictive pericarditis presents as a chronic illness. Its symptoms of dyspnea, fatigue, cachexia, edema, and abdominal distension are often misdiagnosed as cirrhosis of the liver, malignancy, or other chronic disease. Physical exam signs reflect the physiologic abnormalities. Elevation of the neck veins with a prominent *y* descent is virtually a *sine qua non* of constrictive pericarditis and can also be a useful method to distinguish this entity from cirrhosis.[12] Edema and ascites are present in the majority of patients. Auscultatory findings include an absent apical impulse with a pericardial knock. With inspiration, the jugular venous pressure does not decrease normally, either remaining elevated or increasing further (Kussmaul's sign). Pulsus paradox is rare in pure forms of constriction but may be seen in cases of effusive constriction or in the setting of coexisting pulmonary disease.[15]

Physiology of Pericardial Constriction

In pericardial constriction a rigid, unyielding shell encases the heart, creating important hemodynamic consequences.[14,16] First, the constraining pericardium sets a limit to the total volume of blood able to enter the cardiac chambers, seriously affecting ventricular filling during diastole. In early diastole, the ventricle fills briskly. By mid-diastole, however, the volume determined by the rigid pericardium is reached and filling halts abruptly, rapidly raising pressure. In fact, early diastolic filling is more rapid than normal because of the chronically underfilled state of the ventricle. A second important hemodynamic consequence relates to the increase in ventricular interdependence from the constraining pericardium. Without a compliant pericardium to buffer the changes in volume and pressure that occurs during the cardiac and respiratory cycles, volume and pressure changes that occur in one chamber will be reflected in the adjacent chamber. Finally, the rigid, constraining pericardium isolates the pericardial space from changes in intrathoracic pressure during respiration. Thus, inspiration lowers intrathoracic pressure, but not cardiac chamber pressure, increasing venous filling into the thorax but not the right heart chambers. This causes an increase or no change in jugular venous pressure with inspiration instead of the expected decrease (Kussmaul's sign). In addition, inspiration lowers pulmonary venous pressure, but the negative inspiratory pressure is not transmitted to the left ventricle, causing a decrease in the transmitral gradient with inspiration and a corresponding diminished filling of the left ventricle with a drop in LV systolic pressure. Reduced filling of the left ventricle along with increased ventricular interdependence result in a corresponding increase in RV filling and an associated increase in RV systolic pressure. The opposite effects occur with expiration. Accordingly, the normally parallel fall and rise in RV and LV systolic pressure

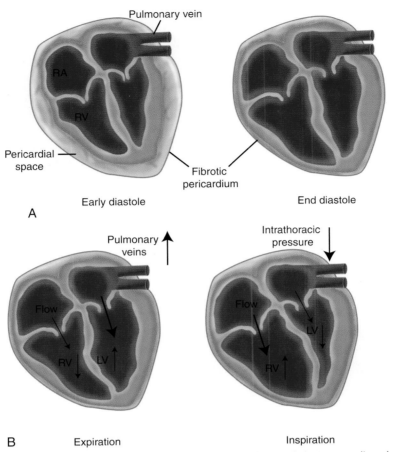

FIGURE 8-15. Schematic representation of the effects of pericardial constriction on cardiac chamber physiology. The rigid pericardium encases the heart and defines the volume able to be accommodated by the cardiac chambers. Early diastolic filling is relatively unimpaired; **(A)** filling abruptly ceases by mid-diastole when the volume determined by the pericardial space has been reached. **B,** The effect of pressure changes during the respiratory cycle in the presence of pericardial constriction. See text for details.

with inspiration and expiration become discordant in constrictive pericarditis. These physiologic effects are summarized in Figure 8-15. The finding of discordance of RV and LV systolic pressures with inspiration is highly sensitive and specific for constrictive pericarditis.[17]

Hemodynamic Findings in Constrictive Pericarditis

The physiologic abnormalities associated with constrictive pericarditis yield several classic hemodynamic findings (Table 8-3). Several abnormalities are

apparent on the RA waveform. The RA pressure shows little respiratory variation. The v wave is often greater than the a wave due to noncompliance of the atrium from the encasing pericardium. The rapid atrial emptying that occurs early in diastole along with increased atrial pressure and the relatively underfilled state of the ventricle cause a rapid y descent on the RA waveform (Figure 8-16). These are often described as an M or W pattern. The ventricular waveforms exhibit a characteristic *square root sign* or dip and plateau during diastole from the abrupt cessation in filling from the constraining

TABLE 8-3.	Summary of Hemodynamic Findings Observed in Constrictive Pericarditis

Elevated right-sided diastolic pressures
M or W pattern on right atrial waveform with rapid y descent
v > a wave due to noncompliance of the right atrium
Little to no respiratory variation in right atrial pressure
Square-root sign or dip-and-plateau pattern on ventricular pressure waves
Failure to separate left and right ventricular diastolic pressures >5 mmHg
Ratio of right ventricular end-diastolic pressure to right ventricular systolic pressure >1:3
Right ventricular (or pulmonary artery) systolic pressure <50 mmHg
Pulmonary capillary wedge pressure decline > left ventricular early diastolic pressure during inspiration
Discordance in left and right ventricular systolic pressure with inspiration

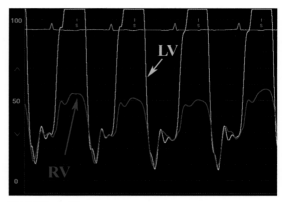

FIGURE 8-17. The right and left ventricular pressure waveforms characteristically demonstrate a diastolic *dip and plateau* or *square root sign* due to unimpeded early diastolic filling followed by a rapid rise in pressure by mid-diastole from pericardial constraint. The right and left ventricular diastolic pressures usually do not separate by more than 5 mmHg in pericardial constriction. These findings are shown in this tracing from a patient with idiopathic constrictive pericarditis.

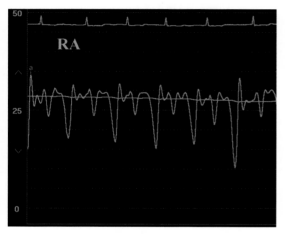

FIGURE 8-16. The right atrial pressure is elevated and the y descent is rapid and prominent in pericardial constriction, as shown from a patient with idiopathic constrictive pericarditis proven at surgery.

TABLE 8-4.	Causes of "Constrictive" Hemodynamics (Pseudoconstriction)

Restrictive cardiomyopathy
Right ventricular infarction
Pulmonary hypertension
Obesity
Severe tricuspid regurgitation
Acute volume overload
Acute heart failure
Acute severe mitral regurgitation

pericardium (Figure 8-17). The LV and RV diastolic pressures do not separate by more than 5 mmHg. Pulmonary hypertension is rare; the pulmonary artery and RV systolic pressures rarely exceed 50 mmHg. None of these hemodynamic abnormalities are specific for constrictive pericarditis. Several other conditions can cause similar findings, termed *constrictive physiology* (Table 8-4). Restrictive cardiomyopathy shares many of these features, and tricuspid regurgitation can be indistinguishable from constriction by these hemodynamic criteria.[18] Examples of *pseudoconstriction* are shown in Figures 8-18 and 8-19.

The most valuable hemodynamic findings for the diagnosis of constrictive pericarditis relate to the dynamic respiratory effects described earlier. Dissociation of intrathoracic and intracardiac pressures can be observed in the cardiac catheterization laboratory by demonstrating respiratory variation in the pressure gradient between the pulmonary capillary wedge pressure (that reflects the pulmonary vein) and the left ventricle

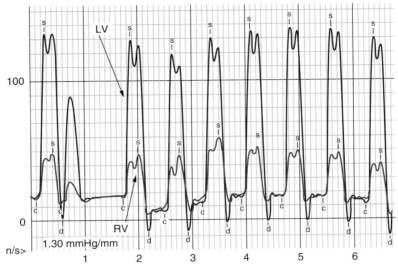

FIGURE 8-18. Some of the hemodynamic findings in constrictive pericarditis may be seen in other disorders. For example, the tracing shown was obtained in a 47-year-old man with severe, end-stage lung disease under evaluation for lung transplantation who had a normal pericardium on CT scan. Pulmonary hypertension is present with pulmonary artery systolic pressure of 50 mmHg. The right and left ventricular diastolic pressures demonstrate a square root sign and diastolic pressures within 5 mmHg. However, concordance exists between the right and left ventricular systolic pressures.

in early diastole. In constriction, because the pulmonary veins sit outside the confines of the pericardial space and are subject to changes in intrathoracic pressure, a fall occurs in the early diastolic gradient with inspiration and a subsequent rise with expiration (Figure 8-20). More importantly, however, is the finding of discordance in LV and RV systolic pressures with inspiration, a sign of increased ventricular interdependence (Figure 8-21). In one study, discordance in LV and RV systolic pressures was the most sensitive (100%) and specific (95%) sign for constrictive pericarditis.[17]

Importantly, these dynamic respiratory effects on ventricular pressure require meticulous attention to detail, high-quality hemodynamic tracings, and a regular rhythm.[19] Ideally, these subtle effects are best assessed with a respirometer to record inspiration and expiration, and high-fidelity, micromanometer catheters, rather than the fluid-filled catheters in clinical use, especially for the demonstration of the LV and pulmonary capillary wedge pressure gradient. Recognizing that

this equipment is not available in most catheterization laboratories, the demonstration of LV-RV systolic discordance remains a valuable clue. Patients with atrial fibrillation or other causes of irregular rhythm should have their rhythm regularized with a temporary pacemaker during the hemodynamic assessment to avoid the confusing effect on pressure with varying R-R intervals.

Ultimately, a final diagnosis of constrictive pericarditis is a clinical one based on incorporation of appropriate signs and symptoms coupled with demonstration of constrictive physiology either by catheterization or by echocardiography.[12,15,16] Imaging modalities are also useful and include CT scan and MRI, demonstrating pericardial thickening. Pericardial calcification on chest X-ray or fluoroscopy is present in only a minority of cases of constriction (Figure 8-22).

Constrictive pericarditis can be treated medically with diuretics if only mild symptoms and relatively low RA pressure are present. Chronic elevations of the RA pressure may lead to hepatic cirrhosis.

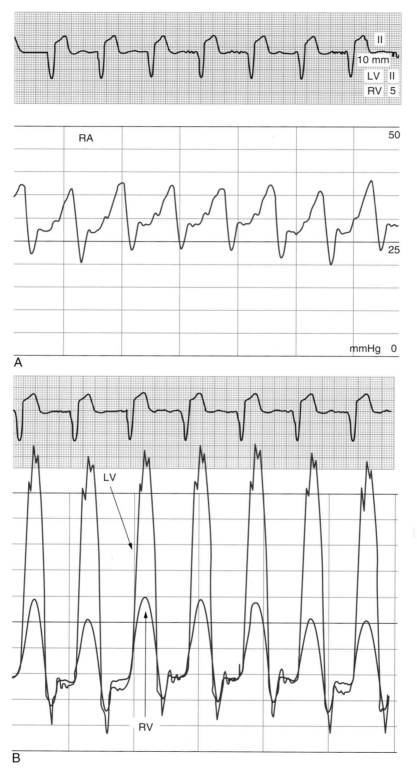

FIGURE 8-19. A, Severe tricuspid regurgitation may lead to hemodynamic findings similar to pericardial constriction with a square root sign, elevated, and equal right and left ventricular diastolic pressures and **(B)** prominent *y* descent on the right atrial waveform. The prominent *y* descent, however, is due predominantly to a large *v* wave.

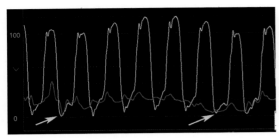

FIGURE 8-20. Demonstration of dissociation of intrathoracic and intracardiac pressures in a patient with pericardial constriction. A fall occurs in the early diastolic gradient between the left ventricle and pulmonary capillary wedge pressure with inspiration and a subsequent rise with expiration.

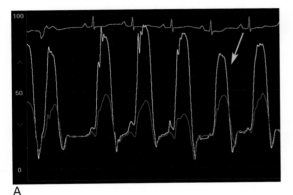

A

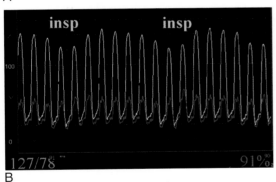

B

FIGURE 8-21. Examples of ventricular interdependence in pericardial constriction. **A,** A drop in left ventricular systolic pressure with inspiration and a rise in right ventricular systolic pressure *(arrow)*. **B,** Part **A** shown over several respiratory cycles.

Therefore, if medical therapy is chosen, it is important to assess the response to therapy by reassessment of RA pressure. Many patients with constriction will require surgical pericardiectomy, a procedure that is effective at lowering RA pressure and improving symptoms.[13]

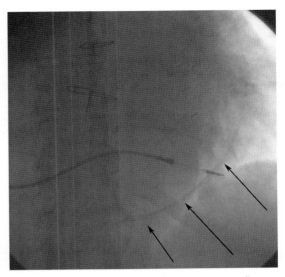

FIGURE 8-22. Pericardial calcification seen on fluoroscopy in a patient with pericardial constriction. Although this is a helpful diagnostic tool, pericardial calcification is only rarely observed.

Effusive-Constrictive Pericarditis

Some patients with pericarditis, initially found to have compressive physiology in the presence of the effusion, continue to have marked hemodynamic abnormalities when the effusion is removed. In pure tamponade, removal of fluid by pericardiocentesis achieves a pericardial pressure of zero or less with a return to normal, right-sided hemodynamics. Persistent elevation in RA pressure, despite removal of all fluid and achievement of a pericardial pressure less than 0 mmHg, suggests continued abnormality of the pericardium, usually due to inflammation and a constricting effect of the visceral pericardium. In addition to the elevation in pressures, the RA waveform typically demonstrates a prominent and rapid *y* descent similar to constriction. This entity is known as *effusive-constrictive* pericarditis and is rare, present in approximately 8% of patients with tamponade who undergo catheterization.[20] Numerous etiologies have been associated with this syndrome, including postoperative pericarditis, neoplastic disease, idiopathic, and infectious pericarditis.[12,20] In many of these patients, the constrictive component resolves as the inflammatory process subsides; however, this syndrome may result in chronic constriction and need for pericardiectomy.[20] The cardinal hemodynamic finding that suggests effusive constrictive pericarditis is shown in Figure 8-23. In this case, acute tamponade complicated post-pericardiotomy syndrome several weeks after mitral valve replacement surgery. Initially, hemodynamics suggested classic tamponade with pericardial pressure equal to RA pressure and blunting

of the y descent on the RA waveform. After removal of all fluid and obtaining a pericardial pressure of zero, the RA pressure remained elevated, now with a rapid and prominent y descent consistent with constriction.

Restrictive Cardiomyopathy

Restrictive cardiomyopathy refers to a group of uncommon disorders of the heart muscle, resulting in impaired ventricular filling with normal systolic function. Increased ventricular stiffness causes noncompliance of the ventricles and

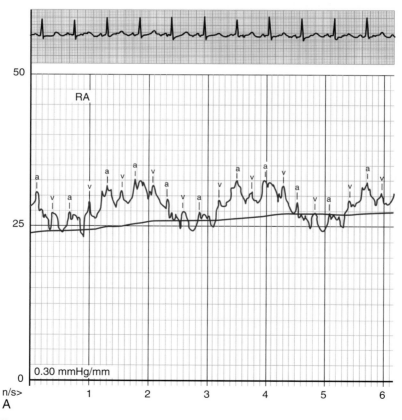

FIGURE 8-23. Effusive constrictive pericarditis in a patient who presents with tamponade from post-pericardiotomy syndrome. **A,** Prior to pericardiocentesis, right atrial pressure was elevated with attenuated x and y descents. Following pericardiocentesis, the pericardial pressure was reduced to 0 mmHg with no residual pericardial fluid discernible on echocardiography.

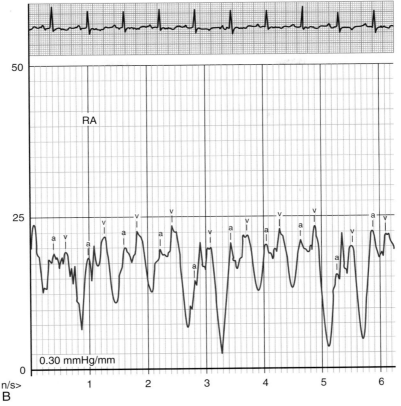

FIGURE 8-23—cont'd. **B,** The post-pericardiocentesis right atrial pressure, however, remained elevated with a prominent *y* descent consistent with effusive constrictive pericarditis.

elevated chamber pressures during diastole with only small increases in volume. The condition can affect either or both ventricles and may not uniformly affect both ventricles.

Amyloidosis and idiopathic restrictive cardiomyopathy are the most common causes outside of the tropics. In tropical regions, the most common cause is endomyocardial fibrosis. Other conditions that lead to restrictive cardiomyopathy are rare (Table 8-5).[21] The clinical presentation and hemodynamic abnormalities are very similar to constrictive pericarditis.[21,22] In fact, many of the hemodynamic findings described for constriction may be present in restrictive cardiomyopathy, particularly the square root sign and the prominent *y* descent on the RA waveform.

TABLE 8-5.	Some Causes of Restrictive Cardiomyopathy
Cardiac amyloidosis	
Idiopathic	
Hypertrophic cardiomyopathy	
Sarcoidosis	
Gaucher's disease	
Fabry's disease	
Glycogen storage disease	
Hypereosinophilia	
Carcinoid	
Transplant rejection	
Prior radiation	
Neoplasm	
Anthracycline toxicity	
Endomyocardial fibroelastosis	

Differentiation between constrictive pericarditis and restrictive cardiomyopathy in the catheterization laboratory may be difficult (Figures 8-24 to 8-26). Features more consistent with restriction

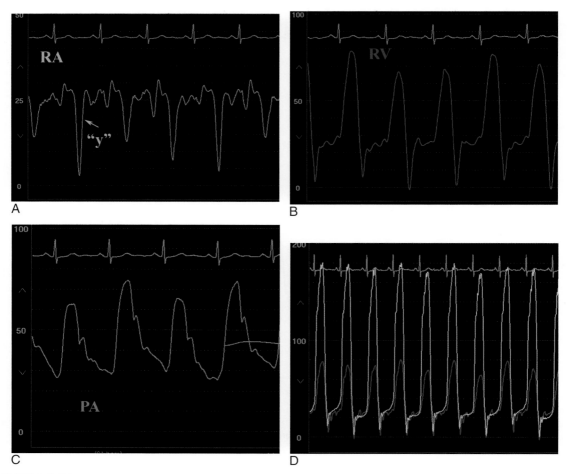

FIGURE 8-24. Hemodynamics obtained from a 47-year-old patient with ascites, edema, and left ventricular hypertrophy on echocardiography with normal systolic blood pressure, normal systolic function, and biatrial enlargement with a normal pericardium on CT scan. Note the **(A)** prominent *y* descent on the right atrial waveform and the **(B)** square root sign on the right ventricular waveform. **C,** The pulmonary artery pressure exceeds 50 mmHg, and, although the left and right ventricular diastolic pressures are within 5 mmHg, there does not appear to be **(D)** ventricular interdependence, as the systolic pressures are concordant.

include separation of the ventricular diastolic pressures >5 mmHg, the presence of pulmonary artery pressure >50 mmHg, and a ratio between RV diastolic pressure and RV systolic pressure of <1:3. As noted earlier, discordance in RV and LV systolic pressures with inspiration is the most valuable method of distinguishing the two entities in the cardiac catheterization laboratory. Some other, clinical features more consistent with restriction include the presence of biatrial enlargement and AV valve regurgitation. The presence of pericardial calcification favors pericardial constriction but is rare. ECG abnormalities, such as low voltage and conduction delay, are more common in restriction than constriction. MRI and CT scans are helpful in identifying the thickened pericardium of constriction. Endomyocardial biopsy might be considered if there is a strong suspicion of restriction with normal findings on biopsy suggestive of constriction. However, constrictive pericarditis and restrictive cardiomyopathy may coexist in patients with sarcoidosis, after radiation therapy, and in hypereosinophilic

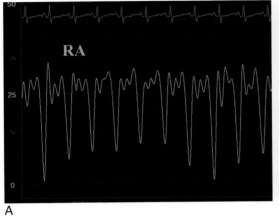

A

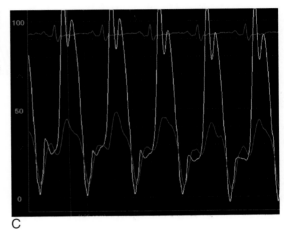

B

FIGURE 8-25. Restrictive hemodynamics in a patient with severe rejection after heart transplantation. **A,** Right atrial pressure is markedly elevated with prominent y descent, and **(B)** right ventricular pressure shows a dip and plateau pattern. **C,** Some separation between left and right ventricular diastolic pressures was apparent and no evidence of ventricular interdependence was present.

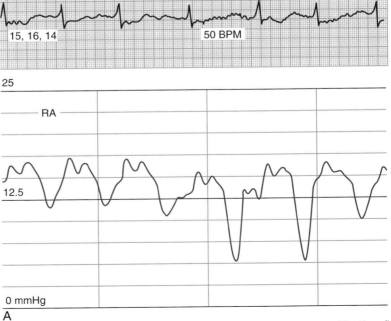

C

FIGURE 8-26. Restrictive cardio-myopathy from biopsy-proven amy-loidosis from multiple myeloma. **A,** Note the prominent y descent on the right atrial waveform.

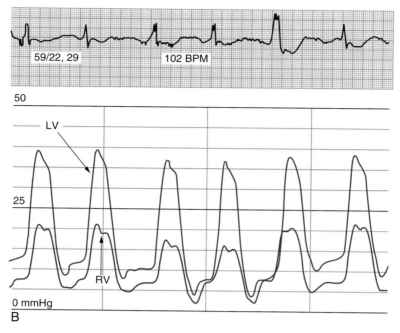

59/22, 29   102 BPM

50

LV

25

RV

0 mmHg

B

FIGURE 8-26—cont'd. **B,** Note the separation between right and left ventricular diastolic pressures.

syndrome. Ventricularization of the RA waveform in the absence of tricuspid regurgitation has been associated with amyloid restrictive cardiomyopathy.[23] Finally, restrictive cardiomyopathy significantly elevates levels of brain natriuretic peptide compared to the normal levels measured in constriction.[24]

References

1. Little WC, Freeman GL. Pericardial disease. *Circulation* 2006;113:1622–1632.
2. Spodick DH. Acute tamponade. *N Engl J Med* 2003;349:684–690.
3. Ewart W. Practical aids in the diagnosis of pericardial effusion, in connection with the question as to surgical treatment. *Br Med J* 1896;1:717–721.
4. Reddy PS, Curtiss EI, Uretsky BF. Spectrum of hemodynamic changes in cardiac tamponade. *Am J Cardiol* 1990;66:1487–1491.
5. Reddy PS, Curtiss EI. Cardiac tamponade. *Cardiol Clin* 1990;8:627–637.
6. Swami A, Spodick DH. Pulsus paradoxus in cardiac tamponade: A pathophysiologic continuum. *Clin Cardiol* 2003;26:215–217.
7. Atwood JE, Lee HJ, Cassimatis DC, et al. Association of pulsus paradoxus with obesity in normal volunteers. *J Am Coll Cardiol* 2006;47:1907–1909.
8. Bommer WJ, Follette D, Pollock M, et al. Tamponade in patients undergoing cardiac surgery; a clinical-echocardiographic diagnosis. *Am Heart J* 1995;130:1216–1223.
9. Antman EM, Cargill V, Grossman W. Low pressure cardiac tamponade. *Ann Intern Med* 1979;91:403–406.
10. Sagrista-Sauleda J, Angel J, Sambola A, et al. Low-pressure cardiac tamponade. Clinical and hemodynamic profile. *Circulation* 2006;114:945–952.
11. Ziskind AA, Pearce AC, Lemmon CC, et al. Percutaneous balloon pericardiotomy for the treatment of cardiac tamponade and large pericardial effusions: Description of technique and report of the first 50 cases. *J Am Coll Cardiol* 1993;21:1–5.
12. Fowler NO. Constrictive pericarditis: Its history and current status. *Clin Cardiol* 1995;18:341–350.
13. Ling LH, Oh JK, Schaff HV, et al. Constrictive pericarditis in the modern era. Evolving clinical spectrum and impact on outcome after pericardiectomy. *Circulation* 1999;100:1380–1386.
14. Killian DM, Furiasse JG, Scanlon PJ, et al. Constrictive pericarditis after cardiac surgery. *Am Heart J* 1989;118:563–568.
15. Myers RB, Spodick DH. Constrictive pericarditis: Clinical and pathophysiologic characteristics. *Am Heart J* 1999;138:219–232.
16. Nishimura RA. Constrictive pericarditis in the modern era: A diagnostic dilemma. *Heart* 2001;86:619–623.

17. Hurrell DG, Nishimura RA, Higano ST, et al. Value of dynamic respiratory changes in left and right ventricular pressures for the diagnosis of constrictive pericarditis. *Circulation* 1996;93:2007–2013.
18. Studley J, Tighe DA, Joelson JM, Flack JE. The hemodynamic signs of constrictive pericarditis can be mimicked by tricuspid regurgitation. *Cardiol Rev* 2003;11:320–326.
19. Higano ST, Azrak E, Tahirkheli NK, Kern MJ. Hemodynamic rounds series II: Hemodynamics of constrictive physiology: Influence of respiratory dynamics on ventricular pressures. *Catheter Cardiovasc Interv* 1999;46:473–486.
20. Sagrista-Sauleda J, Angel J, Sanchez A, et al. Effusive-constrictive pericarditis. *N Engl J Med* 2004; 350:469–475.
21. Kushwaha SS, Fallon JT, Fuster V. Restrictive cardiomyopathy. *N Engl J Med* 1997;336:267–276.
22. Ammash NM, Seward JB, Bailey KR, et al. Clinical profile and outcome of idiopathic restrictive cardiomyopathy. *Circulation* 2000;101:2490–2496.
23. Gowda S, Salem BI, Haikal M. Ventricularization of right atrial wave form in amyloid restrictive cardiomyopathy. *Cathet Cardiovasc Diagn* 1985;11: 483–491.
24. Leya FS, Arab D, Joyal D, et al. The efficacy of brain natriuretic peptide levels in differentiating constrictive pericarditis from restrictive cardiomyopathy. *J Am Coll Cardiol* 2005;45:1900–1902.

CHAPTER 9

Shock, Heart Failure, and Related Disorders

MICHAEL RAGOSTA, MD

Heart failure remains one of the most common cardiovascular disorders, with an estimated prevalence in the United States of over five million cases. Over 500,000 newly diagnosed cases of heart failure are known each year, and the condition accounted for over one million hospital admissions in 2003.[1] Manifestations of the failing heart range from well-compensated left ventricular systolic dysfunction to cardiogenic shock with a wide variety of underlying pathophysiology and hemodynamic manifestations. This chapter will review the pathophysiology and relevant hemodynamics of shock and heart failure syndromes, including the interesting hemodynamic abnormalities associated with the transplanted heart.

Pathophysiology of Shock

Cardiogenic shock represents the most dramatic and deadly manifestation of heart failure. The essence of shock is inadequate tissue perfusion clinically manifest by hypotension, oliguria, mental status changes, peripheral cyanosis, and cool skin and extremities. Inadequate tissue perfusion propagates cardiogenic shock via the compensatory mechanisms intended to raise central blood pressure such as tachycardia and vasoconstriction. Peripheral vasoconstriction causes tissue hypoxia and subsequent acidosis, which further depresses myocardial function, exacerbating shock. A downward spiral

ensues (Figure 9-1). Ultimately, these progressive derangements become irreversible and compensatory mechanisms fail, leading to the patient's demise.

The differential diagnosis of shock is broad. The initial dilemma that faces the physician relates to a determination if shock is due to cardiogenic or noncardiac causes (Table 9-1). This can often be determined by a hemodynamic assessment aimed at measuring the systemic vascular resistance and the filling pressures of the heart.

Systemic vascular resistance, or SVR, is derived from Ohm's law ($V = IR$) and can be calculated from the formula:

$$SVR = \frac{(\text{mean aortic pressure}) - (\text{mean right atrial pressure})}{\text{Cardiac output}}$$

Multiplying the product by 80 achieves resistance units in dynes-sec-cm^{-5}. To calculate the systemic vascular resistance index (SVRI), the cardiac index is substituted for cardiac output in the formula; therefore, the SVRI formula is

$$SVRI = (SVR) \times (\text{body surface area})$$

The normal SVR = 1170 ± 270 dynes-sec-cm^{-5}, and the normal SVRI = 2130 ± 450 dynes-sec-cm^{-5} × m^2.

The SVR is elevated in most cases of cardiogenic shock from excessive vasoconstriction except at the end stages when vasodilatation ensues. Systemic vascular resistance is low in patients with septic shock, anaphylactic shock, and other noncardiogenic causes of shock associated with profound vasodilatation (Addison's crisis, neurogenic, drug, or metabolic).

Elevated right-heart filling pressures, particularly the pulmonary capillary wedge pressure, classically distinguishes the cardiogenic from noncardiogenic causes of shock, with the latter exhibiting

FIGURE 9-1. The initial hemodynamic derangements in cardiogenic shock may be exacerbated by the adverse sequelas of poor perfusion, leading to a progressive, downward spiral.

THE DOWNWARD SPIRAL OF CARDIOGENIC SHOCK

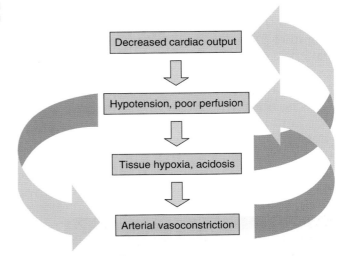

TABLE 9-1. Causes of Shock

Cardiogenic Causes
Acute myocardial infarction
Pump failure
Right ventricular infarction
Ventricular septal rupture
Acute mitral regurgitation
Free wall rupture
Acquired left ventricular outflow tract obstruction
Arrhythmia
Bradycardia
Tachycardia
Acute valvular regurgitation
Aortic regurgitation
Mitral regurgitation
Acute prosthetic valve regurgitation
Obstruction
Decompensated aortic stenosis
Hypertrophic obstructive cardiomyopathy
Acquired left ventricular outflow tract obstruction
Atrial myxoma
Acute prosthetic valve obstruction
Pump failure
Idiopathic
Myocarditis
Rejection
Ischemic
Hypovolemic
Aortic dissection
Ruptured aortic aneurysm
Compressive
Tamponade

Noncardiogenic Causes
Neurogenic
Anaphylaxis
Sepsis
Hypovolemic shock
Toxic/metabolic
Acidosis
Adrenal crisis
Pulmonary embolism
Tension pneumothorax

low pulmonary capillary wedge and right-sided chamber pressures. Naturally, exceptions exist. Advanced stages of septic shock cause myocardial depression and may elevate right-sided pressures. Right ventricular infarction, a cardiogenic cause, may be associated with marked hypotension, low cardiac output, and shock despite a normal pulmonary capillary wedge pressure. Similarly, cardiac tamponade in the setting of hypovolemia may be associated with profound shock despite low-filling pressures.

Hemodynamics of Cardiogenic Shock

Patients with shock usually exhibit arterial hypotension with systolic pressures <90 mmHg. The adequacy of tissue perfusion, however, defines the presence or absence of shock, not an arbitrary blood pressure valve. Thus, shock may be present in patients without overt hypotension. The lowered stroke volume results in reduction in cardiac output despite an associated compensatory tachycardia, and the cardiac index typically measures less than 2.0 L/min/m^2 with a correspondingly low mixed venous saturation (<55%).

The normal aortic waveform appears robust with a pulse pressure of about 40–50 mmHg and ample pulse width (Figure 9-2). In addition to hypotension, patients with cardiogenic shock often exhibit abnormalities in the aortic pressure waveform. The pulse pressure reflects both the strength of contraction and stroke volume; thus, the pulse pressure on the aortic waveform in a patient with cardiogenic shock from pump failure is usually reduced (Figure 9-3).

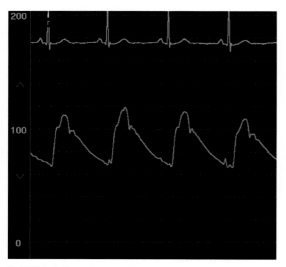

FIGURE 9-2. The robust appearance of a normal aortic waveform.

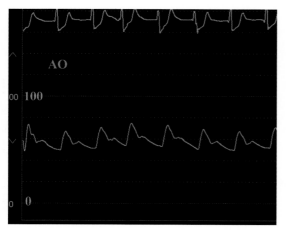

FIGURE 9-3. Example of a patient with a marked reduction in stroke volume from profound pump failure, resulting in a narrow pulse pressure on the aortic waveform.

The pulse width also reflects the stroke volume. Patients in shock with normal or hypercontractile ventricles often have aortic waveforms with narrow pulse widths but normal pulse pressures (Figure 9-4). This finding may be observed, for instance, in patients in shock from non-cardiogenic causes such as anaphylaxis or in patients with cardiogenic causes such as tamponade, acute mitral regurgitation, or post-myocardial infarction ventricular septal defect. The narrow pulse width lends a "spiked" appearance to the aortic pressure waveform with the dicrotic notch appearing low. Importantly, the systolic pressure of this spiked waveform may exceed 90–100 mmHg, falsely reassuring the clinician. The narrow pulse width provides a clue to the low stroke volume and impending cardiovascular collapse (Figure 9-5).

Additional hemodynamic findings reflect the underlying pathology that causes cardiogenic shock. For example, although neither specific nor sensitive, a large v wave on the pulmonary capillary wedge pressure tracing suggests shock from acute, severe mitral regurgitation. Cardiac tamponade characteristically causes elevated and equalized diastolic pressures with loss of the y descent on the right atrial waveform. The right atrial and right ventricular diastolic pressures are markedly elevated with a normal pulmonary capillary wedge pressure in cases of cardiogenic shock from right ventricular infarction. A left-to-right shunt at the level of the right ventricle identifies an acute ventricular septal defect.

Treatment of cardiogenic shock is based on efforts to maintain adequate tissue perfusion and reverse the downward spiral of hemodynamic derangements.[2] Vasopressor and inotropic agents are the mainstay of pharmacologic therapy. Aggressive treatment of acidosis and hypoxia prevents additional myocardial depression. Specific therapy is directed at

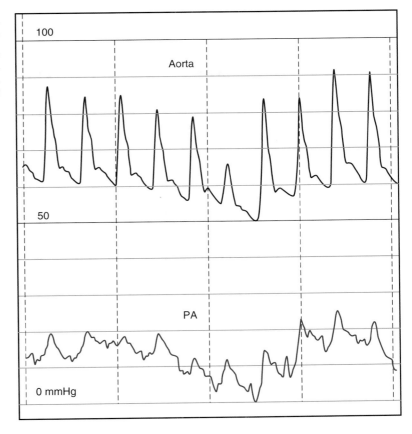

FIGURE 9-4. Aortic and pulmonary artery (PA) pressure tracing in a patient with anaphylactic shock. Note the normal pulmonary artery pressure and the presence of hypotension with a narrow pulse width, lending a *spike* appearance to the aortic pressure tracing.

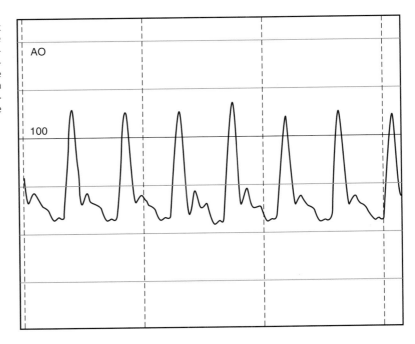

FIGURE 9-5. Example of a patient in cardiogenic shock from acute ventricular septal rupture post-myocardial infarction demonstrating normal peak systolic pressure but a very narrow pulse width and a *spiked* appearance to the aortic pressure. Note also the location of the dicrotic notch.

the underlying cause (for example, reperfusion therapy for acute myocardial infarction or pericardiocentesis for tamponade). Finally, the intra-aortic balloon pump is an invaluable therapeutic adjunct.

Intra-Aortic Balloon Counterpulsation in Cardiogenic Shock

The intra-aortic balloon pump improves many of the hemodynamic abnormalities in cardiogenic shock.[3,4] The balloon catheter is inserted percutaneously and positioned in the descending aorta (Figure 9-6). The balloon is timed to inflate during diastole against a closed aortic valve displacing aortic blood (30–50 mL, depending on the balloon volume) and increasing the diastolic pressure within the aorta *(diastolic augmentation)*. The balloon rapidly deflates at the end of diastole, just prior to aortic ejection, creating a potential space of 30–50 mL within the aorta,

lowering the impedance of the aorta and reducing end-diastolic pressure and resulting in afterload reduction. Thus, the intra-aortic balloon pump provides two major beneficial effects in cardiogenic shock: improved tissue perfusion by diastolic augmentation of aortic pressure and enhancement of ventricular function by reducing afterload.

The hemodynamic benefits of an intra-aortic balloon pump are summarized in Table 9-2. In the hypotensive patient with cardiogenic shock, diastolic pressure increases because of diastolic augmentation and generally exceeds systolic pressure. The systolic pressure may, in fact, decrease further because of the afterload reduction afforded by the balloon pump. The net effect, however, is an increase in the mean arterial pressure, thereby improving tissue perfusion. Cardiac output and stroke volume generally increase while heart rates are either unaffected or may decrease slightly as a consequence of improved hemodynamics.

One of the presumed hemodynamic benefits of the intra-aortic balloon pump relates to the potential enhancement of coronary blood flow, a mostly diastolic phenomenon. However, the effect on coronary blood flow varies depending on the underlying hemodynamics and the degree of coronary arterial narrowing. Using the Doppler flow wire in human subjects, studies suggest that aortic counterpulsation increases coronary blood flow velocity in the proximal, prestenotic segment of the coronary artery

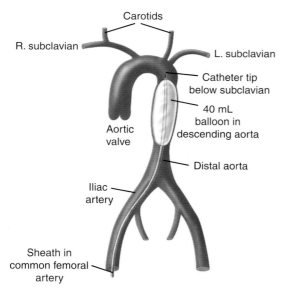

FIGURE 9-6. Schematic representation of proper placement of an intra-aortic balloon pump in the descending aorta via the right femoral artery. The tip of the catheter should be below the subclavian, usually achieved by placing this at the tracheal bifurcation.

TABLE 9-2.	Effects of Intra-Aortic Balloon Pump in Cardiogenic Shock
HEMODYNAMIC VARIABLE	**EFFECT**
Diastolic pressure, aorta	+ + + +
Systolic pressure, aorta	− −
Mean pressure, aorta	+ +
Cardiac output	+ +
Heart rate	− or no change
Coronary blood flow	+ or no change

and in the distal artery, only if no significant stenosis is present. However, in the presence of a severe coronary stenosis, coronary blood flow velocity in the distal artery does not increase with the intra-aortic balloon pump. This suggests that the dramatic relief of ischemia afforded by the balloon pump in patients with critical coronary stenoses is from afterload and preload reduction, thereby decreasing myocardial oxygen demand, rather than via a direct increase in coronary blood flow.[5–8]

The hemodynamic benefits vary in an individual and depend upon the degree of ventricular impairment, the underlying cardiac rhythm, the systemic vascular resistance, and the timing and volume of balloon inflation. The balloon pump should be thought of as a support device and not an artificial heart; it augments cardiac output and is less effective in patients with profoundly depressed cardiac output. Similarly, patients with excessive tachycardia have diminished diastolic filling times, decreasing the efficacy of the device. Patients with cardiogenic shock and low systemic vascular resistance will have little or no additional afterload reduction and are unlikely to achieve any diastolic pressure augmentation. For this reason, the intra-aortic balloon pump is not an effective treatment for septic shock or other, noncardiogenic causes associated with low systemic vascular resistance. Finally, the optimal benefits are seen only when the timing of inflation and deflation are correct and when the appropriate volume of inflation is used; improper timing or inadequate inflation volumes may not provide beneficial effects and may, in the event of improper timing, be detrimental.

Timing of inflation and deflation can best be accomplished by placing the pump on a 1:2 mode (inflated once for every two cycles) (Figure 9-7). Onset of inflation optimally occurs just after the

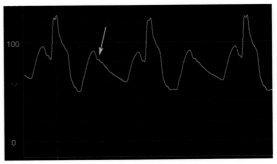

FIGURE 9-7. Proper timing of inflation and deflation of an intra-aortic balloon pump. The pump is set at a 1:2 ratio, meaning that it is set to inflate and deflate during one of two cardiac cycles. The balloon inflates just after the dicrotic notch on the aortic pressure waveform *(arrow)*. Deflation should be completed before aortic ejection begins on the next cardiac cycle, which is evident by a lower end-diastolic pressure of the augmented beat as compared to the unaugmented beat.

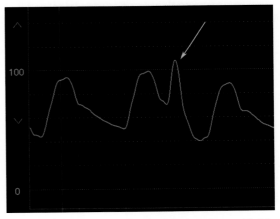

FIGURE 9-8. Example of early deflation along with late inflation. The balloon timing is set at a 1:2 ratio. Note the asthenic appearance of the augmented beat *(arrow)* providing little additional perfusion.

dicrotic notch. Deflation should be completed prior to the beginning of aortic ejection, as evidenced by a lower end-diastolic pressure for the augmented compared to the unaugmented beat. Recognizing faulty timing is important because improper timing may, at minimal, fail to achieve a therapeutic effect or worse—clinical deterioration (Figures 9-8 to 9-10). Early deflation or late inflation of the balloon causes inadequate augmentation and either no or poor additional perfusion pressure. Late deflation or early inflation may be harmful.

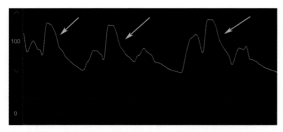

FIGURE 9-9. Example of late deflation. The balloon timing is set at a 1:2 ratio. The arrows point to the augmented beat. Note that the end-diastolic pressure of the augmented beat is much higher than that of the unaugmented beat. This indicates that the balloon pump remains partially inflated at the beginning of aortic ejection, increasing afterload with potentially detrimental effects.

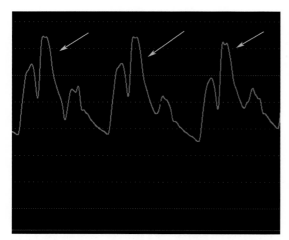

FIGURE 9-10. Example of early inflation and late deflation. The balloon timing is set at a 1:2 ratio. The arrows point to the augmented beat. Balloon inflation is occurring prior to the dicrotic notch. Also, the end-diastolic pressure of the augmented beat is higher than that of the unaugmented beat consistent with late deflation.

In the case of late deflation, increased impedance and increased afterload are present because of ejection against a partially inflated balloon. In the event of early inflation, the aortic valve has not yet closed; the inflating balloon may cause aortic regurgitation and increased impedance with adverse consequences.

The intra-aortic balloon pump is indicated for most causes of cardiogenic shock and is effective at stabilizing hemodynamics in patients with mechanical complications of acute myocardial infarction (acute mitral regurgitation and ventricular septal defect).[9,10] It may not benefit patients with shock from right ventricular infarction, unless associated with a large left ventricular infarction and elevation in pulmonary capillary wedge pressure that causes increased right ventricular afterload. The balloon pump improves the hemodynamic and rhythm status of patients with shock from malignant ventricular arrhythmia.[11] In cardiogenic shock from ischemic pump failure, the balloon pump improves clinical stability but appears most useful when coupled with revascularization.[12,13] Patients with decompensated aortic stenosis or shock from acute mitral regurgitation also improve and, in patients with end-stage heart failure, the balloon pump provides a bridge to transplantation or a ventricular assist device.

The balloon pump is contraindicated in patients with significant aortic regurgitation and in patients with aortic dissection. The device is relatively contraindicated in the setting of peripheral vascular disease, aortic aneurysm, and in those without a clear end point such as a coronary revascularization procedure, transplantation, or a ventricular assist device. Severe iliac tortuosity may not allow passage of the relatively stiff device. The numerous potential complications of an intra-aortic balloon pump have been reviewed.[3,4]

Chronic Left Ventricular Failure

Chronic left ventricular dysfunction is caused either by chronic ischemic heart disease or from numerous nonischemic etiologies such as idiopathic, viral, alcoholic, or hypertensive cardiomyopathy.[14] Left ventricular dilatation and several other compensatory mechanisms ensue regardless of the inciting cause of left-heart failure. The hemodynamic findings in dilated cardiomyopathy are relatively nonspecific. They may be entirely normal if the patient is well compensated. With decompensation, the left ventricular end-diastolic pressure elevates, resulting in elevation of the pulmonary capillary wedge pressure and passive elevations in the pulmonary artery, right ventricular, and right atrial pressures. The cardiac output is usually normal or mildly reduced with the potential for marked reduction in cardiac output and a correspondingly low mixed venous saturation in severe cases.

The intact pericardium plays an important role in the hemodynamics of both acute and chronic heart failure. With acute heart failure, the abrupt increase in cardiac chamber volume within the confines of a relatively inelastic pericardium may cause a hemodynamic finding similar to constrictive pericarditis.[15] In chronic heart failure with left ventricular enlargement, the constraining effect of the pericardium couples the ventricles via the intraventricular septum. In other words, changes in volume in one chamber influence the opposing chamber. This phenomenon is used to explain the mechanism by which diuresis improves left ventricular stroke volume in chronic heart failure. The Frank-Starling mechanism states that a decrease in chamber volume (preload) would *decrease* stroke volume; however, diuresis *improves* stroke volume when there is cardiac chamber enlargement and high filling pressures because diuresis decreases right ventricular chamber volume; this allows an increase in left ventricular diastolic volume, thereby improving left ventricular stroke volume.[16]

Severe left ventricular dysfunction is associated with several abnormalities on the left ventricular pressure waveform. In patients with normal systolic function, left ventricular upstroke (or Dp/Dt) is brisk with a rapid decline after reaching peak systolic pressure. With the onset of diastole, left ventricular pressure is

normally very low (zero or even negative) and rises throughout diastole to reach an end-diastolic pressure of 10–12 mmHg. Patients with severe left ventricular dysfunction may show a slow rise in left ventricular pressure due to poor contractility that yields a triangular appearance to the left ventricular waveform (Figure 9-11). In addition, left ventricular diastolic pressure is high early in diastole, with left ventricular end-diastolic pressure reaching very high levels (40–50 mmHg). A prominent *a* wave is often seen on the left ventricular tracing due to atrial contraction against an already high end-diastolic volume within a noncompliant ventricle (Figure 9-12). In patients with heart failure, the left ventricular end-diastolic pressure is often used as a surrogate for mean left atrial pressure; however, a prominent *a* wave may interfere with accurate estimation of left atrial pressure. In such cases, the left ventricular pre-*a* wave pressure, or the mean left ventricular diastolic pressure, correlates well with mean left atrial pressure.[17]

A large *v* wave may be seen on the pulmonary capillary wedge pressure tracing in severe heart failure without associated mitral regurgitation. Normally, at low pressures and volumes, the small additional increase in volume that occurs during passive left atrial filling when the mitral valve is closed causes just a small rise in pressure and a physiologic *v* wave. In heart failure, the distended volumes of the left atrium shift the compliance curve to the right so that the additional volume from passive atrial filling causes a large increase in pressure, generating a substantial *v* wave (Figure 9-13).

Pulsus alternans represents an unusual and interesting hemodynamic sign of a failing heart. The sign is manifest by an alternating rise and fall in aortic systolic pressure from beat to beat while the patient is in a regular cardiac rhythm

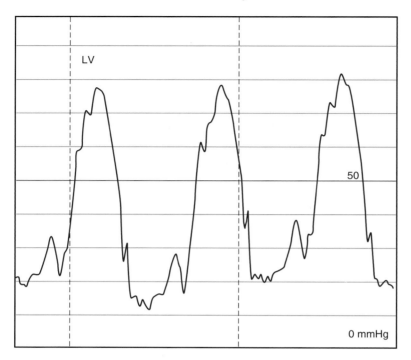

FIGURE 9-11. Left ventricular pressure waveform in a patient with severe left ventricular dysfunction with a delayed upstroke and pressure decay lending a triangular appearance.

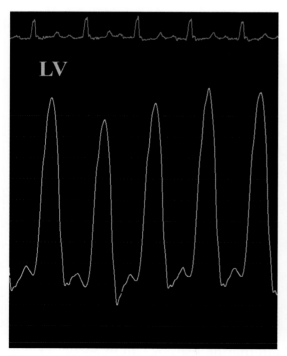

FIGURE 9-12. Example of a large *a* wave on a left ventricular *(LV)* pressure waveform in a patient with heart failure.

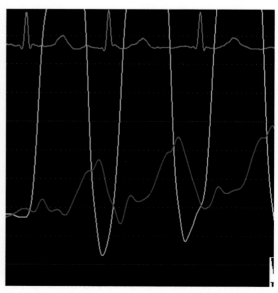

FIGURE 9-13. Prominent *v* wave on a pulmonary capillary wedge pressure tracing in a patient with heart failure from severe left ventricular systolic dysfunction and no mitral regurgitation.

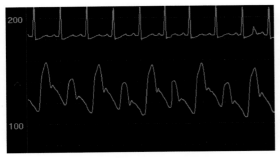

FIGURE 9-14. Example of pulsus alternans present on an aortic pressure tracing in a patient with severe left ventricular dysfunction.

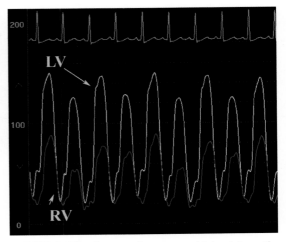

FIGURE 9-15. These tracings were obtained from the same patient shown in Figure 9-14 and demonstrate pulsus alternans on the right (green) and left ventricular (LV) pressure tracings.

(Figure 9-14). This case is different from a *pulsus bigeminus*, which is seen with an atrial or ventricular bigeminal rhythm, or a *pulsus paradoxus,* in which the rise and fall of aortic systolic pressure is related to the respiratory cycle. Pulsus alternans usually implies serious underlying myocardial disease. It occurs in association with severe aortic stenosis, cardiomyopathy, and severe coronary artery disease. However, it has been described in normal hearts after termination of a supraventricular tachycardia. It may be accentuated by decreasing venous return such as what occurs with inferior vena caval occlusion and may become more apparent after a premature ventricular beat. The pattern of alternating rise and fall in systolic pressure may be seen on the left ventricular, right ventricular, and pulmonary artery waveforms, in addition to the aortic waveform (Figure 9-15). Both right ventricular and pulmonary arterial pulsus alternans may be seen independent of left-sided pulsus alternans if there is isolated right-heart failure. Isolated atrial alternans has also been described. The cause of pulsus alternans is not entirely clear. One explanation suggests that it might be due to alternation of myocardial contractility on a beat-to-beat basis due to a loss of the number of cells that contract on alternate beats because of

abnormal intracellular calcium cycling—that is, a form of *localized* electrical mechanical dissociation.[18]

Pulmonary Hypertension in Chronic Heart Failure

Secondary pulmonary hypertension may complicate the clinical course of patients with chronic heart failure, reducing exercise capacity, accentuating the propensity for right-heart failure, and increasing mortality. Elevations in pulmonary artery, or PA, pressure may be seen in patients with chronic heart failure simply because the circuit composed by the left ventricle, left atrium, pulmonary veins, and pulmonary arteries is in a series, and thus a rise in left atrial pressure (and thus the pulmonary capillary wedge pressure, or PCWP) will passively elevate the pulmonary artery systolic pressure. In such cases, pulmonary vascular resistance is normal. Based on Ohm's law, pulmonary vascular resistance (or PVR) in Wood units is calculated as follows:

$$PVR = \frac{(Mean\ PA) - (Mean\ PCWP)}{Cardiac\ output}$$

Multiplying the PVR in Wood units by 80 converts this measurement to the resistance units of dynes-sec-cm^5; a normal pulmonary artery systolic pressure is 20–25 mmHg, and normal PVR is about 70 dynes-sec-cm^5. In patients with chronic heart failure, abnormal pulmonary vascular resistance is present when PVR is >2 Wood units or the transpulmonary gradient (mean PA – mean PCWP) exceeds 15 mmHg.

Pulmonary hypertension with increased pulmonary vascular resistance may be caused either by excessive pulmonary vascular tone or from chronic structural changes in the pulmonary vasculature. Dysregulation of vascular tone in chronic heart failure is attributed to endothelial dysfunction.[19,20] The pulmonary vascular endothelium produces both nitric oxide (NO), an important vasodilator of pulmonary vessels, and endothelin, a vasoconstrictor. A fine balance between these opposing agents maintains normal vascular tone. Pulmonary vascular endothelial dysfunction in chronic heart failure decreases NO and increases endothelin, tipping the balance toward vasoconstriction, causing pulmonary hypertension. This mechanism is readily reversible with administration of vasodilator agents. However, NO also inhibits vascular smooth muscle cell proliferation and hypertrophy; therefore, a decrease in NO contributes to more permanent structural changes in the pulmonary vasculature, including intimal fibrosis and medial hypertrophy, which are much slower to reverse and are not responsive to vasodilator agents.

Administration of vasodilator agents assists the physician to decide whether increased pulmonary vascular resistance in patients with secondary pulmonary hypertension from chronic heart failure is reversible. This represents an important determination for patients considered for heart transplantation, because the unaccustomed right ventricle of the transplanted heart may fail in patients with *fixed* pulmonary hypertension.

Proposed methods of determining whether increased pulmonary resistance is reactive or fixed involve the administration of various vasodilator agents, including inhaled NO,[21] prostacyclin,[22] and nitroprusside.[23] Many cardiac catheterization laboratories use nitroprusside infusion based on their familiarity with the drug and its relatively easy means of administration. At the University of Virginia, patients with chronic heart failure who undergo evaluation for heart transplantation are given nitroprusside infusion if the pulmonary artery systolic pressure exceeds 50 mmHg, if pulmonary vascular resistance exceeds 4 Wood units, or if the transpulmonary gradient is more than 15 mmHg. Arterial pressure is monitored continuously with infusion of nitroprusside beginning at 0.25 μg/kg/min, increasing every 2 minutes by 0.25-μg increments until systemic arterial blood pressure drops by at least 15% from baseline.

Using a similar protocol, investigators at Stanford reported a 3-month mortality after transplantation of only 3.8% for patients found to have reversible pulmonary hypertension with nitroprusside compared to 40.6% for patients whose pulmonary vascular resistance remained >2.5 Wood units despite nitroprusside and 27.5% for those whose pulmonary vascular resistance dropped below 2.5 Wood units but at the expense of systemic hypotension.[23] Thus, this fairly simple technique provides useful information in the evaluation of patients with heart failure and secondary pulmonary hypertension. An example of the use of nitroprusside infusion to determine reversibility of pulmonary hypertension in a patient under evaluation for heart transplantation is shown in Figure 9-16.

Heart failure patients with secondary pulmonary hypertension develop compensatory right ventricular hypertrophy, resulting in noncompliance of the right ventricle. This may manifest by a prominent *a* wave on the right ventricular waveform (Figure 9-17). Ultimately, chronic heart failure with secondary pulmonary hypertension causes right-heart failure with annular dilatation and tricuspid regurgitation, notable on a right atrial waveform by a prominent *v* wave (Figure 9-18).

Cardiac-Transplantation Hemodynamics

Several interesting hemodynamic findings occur following heart transplantation. In patients without severe, fixed pulmonary hypertension, pulmonary pressures fall to near normal within 2 weeks of transplantation.[24] However, the donor right ventricle dilates early after transplantation in response to the recipient's abnormal pulmonary vasculature and may remain dilated despite the rapid fall in pulmonary pressures. Accordingly, tricuspid regurgitation from annular dilatation is common in the transplanted heart.

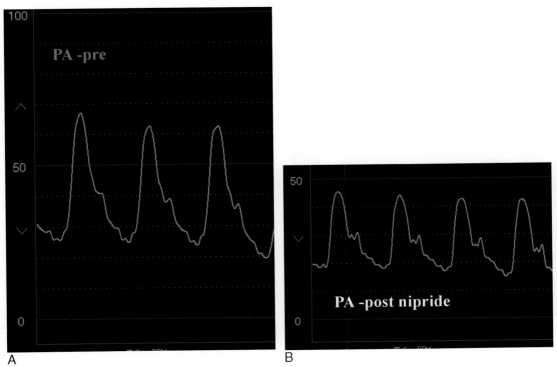

A   B

FIGURE 9-16. These tracings demonstrate reversible pulmonary hypertension in a patient with chronic heart failure and left ventricular dysfunction with pulmonary hypertension. **A,** At baseline, the pulmonary artery pressure was 67/22 mmHg with a mean pressure of 37 mmHg. The mean pulmonary capillary wedge pressure was 25 mmHg with a cardiac output of 3.3 L/min. Thus, the transpulmonary gradient was 37–25, or 12 mmHg, and the pulmonary vascular resistance = 12/3.3 = 3.6 Wood units. Nitroprusside was infused until the arterial blood pressure decreased from 124/78 to 103/64 mmHg. Pressures were remeasured at peak nitroprusside infusion. The cardiac output increased to 5.1 L/min and **(B)** the pulmonary artery pressure decreased to 43/15 mmHg with a mean pressure of 25 mmHg. The mean pulmonary capillary wedge pressure decreased to 16 mmHg. This resulted in a pulmonary vascular resistance of 9/5.1, or 1.8 Wood units.

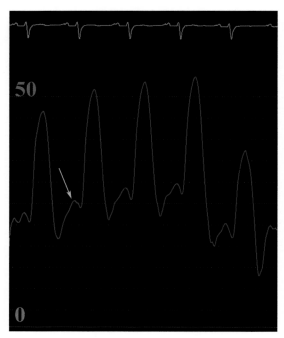

FIGURE 9-17. Patient with pulmonary hypertension who demonstrates a large *a* wave *(arrow)* on the right ventricular pressure waveform.

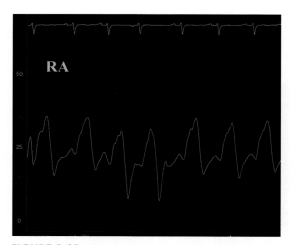

FIGURE 9-18. Prominent *v* waves on the right atrial *(RA)* pressure waveform consistent with tricuspid regurgitation in a patient with severe pulmonary hypertension.

The transplanted heart often exhibits abnormal right-heart hemodynamics consistent with restrictive physiology. The early pioneers of cardiac transplantation observed prominent *a* and *v* waves and rapid *y* descent upon physical examination of the jugular venous pulse,

similar to individuals with restrictive disease, in patients experiencing acute rejection.[25] Restrictive abnormalities include (1) elevation of right atrial pressure, (2) prominence of the *y* descent, and (3) elevated right ventricular end-diastolic pressure with an early diastolic dip followed by an exaggerated and abrupt rise in right ventricular diastolic pressure prior to the *a* wave. These restrictive abnormalities occur commonly in nearly all patients in the early posttransplantation period, resolving by 9 weeks in the absence of rejection (Figure 9-19).[26] In patients without histological rejection, a mean right atrial pressure of 10 mmHg and a *y* descent of >7 mmHg recorded in the first few weeks after transplantation decreased to a mean right atrial pressure of 4 mmHg and a *y* descent <5 mmHg.[26] Many of these early abnormalities are attributed to the adaptation of the donor right heart to the recipient's abnormal pulmonary vasculature.

Persistence of restrictive hemodynamics, long-term after transplantation, has been observed in at least 15% of patients studied in average of 5 years after transplant and was associated with more rejection episodes than patients without this hemodynamic finding.[27] Furthermore, the return of a restrictive pattern on right-heart pressure waveforms correlates with the presence of acute rejection by histology (Figure 9-20). This finding is a specific but not very sensitive indicator of rejection. One study found a right atrial mean pressure >11 mmHg or a *y* descent >10 mmHg to be 94% and 96% specific, respectively, for moderate rejection on histology but only associated with a sensitivity of 41% and 52%, respectively.[26] These abnormalities often improve with treatment of rejection, but right ventricular diastolic pressures may remain elevated >10 mmHg despite resolution of rejection.[28] The cause of these persisting abnormalities is not known

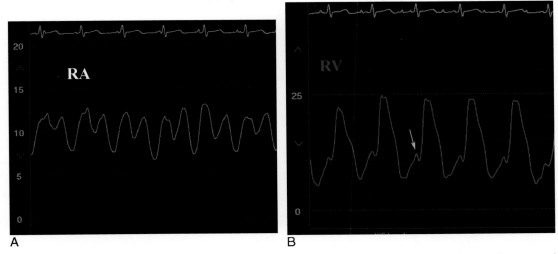

FIGURE 9-19. Restrictive pattern in a patient early after heart transplantation. **A,** Note the prominent *y* descent on the right atrial *(RA)* waveform. **B,** Elevation of the right ventricular *(RV)* end-diastolic pressure and a prominent *a* wave *(arrow)*.

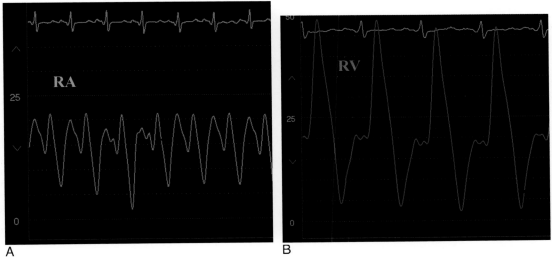

FIGURE 9-20. Hemodynamics obtained during an episode of acute rejection after cardiac transplantation. **A,** Elevation of the right atrial (RA) pressure with prominent *y* descent. **B,** The right ventricular (RV) waveform shows a *dip and plateau* or *square-root pattern* with elevation of the end-diastolic pressure to 20 mmHg.

and likely represents myocardial fibrosis or right ventricular remodeling.

Most cases of rejection have modest effects on right-heart pressures. Rarely, severe, acute rejection may cause striking hemodynamic abnormalities. *Atrialization* of the right ventricular pressure waveform thought secondary to transient adynamic function of the right ventricle has been reported in acute severe rejection (Figure 9-21).[29] This unusual finding has been noted in Uhl's anomaly (absence of the myocardium of the right ventricle) and endomyocardial fibrosis but, interestingly, not in right ventricular infarction.

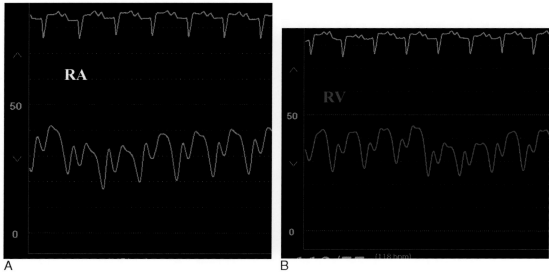

FIGURE 9-21. An unusual hemodynamic abnormality that occurs during an episode of acute, severe rejection after heart transplantation. **A,** The right atrial (RA) pressure is elevated with a prominent *y* descent. **B,** The right ventricular *(RV)* pressure waveform appears similar to the right atrial waveform consistent with *atrialization* of the right ventricle.

References

1. Thom T, Haase N, Rosamond W, et al. Heart disease and stroke statistics—2006 update. A report from the American Heart Association Statistics Committee and Stroke Statistics Subcommittee. *Circulation* 2006;113:85–151.
2. Kellum JA, Pinsky MR. Use of vasopressor agents in critically ill patients. *Curr Opin Crit Care* 2002; 8:236–241.
3. Trost JC, Hillis LD. Intra-aortic balloon counterpulsation. *Am J Cardiol* 2006;97:1391–1398.
4. Santa-Cruz RA, Cohen MG, Ohman EM. Aortic counterpulsation: A review of the hemodynamics and indications for use. *Catheter Cardiovasc Interv* 2006;67:68–77.
5. Kern MJ, Aguirre FV, Tatineni S, et al. Enhanced coronary blood flow velocity during intra-aortic balloon counterpulsation in critically ill patients. *J Am Coll Cardiol* 1993;21:359–368.
6. Kern MJ, Aguirre F, Bach R, et al. Augmentation of coronary blood flow by intra-aortic balloon pumping in patients after coronary angioplasty. *Circulation* 1993;87:500–511.
7. Ryan EW, Foster E. Augmentation of coronary blood flow with intra-aortic balloon pump counter-pulsation. *Circulation* 2000;102:364–365.
8. Kimura A, Toyota E, Songfang L, et al. Effects of intra-aortic balloon pumping on septal arterial blood flow velocity waveform during severe left main coronary artery stenosis. *J Am Coll Cardiol* 1996;27:810–816.
9. Gold HK, Leinbach RC, Sanders CA, et al. Intra-aortic balloon pumping for ventricular septal defect or mitral regurgitation complicating acute myocardial infarction. *Circulation* 1973;47:1191–1196.
10. Thiele H, Lauer B, Hambrecht R, et al. Short- and long-term hemodynamic effects of intra-aortic balloon support in ventricular septal defect complicating acute myocardial infarction. *Am J Cardiol* 2003;92:450–454.
11. Fotopoulos GD, Mason MJ, Walker S, et al. Stabilisation of medically refractory ventricular arrhythmia by intra-aortic balloon counterpulsation. *Heart* 1999;82:96–100.
12. Sanborn TA, Sleeper LA, Bates ER, et al. for the SHOCK Investigators. Impact of thrombolysis, intra-aortic balloon pump counterpulsation, and their combination in cardiogenic shock complicating acute myocardial infarction: A report from the SHOCK Trial Registry. *J Am Coll Cardiol* 2000;36:1123–1129.
13. Anderson RD, Ohman EM, Holmes DR Jr, et al. Use of intra-aortic balloon counterpulsation in patients presenting with cardiogenic shock: Observations from the GUSTO-I Study. Global utilization of streptokinase and TPA for occluded coronary arteries. *J Am Coll Cardiol* 1997;30:708–715.
14. Follath F. Nonischemic heart failure: Epidemiology, pathophysiology, and progression of disease. *J Cardiovasc Pharmacol* 1999;33(Suppl 3):S31–S35.
15. Applegate RJ, Johnston WE, Vinten-Johansen J, et al. Restraining effect of intact pericardium during acute volume loading. *Am J Physiology* 1992;262: H1725–H1733.
16. Atherton JJ, Moore TD, Lele SS, et al. Diastolic ventricular interaction in chronic heart failure. *Lancet* 1997;349:1720–1724.
17. Yamamoto K, Nishimura RA, Redfield MM. Assessment of mean left atrial pressure from the left ventricular pressure tracing in patients with cardiomyopathies. *Am J Cardiol* 1996;78:107–110.
18. Lab MJ, Lee JA. Changes in intracellular calcium during mechanical alternans in isolated ferret ventricular muscle. *Circulation Res* 1990;66:585–595.
19. Moraes DL, Colucci WS, Givertz MM. Secondary pulmonary hypertension in chronic heart failure. The role of the endothelium in pathophysiology and management. *Circulation* 2000;102:1718–1723.

20. Ooi H, Colucci WS, Givertz MM. Endothelin mediates increased pulmonary vascular tone in patients with heart failure. Demonstration by direct intrapulmonary infusion of sitaxsentan. *Circulation* 2002;106:1618–1621.
21. Fojon S, Fernandez-Gonzalez C, Sanchez-Andrade J, et al. Inhaled nitric oxide through a non-invasive ventilation device to assess reversibility of pulmonary hypertension in heart transplant. *Transplant Proc* 2005;37:4028–4030.
22. Montalescot G, Drobinski G, Meurin P, et al. Effects of prostacyclin on the pulmonary vascular tone and cardiac contractility of patients with pulmonary hypertension secondary to end-stage heart failure. *Am J Cardiol* 1998;82:749–755.
23. Costard-Jackle A, Fowler MB. Influence of preoperative pulmonary artery pressure on mortality after heart transplantation: Testing of potential reversibility of pulmonary hypertension with nitroprusside is useful in defining a high risk group. *J Am Coll Cardiol* 1992;19:48–54.
24. Bhatia SJ, Kirshenbaum JM, Shemin RJ, et al. Time course of resolution of pulmonary hypertension and right ventricular remodeling after orthotopic cardiac transplantation. *Circulation* 1987;76:819–826.
25. Shroeder JS, Popp RL, Stinson EB, et al. Acute rejection following cardiac transplantation: Phonocardiographic and ultrasound observations. *Circulation* 1969;40:155–164.
26. Wilensky RL, Bourdillon PD, O'Donnell JA, et al. Restrictive hemodynamic patterns after cardiac transplantation: Relationship to histologic signs of rejection. *Am Heart J* 1991;122:1079–1087.
27. Valentine HA, Appleton CP, Hatle LK, et al. A hemodynamic and Doppler echocardiographic study of ventricular function in long-term cardiac allograft recipients. Etiology and prognosis of restrictive-constrictive physiology. *Circulation* 1989;79:66–75.
28. Skowronski EW, Epstein M, Ota D, et al. Right and left ventricular function after cardiac transplantation. Changes during and after rejection. *Circulation* 1991;84:2409–2417.
29. de Marchena E, Madrid W, Wozniak P, et al. Atrialization of right ventricular pressure during acute cardiac allograft rejection. *Cathet Cardiovasc Diagn* 1990;19:53–55.

Chapter 10

Complications of Acute Myocardial Infarction

Brandon Brown, MD

Despite improvements in recognition, prevention, and treatment, coronary heart disease and acute myocardial infarction (AMI) are responsible for roughly one in five deaths and remain significant public health problems in the United States. Many of these are sudden and due to ventricular arrhythmia. In addition to severe pump failure, the mechanical complications, including ventricular septal rupture, papillary muscle rupture, right ventricular infarction, and free wall rupture account for a significant proportion of post-MI deaths, even though the incidence of these complications has decreased in recent years.[1] This chapter will review the clinical features, pathophysiology, and hemodynamics of each of these complications.

Cardiogenic Shock Post-Myocardial Infarction

The inability of the heart to deliver adequate blood flow to tissues to meet metabolic demands defines cardiogenic shock. Clinically, cardiogenic shock is diagnosed by hypotension combined with evidence of poor perfusion (oliguria, cyanosis, cool extremities, and altered mentation). Cardiogenic shock complicates AMI in nearly 10% of cases.[2] Four clinical variables predict the development of cardiogenic shock after MI: patient age, systolic blood pressure, heart rate, and Killip class.[3] Historically, the mortality of shock that complicates MI has been as high as 80%–90%.[4] However, lower rates of mortality have been observed in more contemporary series, ranging from 56%–74%.[5,6] Angiographic and pathologic studies have demonstrated a higher incidence of left anterior descending artery occlusion, multivessel coronary artery disease, and persistent occlusion of the infarct-related artery among those with cardiogenic shock.

In the setting of AMI, cardiogenic shock is most often the consequence of an extensive infarction that causes pump failure. At least 40% of the left ventricular myocardial mass must be lost to cause pump failure.[7] Right ventricular infarction, mechanical complications, and arrhythmias (tachy or brady) account for many of the other causes of cardiogenic shock in AMI. A very unusual cause of cardiogenic shock in AMI is from obstruction of the left ventricular outflow tract due to systolic anterior motion of the mitral valve, induced from distortion of the ventricular chamber from infarction and the presence of hypercontractile, noninfarcted, adjacent segments (see Chapter 6).

Cardiogenic shock is often described as a "vicious cycle." Hypotension initially occurs from reduced stroke volume. In an attempt to maintain tissue perfusion, several compensatory mechanisms primarily involving the sympathetic nervous system are activated. The heart rate increases, inotropic stimulation increases, and the peripheral arterial beds vasoconstrict. Fluids shift into the intravascular space. The kidneys play an important role in compensation. Reduced renal perfusion pressure activates the renin-angiotensin system, and aldosterone secretion results in sodium and water absorption by the kidneys. Antidiuretic hormone is released as a result of hypotension and contributes to renal water resorption. Atrial stretch stimulates natriuretic peptide release, promoting renal excretion of sodium and water that counteracts the actions of angiotensin II. Blood is redistributed away from nonvital organs such as skin, intestines, and skeletal muscle. With continued tissue hypoperfusion, metabolic acidosis further depresses myocardial contractility and worsens stroke volume, contributing to the downward spiral. Eventually, compensatory mechanisms are overwhelmed, vasodilation ensues, and cardiovascular collapse results.

One challenge in the diagnosis of cardiogenic shock is its differentiation from other, noncardiogenic causes of shock. This can usually be accomplished by defining the hemodynamic derangements. Low systolic blood pressure (<90 mmHg) coupled with decreased cardiac index (<2.2 L/min/m^2), elevated pulmonary capillary wedge pressure, and elevated systemic vascular resistance (SVR) characterizes cardiogenic shock (see Chapter 9). Although the SVR is elevated in most cases due to excessive vasoconstriction, this paradigm has been challenged by data from patients with confirmed cardiogenic shock in the SHOCK trial in which the SVR varied widely and on average was not elevated despite the use of vasopressors.[8] This may be explained by the induction of systemic inflammation and a vasodilated state similar to sepsis. Similarly, although elevation of the pulmonary capillary wedge pressure helps distinguish cardiogenic from other forms of shock, exceptions exist. For example, myocardial depression may complicate septic shock and elevate the wedge pressure. In addition, elevation of the wedge pressure is often present in patients with infarction, with or without pulmonary congestion.[9] Although arterial hypotension is the hemodynamic hallmark of cardiogenic shock, blood pressure may be maintained despite poor tissue perfusion.[9] Examination of the aortic waveform may provide

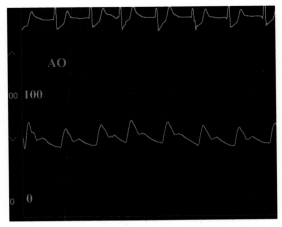

FIGURE 10-1. This aortic pressure tracing obtained in a patient with cardiogenic shock demonstrates a low systolic pressure and a reduced pulse pressure.

important clues. Often, a reduced pulse pressure is apparent due to a reduction in the strength of contraction and diminished stroke volume (Figure 10-1).

Intra-Aortic Balloon Pump Hemodynamics

Intra-aortic balloon pump (IABP) counterpulsation, first introduced in 1962, represents a vital tool in the management of cardiogenic shock that complicates AMI, particularly when used in conjunction with revascularization.[10–12] In addition to improving the hemodynamic status of patients with profound pump failure from extensive infarction, the IABP also stabilizes hemodynamics in patients with mechanical complications such as ventricular septal rupture and acute mitral regurgitation.[13,14] Its role in stabilizing patients with right ventricular infarction is less clear.

The IABP is inserted percutaneously over a guidewire through the femoral artery into the descending aorta distal to the left subclavian artery. The balloon is timed to inflate during diastole against a closed aortic valve, displacing 30–50 mL of blood volume (depending on balloon size), and increasing the aortic diastolic pressure *(diastolic augmentation)*. At the end of diastole, the balloon rapidly deflates, creating a potential space of 30–50 mL within the aorta. This reduces aortic impedance, resulting in a reduction of aortic end-diastolic pressure and afterload reduction. The hemodynamic effects of IABP counterpulsation have been described in detail in Chapter 9. A summary of the hemodynamic benefits of the IABP in cardiogenic shock is presented in Table 10-1. The safety of these devices has improved in recent years, and the incidence of vascular complications, once reported to be as high as 5%–20%, has declined with the introduction of smaller sheaths and sheathless insertion techniques.[15–17] Contraindications include severe aortic regurgitation, aortic dissection, abdominal aortic aneurysm, and severe peripheral arterial disease.

The timing and volume of balloon inflation affect the hemodynamic response. Inflation should occur early in diastole and timed with the dicrotic notch. Deflation occurs just prior to systole, resulting in a lower end-diastolic pressure for the augmented cycle compared to the unaugmented cycle (Figure 10-2). IABP triggering is typically based on the R-wave on the electrocardiogram but can be set according to AV pacing, internal timing, or the aortic pressure wave. Recognizing incorrect timing of inflation and deflation is crucial, because it may lead to a lack of hemodynamic benefit or even clinical deterioration (see Chapter 9).

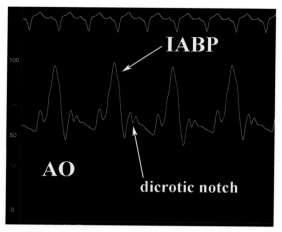

FIGURE 10-2. Example of proper timing of an intra-aortic balloon pump placed in a patient with cardiogenic shock. The pump is set to a 1:2 ratio, so it inflates once for every two cardiac cycles. Inflation occurs on the dicrotic notch, producing a large augmentation wave that provides perfusion pressure. Deflation should occur before the next systole, indicated by a lower end-diastolic pressure for the augmented beat compared to the unaugmented beat because of afterload reduction.

Right Ventricular Infarction

Infarction of the right ventricle may present with dramatic hemodynamic consequences and is one of the major causes of cardiogenic shock in patients with acute infarction. Initially described as a distinct clinical entity in 1974, it usually occurs in association with between one third and one half of all inferior wall MIs.[18,19] Occlusion of the right coronary artery proximal to the right ventricular marginal branches is the most common cause, but right ventricular infarction may also occur with occlusion of the left circumflex or even the left anterior descending in a minority of patients.[19,20] Rarely, it may occur in isolation (i.e., without associated left ventricular infarction) from occlusion of a nondominant right coronary artery or right ventricular marginal branch.

Interestingly, not all cases of proximal right coronary occlusion cause right ventricular infarction. This may be explained by several mechanisms. Oxygen demand

TABLE 10-1.	Effects of Intra-Aortic Balloon Pump in Cardiogenic Shock
HEMODYNAMIC VARIABLE	**EFFECT**
Diastolic pressure, aorta	+ + + +
Systolic pressure, aorta	− −
Mean pressure, aorta	+ +
Cardiac output	+ +
Heart rate	− or no change
Coronary blood flow	+ or no change

is much lower in the right ventricle given its smaller muscle mass. Accordingly, the susceptibility of the right ventricle to infarction and ischemia is increased in patients with right ventricular hypertrophy. Other protective mechanisms include collateral supply of the right ventricle and, possibly, perfusion of the right ventricular myocardium directly from the blood in the ventricular cavity via the thebesian veins. Also, each of these factors is felt to explain the high likelihood of recovery of right ventricular function following infarction. Early recognition of right ventricular infarction remains important because, although the long-term prognosis of right ventricular infarction is good, the in-hospital morbidity and mortality is high.[21,22]

The clinical consequences of right ventricular infarction vary from no apparent hemodynamics abnormality to profound shock and cardiovascular collapse. This wide spectrum of clinical presentations is because the pathophysiology of right ventricular infarction depends on many complex factors (Table 10-2). Each factor plays varying roles in any given patient, explaining the variety of hemodynamic findings observed in this condition.

The pathophysiology of right ventricular infarction is complex. Acute ischemia of the right ventricle results in profound *systolic dysfunction,* which decreases right ventricular stroke volume and peak systolic pressure and thus left ventricular preload. Cardiac output falls. The right ventricle acutely dilates. Acute ischemia also results in *diastolic dysfunction.* This elevates right-sided filling pressures during diastole and increases resistance to early filling. The pericardial space becomes filled with the acutely dilated right ventricle, which increases intrapericardial pressure, further impairing right ventricular and left ventricular filling. Furthermore, the effect of *pericardial constraint* also facilitates *systolic ventricular*

TABLE 10-2.	Important Variables That Impact the Pathophysiology of Right Ventricular Infarction

Right Ventricular Systolic Dysfunction
Decreased left-sided preload
Right ventricular dilatation

Right Ventricular Diastolic Dysfunction
Diminished compliance of right ventricle
Elevated filling pressures

Pericardial Constraint
Increases right-sided filling pressures
Enhances systolic ventricular interactions via the
  septum

Systolic Ventricular Interactions via the Septum
Impaired left ventricular function
Dependence on left ventricular function to enhance
  pulmonary blood flow

Right Atrial Function
Maintains preload
Loss of atrial function more important than other
  infarctions

interactions mediated by the septum by shifting the interventricular septum toward the preload-deprived left ventricle, further decreasing left ventricular filling and cardiac output. Left ventricular contraction may cause septal bulging to the right, which may be sufficient to generate systolic force and augment pulmonary blood flow. Thus, if an associated large left ventricular infarction is present, this force may be lost and cause further worsening of hemodynamics. Finally, the *right atrium* plays an extremely important role in maintaining adequate right ventricular preload. If an extensive associated right atrial infarction is present, or if loss of AV synchrony from heart block or atrial fibrillation occurs, significant hemodynamic deterioration may ensue.

The net effect of right ventricular infarction is that left-sided filling pressure may be low, despite elevated right-sided pressure, which is clinically apparent by the triad of hypotension, clear lung fields, and elevated jugular venous pressure. The physical exam may also reveal Kussmaul's sign (paradoxical distension of the neck veins with inspiration), a feature that is both sensitive and specific for right ventricular infarction.[23] The physical findings may be confused with pericardial disease because right ventricular infarction mimics both tamponade and constrictive pericarditis.

Possible hemodynamic findings of right ventricular infarction include elevated right atrial pressure typically exceeding the pulmonary capillary wedge pressure. The right atrial pressure often exceeds 10 mmHg, and the ratio of right atrial pressure to pulmonary capillary wedge pressure is >0.8.[18] These hemodynamic findings may be masked by intravascular volume depletion and only emerge with volume loading.[24] The condition in which right atrial pressure exceeds left atrial pressure may cause right-to-left shunting in the presence of a patent foramen ovale. This unusual scenario should be suspected in the event of unexplained hypoxia not corrected with oxygen administration in the setting of right ventricular infarction.

Elevated right atrial pressure is primarily from right ventricular diastolic dysfunction, but pericardial constraint and right ventricular failure also contribute. Impaired filling of the right ventricle is evidenced by a blunted *y* descent on the right atrial waveform (Figure 10-3). The *a* wave on the right atrial tracing reflects the strength of contraction of the right atrium. In right ventricular infarction, right atrial contraction is enhanced by the increased preload, resulting in augmentation in the height of the *a* wave. The *x* descent may be steep because of enhanced atrial relaxation. This may be seen as a W pattern on the right atrial waveform (Figure 10-4). These features benefit right ventricular filling. However, if infarction involves the right atrium, then the *a* wave and *x* descents are

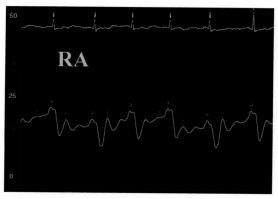

FIGURE 10-3. Right atrial waveform from a patient with right ventricular infarction, demonstrating a large *a* wave with prominent *x* descent and a blunted *y* descent.

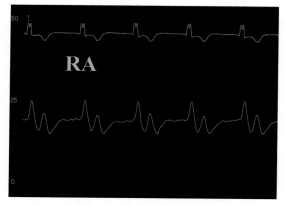

FIGURE 10-4. Example of the W pattern seen on a right atrial waveform in a patient with right ventricular infarction. Note the prominent *a* wave.

depressed. This produces a characteristic M pattern. Thus, two hemodynamic subtypes exist based on the status of the right atrium, with both having a relatively blunted *y* descent. The first, or W pattern, is usually associated with right coronary artery occlusion proximal to the right ventricular branches but distal to the right atrial branches and is associated with better hemodynamics than the second, or M pattern, associated with occlusion of the right coronary artery proximal to the right atrial branches and worse hemodynamics. Although the hemodynamics are better in those with a W pattern than those with an M pattern, those with a W pattern can decompensate quickly when they lose A-V synchrony.

Right ventricular systolic dysfunction results in a right ventricular pressure tracing characterized by a broad upstroke that reflects a depressed upstroke, reduced peak pressure, and delayed relaxation. The diastolic portion of the right ventricular pressure curve has been described as a *dip and plateau* that reflects decreased compliance as well as the constraining forces of the pericardium (Figure 10-5). This constraint imparted by the pericardium may also produce equalization of left and right ventricular diastolic pressures similar to constrictive pericarditis (Figure 10-6).

The treatment of right ventricular infarction includes prompt reperfusion, maintenance of right ventricular preload, reduction of right ventricular afterload, and inotropic support of the failing ventricle. The benefit of reperfusion in the setting of right ventricular infarction has not been well defined, but several studies have shown lower rates of right ventricular infarction and more rapid recovery in right ventricular function in patients who undergo successful reperfusion of the infarct-related artery.[21,25] Because of preload dependence, volume infusion improves hypotension and low cardiac output associated with right ventricular infarction, often requiring several liters of normal saline. Once a patient is euvolemic, however, there is little additional benefit of volume infusion in improving cardiac output, and more aggressive infusion of volume may lead to pulmonary edema, particularly if there is a large, associated left ventricular infarction that impairs left ventricular function. Recognition of preload dependence is

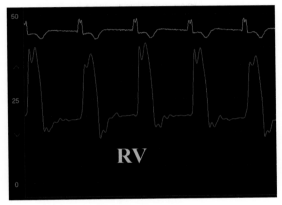

FIGURE 10-5. Right ventricular waveform in a patient with right ventricular infarction, demonstrating the *square root* sign or *dip and plateau* during diastole.

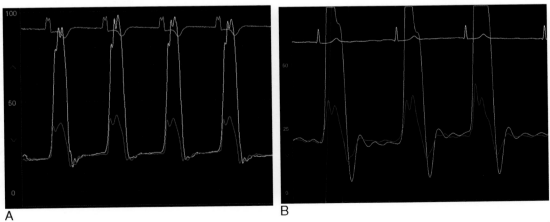

A   B

FIGURE 10-6. **A–B,** Examples of equalization of the right ventricular and left ventricular diastolic pressures or *pseudo-constriction* pattern. **B,** Note how the early left ventricular diastolic pressure is lower than right ventricular diastolic pressure due to impaired left ventricular filling and reduced preload.

important because many of the drugs typically used to treat patients with AMI such as nitrates or diuretics may produce deleterious hemodynamic effects if right ventricular infarction is also present. If volume replacement fails to improve cardiac output and blood pressure, then inotropic support with dobutamine should be instituted. Dobutamine may also improve forward flow by reducing pulmonary vascular resistance and therefore right ventricular afterload. Right ventricular afterload may also be increased when left ventricular dysfunction accompanies right ventricular infarction by increasing pulmonary venous pressures. In this setting, afterload-reducing drugs such as nitroprusside may be beneficial. An IABP may be beneficial. Maintenance of atrioventricular synchrony is extremely important because the loss of atrial contraction may have dramatic hemodynamic consequences in right ventricular infarction. Cardioversion of atrial fibrillation should be performed promptly at the first sign of hemodynamic deterioration and AV pacing considered if heart block develops.

Ventricular Septal Rupture Post-Myocardial Infarction

Rupture of the interventricular septum is a relatively rare mechanical complication that occurs 3 to 5 days following infarction but may appear within the first 24 hours or on presentation, particularly in patients treated with thrombolytic therapy.[26] The incidence has been reduced from 2.0% to 0.2% in the reperfusion era.[26] Risk factors for rupture in the modern era include advanced age and female gender.[27] Pre-infarct angina and the development of coronary collaterals in the infarct-related artery are associated with reduced risk of rupture.[28] Ventricular septal rupture is seen more frequently in anterior infarctions where the defect is located in the apical septum; with inferior infarcts, the defect is located in the basal inferoposterior septum. Rupture occurs at the margin of necrotic and healthy myocardium and may be a discrete defect that ranges from a few millimeters to several centimeters wide or the rupture may be an irregular and serpiginous connection. Associated right ventricular infarction is common, and when right ventricular dysfunction is present, prognosis is significantly worsened.[29,30]

Patients with a ruptured ventricular septum present with abrupt onset of hemodynamic collapse characterized by hypotension, shock, dyspnea, chest pain, and a harsh, holosystolic murmur. A thrill may be detected in up to 50% of patients. Unlike acute mitral regurgitation from papillary muscle rupture, pulmonary congestion is distinctly unusual in ventricular septal rupture, leading to the adage, "A new murmur with the patient lying flat is ventricular septal rupture and a new murmur with the patient sitting bolt upright short of breath is acute mitral regurgitation."

The major hemodynamic findings relate to the left-to-right shunt created from the ruptured septum. A significant left-to-right shunt causes an acute increase in pulmonary blood flow and overload of the left heart. An oxygen step-up at the ventricular level is detectable by the use of a pulmonary artery catheter, and the shunt size can be calculated by oximetry (see Chapter 3) (Figure 10-7). Multiple factors determine the degree of shunting, including the size of the defect, pulmonary and systemic vascular resistances, and left and right ventricular systolic function. As left ventricular systolic function deteriorates and cardiac output diminishes, compensatory vasoconstriction leads to increased systemic vascular resistance, increasing the left-to-right shunt.

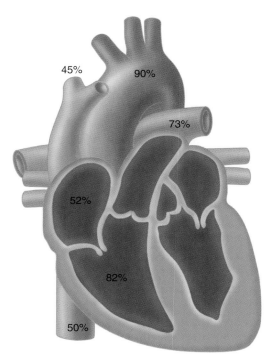

FIGURE 10-7. These oximetry data were obtained in a patient with an inferior wall MI and a post-MI ventricular septal rupture. The low oxygen saturations in the inferior and superior vena cava are consistent with low cardiac output. A large step-up is apparent from the right atrium to the right ventricle. A shunt calculation determined the Qp/Qs = 1.5 to 1.0.

In addition to the usual hemodynamic findings associated with shock and the oxygen step-up at the right ventricular level, ventricular septal rupture causes moderate elevations in the pulmonary artery pressure and may cause elevations in right atrial and right ventricular diastolic pressures, particularly if an associated right ventricular infarction is present. The right atrial pressure may be markedly elevated and equal to that of the pulmonary capillary wedge pressure in patients with large shunts.[31] Because pulmonary blood flow increases, left atrial filling is increased, and a large *v* wave may be inscribed on the pulmonary capillary wedge pressure tracing (Figure 10-8).[32] Therefore, this finding, typically associated with severe mitral regurgitation, is not reliable to differentiate ventricular septal defect from acute, severe mitral regurgitation in a patient with a new systolic murmur and cardiogenic shock following MI.

Ventricular septal rupture is a medical emergency. Initial treatment includes

FIGURE 10-8. Prominent *v* wave on the pulmonary capillary wedge pressure tracing in a patient with a post-MI ventricular septal defect.

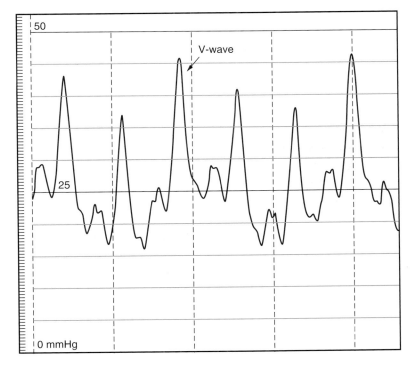

support with intra-aortic balloon counter-pulsation, intravenous inotropic agents, and afterload reduction with sodium nitroprusside to reduce left-to-right-shunt. Early surgical repair is recommended for patients who are surgical candidates.[33] Mortality remains high, especially in patients with cardiogenic shock, but is lower than in patients treated medically.[26] Percutaneous closure of the septal rupture has been reported successfully as an alternative to surgical repair, although the role of this new technology in this disease entity remains undefined.[34]

Papillary Muscle Rupture Post-Myocardial Infarction

Acute mitral regurgitation due to rupture of a papillary muscle is a life-threatening complication of MI that occurs between 2 and 7 days after infarction. The papillary muscles are mostly subendocardial and are thus susceptible to ischemia as a result of the increasing pressure gradient from epicardium to endocardium, lowering subendocardial perfusion. The anterolateral head receives dual blood supply from both the left anterior descending and left circumflex arteries, making it less vulnerable to ischemia and subsequent rupture than the posteromedial papillary muscle that receives its blood from a sole source: the right coronary artery (Figure 10-9). Thus, papillary muscle rupture is more commonly a complication of inferior infarction and right coronary occlusion. Often, the infarct is small, and autopsy studies demonstrate that papillary muscle rupture occurs most often in the setting of first MI, suggesting that a relative lack of collateral circulation may play a role in the pathogenesis.[35]

Papillary muscle rupture causes severe, acute mitral regurgitation. The left atrium is normally noncompliant (unless preexisting mitral regurgitation is present), and the sudden increase in left atrial volume rapidly raises left atrial pressure. This increased pressure transmits to the pulmonary venous circulation, causing acute pulmonary edema. Because the left atrium is a low-pressure chamber, most blood ejected from the left ventricle is directed toward the left atrium, and forward stroke volume is markedly diminished. Despite a compensatory tachycardia, cardiac output plummets precipitating hypotension and shock. The increase in systemic vascular resistance due to the neurohormonal compensatory response to shock only serves to worsen the amount of regurgitation.

Papillary muscle rupture presents with the sudden onset of shortness of breath

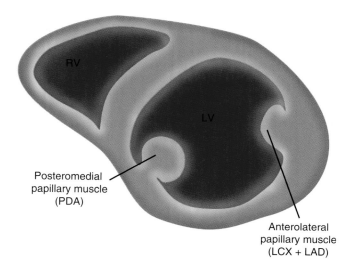

FIGURE 10-9. Papillary muscles and their blood supply. The posterior descending coronary artery *(PDA)*, typically originating from the right coronary artery, supplies the posteromedial papillary muscle, and both the left circumflex *(LCX)* and left anterior descending *(LAD)* coronary arteries supply the anterolateral papillary muscle.

Posteromedial
papillary muscle
(PDA)

Anterolateral
papillary muscle
(LCX + LAD)

RV

LV

due to acute pulmonary edema, hypotension, and a new systolic murmur. The murmur of acute mitral regurgitation is best heard at the left sternal border and may radiate to the back. The murmur is typically soft, low-pitched, and decrescendo as the pressure in the left atrium rises to that of the left ventricle in end-systole, diminishing the pressure gradient between the two chambers. The murmur may be completely inaudible due to the presence of very high left atrial pressures and low ventricular systolic pressures from shock (Figure 10-10). A suspected diagnosis of papillary muscle rupture is easily confirmed by echocardiography; transesophageal echocardiography may be needed in the rare instances in which acoustic windows are poor or the ruptured head of the papillary muscle does not prolapse into the left atrium.

The hemodynamic findings are similar to acute mitral regurgitation seen in association with other conditions (see Chapter 4). Hypotension with diminished pulse pressure, low cardiac output, and marked abnormalities of right heart pressures are usually present. A giant *v* wave may be present on the pulmonary capillary wedge pressure, although this depends on the compliance properties of the atrium (Figures 10-11 and 10-12). In addition, a large *v* wave is not specific for mitral regurgitation and may be due to other conditions in the setting of an acute infarction such as ventricular septal defect or severe left-sided heart failure.

Acute mitral regurgitation from papillary muscle rupture is a medical emergency; surgery is the definitive treatment. Medical therapy plays an important supportive role to stabilize the patient prior to surgery. An intra-aortic balloon pump often coupled with inotropic support and vasodilators, such as nitroprusside, improve hemodynamics that allows emergency surgery. Although operative mortality is as high as 20%–25%, outcomes with medical therapy are dismal.[36] Risk factors for a poor outcome with surgery include advanced age, female gender, and poor left ventricular systolic function.[37] Mitral valve repair is favored, and concomitant coronary artery bypass grafting should be performed as indicated at the time of valve surgery because this may improve outcomes.[38,39]

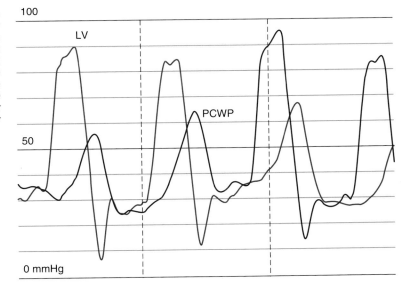

FIGURE 10-10. Example of a large *v* wave on the pulmonary capillary wedge pressure tracing and low left ventricular systolic pressure in a patient with acute, severe mitral regurgitation from papillary muscle rupture. Note the small difference between the peak of the *v* wave and the peak systolic pressure. For this reason, a systolic murmur may be absent.

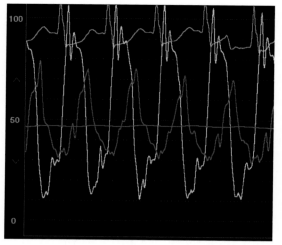

FIGURE 10-11. Example of a large *v* wave on the pulmonary capillary wedge pressure tracing in a patient with severe mitral regurgitation from papillary muscle rupture.

Left Ventricular Free Wall Rupture Post-Myocardial Infarction

Free wall rupture is a dramatic and often fatal mechanical complication post-MI. A review of 350,755 patients included in the National Registry of Myocardial Infarction revealed an incidence of less than 1%.[40] However, rupture of the left ventricular free wall is a relatively common cause of death in patients with AMI, accounting for 8%–26% of deaths post MI.[41,42] Traditionally, rupture occurs within 5 days of infarction. Patients are typically elderly, female, present late, and likely have little to no collateral flow, as evidenced by the observation

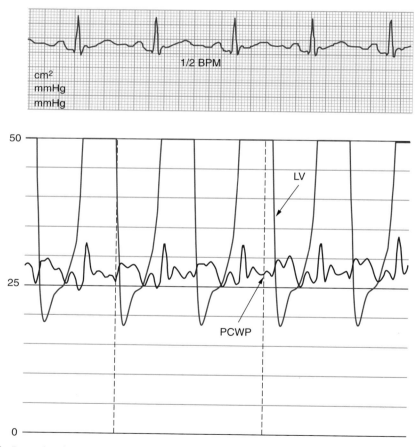

FIGURE 10-12. Example of a normal *v* wave on the pulmonary capillary wedge pressure tracing in a patient with severe mitral regurgitation from papillary muscle rupture. The compliance of the left atrium determines the presence of a *v* wave.

that the infarction is often the patient's first event, is completely transmural, and is usually without an antecedent history of angina pectoris. Left ventricular free wall rupture is less common in patients with a patent infarct-related artery.[43] Thrombolytic therapy is associated with a lower incidence of rupture, except in patients greater than age 75 who may have a greater likelihood of rupture following thrombolytic therapy.[44,45] Despite initial concerns that suggest an increased risk of rupture, late administration of thrombolytics does not appear to increase the risk of rupture, but it does accelerate its time of onset.[40] The incidence may be lower in patients treated with percutaneous coronary intervention as opposed to thrombolytic therapy.[46]

The pathology of free wall rupture differs depending on its time of occurrence.[47] Rupture that occurs within 72 hours of coronary occlusion is characterized by a slit-like tear in the infarcted region of myocardium, whereas cases that present later (>4 days) are characterized by rupture within an infarct expansion. Rupture tends to preferentially affect the left ventricle and occurs at the junction of infarcted and normal myocardium.

According to the type of presentation, rupture may be classified as acute or subacute. Acute rupture is often associated with sudden death. In some patients, rupture presents as an abrupt collapse from electromechanical dissociation, resulting from pericardial tamponade. Thus, the hemodynamic findings are those characteristic of tamponade (Chapter 8). Often present is an unheralded vagal event, perhaps associated with chest pain, followed by cardiovascular collapse. The presence of pulseless electrical activity in a patient with a first MI has a high predictive accuracy for free wall rupture.[48] Echocardiography may confirm the diagnosis by demonstrating

a pericardial effusion or echogenic material in the pericardial space. Rarely, the actual tear may be visualized. Pericardiocentesis yields blood and may temporarily improve the patient's hemodynamics to allow a heroic surgeon to definitely repair the rent in the myocardium, thus saving the patient's life. This rarely occurs, however.

Subacute rupture accounts for one-third of all cases of in-hospital free wall rupture and occurs when organized thrombus and the pericardium are able to seal the perforation. This results in a pseudoaneurysm and is often clinically silent and may be revealed only by a routine post-infarction echocardiogram or left ventriculogram. In fact, any significant effusion seen by echocardiography post-MI should alert the physician to the presence of a subacute rupture as pericardial effusion. A patient with subacute rupture or ventricular pseudo-aneurysm may unpredictably progress to complete rupture and tamponade. Surgery is usually indicated once these are identified. Surgery is most often performed with a pericardial patch placement, using epicardial sutures of biological glue. Other surgical techniques include infarctectomy with patch placement and ventricular wall reconstruction. With prompt recognition and surgical intervention, a survival rate of 76% may be attained with a long-term survival of 48% in one series of patients with subacute left ventricular free wall rupture.[49]

References

1. Nakatani D, Sato H, Kinjo K, et al. Effect of successful late reperfusion by primary coronary angioplasty on mechanical complications of acute myocardial infarction. *Am J Cardiol* 2003;92(7): 785–788.
2. Babaev A, Frederick PD, Pasta DJ, et al. Trends in management and outcomes of patients with acute myocardial infarction complicated by cardiogenic shock. *JAMA* 2005;294(4):448–454.

3. Hasdai D, Califf RM, Thompson TD, et al. Predictors of cardiogenic shock after thrombolytic therapy for acute myocardial infarction. *J Am Coll Cardiol* 2000;35(1):136–143.

4. Goldberg RJ, Gore JM, Alpert JS, et al. Cardiogenic shock after acute myocardial infarction. Incidence and mortality from a community-wide perspective, 1975 to 1988. *N Engl J Med* 1991;325(16): 1117–1122.

5. Goldberg RJ, Gore JM, Thompson CA, et al. Recent magnitude of and temporal trends (1994–1997) in the incidence and hospital death rates of cardiogenic shock complicating acute myocardial infarction: The second national registry of myocardial infarction. *Am Heart J* 2001;141(1):65–72.

6. Holmes DR Jr, Bates ER, Kleiman NS, et al. Contemporary reperfusion therapy for cardiogenic shock: the GUSTO-I trial experience. The GUSTO-I Investigators. Global Utilization of Streptokinase and Tissue Plasminogen Activator for Occluded Coronary Arteries. *J Am Coll Cardiol* 1995;26(3): 668–674.

7. Alonso DR, Scheidt S, Post M, et al. Pathophysiology of cardiogenic shock. Quantification of myocardial necrosis, clinical, pathologic and electrocardiographic correlations. *Circulation* 1973;48(3): 588–596.

8. Hochman JS. Cardiogenic shock complicating acute myocardial infarction: Expanding the paradigm. *Circulation* 2003;107(24):2998–3002.

9. Menon V, Slater JN, White HD, et al. Acute myocardial infarction complicated by systemic hypoperfusion without hypotension: Report of the SHOCK trial registry. *Am J Med* 2000;108(5):374–380.

10. Mouloupoulos SD, Topaz S, Kolff WJ. Diastolic balloon pumping (with carbon dioxide) in the aorta—a mechanical assistance to the failing circulation. *Am Heart J* 1962;63:669–675.

11. Hochman JS, Sleeper LA, Webb JG, et al. Early revascularization in acute myocardial infarction complicated by cardiogenic shock. SHOCK Investigators. Should we emergently revascularize occluded coronaries for cardiogenic shock? *N Engl J Med* 1999;341(9):625–634.

12. Sanborn TA, Sleeper LA, Bates ER, et al. Impact of thrombolysis, intra-aortic balloon pump counterpulsation, and their combination in cardiogenic shock complicating acute myocardial infarction: A report from the SHOCK Trial Registry. Should we emergently revascularize occluded coronaries for cardiogenic shock? *J Am Coll Cardiol* 2000;36 (3 Suppl A):1123–1129.

13. Gold HK, Leinbach RC, Sanders CA, et al. Intraaortic balloon pumping for ventricular septal defect or mitral regurgitation complicating acute myocardial infarction. *Circulation* 1973;47(6): 1191–1196.

14. Thiele H, Lauer B, Hambrecht R, et al. Short- and long-term hemodynamic effects of intra-aortic balloon support in ventricular septal defect complicating acute myocardial infarction. *Am J Cardiol* 2003;92(4):450–454.

15. Goldberger M, Tabak SW, Shah PK. Clinical experience with intra-aortic balloon counterpulsation in 112 consecutive patients. *Am Heart J* 1986;111(3): 497–502.

16. Nash IS, Lorell BH, Fishman RF, et al. A new technique for sheathless percutaneous intraaortic balloon catheter insertion. *Cathet Cardiovasc Diagn* 1991;23(1):57–60.

17. Tatar H, Cicek S, Demirkilic U, et al. Vascular complications of intra-aortic balloon pumping: Unsheathed versus sheathed insertion. *Ann Thorac Surg* 1993;55(6):1518–1521.

18. Cohn JN, Guiha NH, Broder MI, et al. Right ventricular infarction. Clinical and hemodynamic features. *Am J Cardiol* 1974;33(2):209–214.

19. Andersen HR, Falk E, Nielsen D. Right ventricular infarction: Frequency, size and topography in coronary heart disease: A prospective study comprising 107 consecutive autopsies from a coronary care unit. *J Am Coll Cardiol* 1987;10(6):1223–1232.

20. Cabin HS, Clubb KS, Wackers FJ, et al. Right ventricular myocardial infarction with anterior wall left ventricular infarction: An autopsy study. *Am Heart J* 1987;113(1):16–23.

21. Berger PB, Ruocco NA, Ryan TJ, et al. Frequency and significance of right ventricular dysfunction during inferior wall left ventricular myocardial infarction treated with thrombolytic therapy (results from the thrombolysis in myocardial infarction [TIMI] II trial). The TIMI Research Group. *Am J Cardiol* 1993;71(13):1148–1152.

22. Zehender M, Kasper W, Kauder E, et al. Right ventricular infarction as an independent predictor of prognosis after acute inferior myocardial infarction. *N Engl J Med* 1993;328(14):981–988.

23. Cintron GB, Hernandez E, Linares E, et al. Bedside recognition, incidence and clinical course of right ventricular infarction. *Am J Cardiol* 1981;47(2): 224–227.

24. Dell'Italia LJ, Starling MR, Crawford MH, et al. Right ventricular infarction: Identification by hemodynamic measurements before and after volume loading and correlation with noninvasive techniques. *J Am Coll Cardiol* 1984;4(5): 931–939.

25. Bowers TR, O'Neil WW, Grines C, et al. Effect of reperfusion on biventricular function and survival after right ventricular infarction. *N Engl J Med* 1998;338(14):933–940.

26. Crenshaw BS, Granger CB, Birnbaum Y, et al. Risk factors, angiographic patterns, and outcomes in patients with ventricular septal defect complicating acute myocardial infarction. GUSTO-I (Global Utilization of Streptokinase and TPA for Occluded Coronary Arteries) Trial Investigators. *Circulation* 2000;101(1):27–32.

27. Skehan JD, Carey C, Norrell MS, et al. Patterns of coronary artery disease in post-infarction ventricular septal rupture. *Br Heart J* 1989;62(4):268–272.

28. Pretre R, Rickli H, Ye Q, et al. Frequency of collateral blood flow in the infarct-related coronary artery in rupture of the ventricular septum after acute myocardial infarction. *Am J Cardiol* 2000;85(4): 497–499A10.

29. Cummings RG, Reimer KA, Califf R, et al. Quantitative analysis of right and left ventricular infarction in the presence of postinfarction ventricular septal defect. *Circulation* 1988;77(1): 33–42.

30. Moore CA, Nygaard TW, Kaiser DL, et al. Postinfarction ventricular septal rupture: The importance of location of infarction and right ventricular function in determining survival. *Circulation* 1986;74(1):45–55.

31. Drobac M, Schwartz L, Scully HE, et al. Giant left atrial V-waves in post-myocardial infarction ventricular septal defect. *Ann Thorac Surg* 1979;27(4): 347–349.

32. Heikkila J, Karesoja M, Luomanmaki K. Ruptured interventricular septum complicating acute myocardial infarction. Clinical spectrum and hemodynamic evaluation with rapid bedside cardiac catheterization. *Chest* 1974;66(6):675–681.

33. Antman EM, Anbe DT, Armstrong PW, et al. ACC/AHA guidelines for the management of patients with ST-elevation myocardial infarction: A report of the American College of Cardiology/American Heart Association Task Force on Practice Guidelines (Committee to Revise the 1999 Guidelines for the Management of patients with acute myocardial infarction). *J Am Coll Cardiol* 2004;44(3):E1–E211.

34. Szkutnik M, Bialkowski J, Kulsa J, et al. Postinfarction ventricular septal defect closure with Amplatzer occluders. *Eur J Cardiothorac Surg* 2003; 23(3):323–327.

35. Barbour DJ, Roberts WC. Rupture of a left ventricular papillary muscle during acute myocardial infarction: Analysis of 22 necropsy patients. *J Am Coll Cardiol* 1986;8(3):558–565.

36. Kishon Y, Oh JK, Schaff HV, et al. Mitral valve operation in postinfarction rupture of a papillary muscle: Immediate results and long-term follow-up of 22 patients. *Mayo Clin Proc* 1992;67(11):1023–1030.

37. DiSesa VJ, Cohn LH, Collins JJ, et al. Determinants of operative survival following combined mitral valve replacement and coronary revascularization. *Ann Thorac Surg* 1982;34(5):482–489.

38. David TE. Techniques and results of mitral valve repair for ischemic mitral regurgitation. *J Cardiol Surg* 1994;9(2 Suppl):274–277.

39. Chevalier P, Burri H, Fahrat F, et al. Perioperative outcome and long-term survival of surgery for acute post-infarction mitral regurgitation. *Eur J Cardiothorac Surg* 2004;26(2):330–335.

40. Becker RC, Gore JM, Lambrew C, et al. A composite view of cardiac rupture in the United States National Registry of Myocardial Infarction. *J Am Coll Cardiol* 1996;27(6):1321–1326.

41. Reddy SG, Roberts WC. Frequency of rupture of the left ventricular free wall or ventricular septum among necropsy cases of fatal acute myocardial infarction since introduction of coronary care units. *Am J Cardiol* 1989;63(13):906–911.

42. Stevenson WG, Linssen WG, Havenith MG, et al. The spectrum of death after myocardial infarction: A necropsy study. *Am Heart J* 1989;118(6): 1182–1188.

43. Cheriex EC, de Swart H, Dijkman LW, et al. Myocardial rupture after myocardial infarction is related to the perfusion status of the infarct-related coronary artery. *Am Heart J* 1995;129(4):644–650.

44. Gertz SD, Kragel AH, Kalan JM, et al. Comparison of coronary and myocardial morphologic findings in patients with and without thrombolytic therapy during fatal first acute myocardial infarction. The TIMI Investigators. *Am J Cardiol* 1990;66(12): 904–909.

45. Keeley EC, de Lemos JA. Free wall rupture in the elderly: Deleterious effect of fibrinolytic therapy on the ageing heart. *Eur Heart J* 2005;26(17): 1693–1694.

46. Moreno R, Lopez-Sendon J, Garcia E, et al. Primary angioplasty reduces the risk of left ventricular free wall rupture compared with thrombolysis in patients with acute myocardial infarction. *J Am Coll Cardiol* 2002;39(4):598–603.

47. Nakatsuchi Y, Minamino T, Fuji K, et al. Clinicopathological characterization of cardiac free wall rupture in patients with acute myocardial infarction: Difference between early and late phase rupture. *Int J Cardiol* 1994;47(1 Suppl):S33–S38.

48. Figueras J, Curos A, Cortadellas J, et al. Reliability of electromechanical dissociation in the diagnosis of left ventricular free wall rupture in acute myocardial infarction. *Am Heart J* 1996;131(5):861–864.

49. Lopez-Sendon J, Gonzalez A, Lopez de Sa E, et al. Diagnosis of subacute ventricular wall rupture after acute myocardial infarction: Sensitivity and specificity of clinical, hemodynamic and echocardiographic criteria. *J Am Coll Cardiol* 1992;19(6): 1145–1153.

CHAPTER 11

Congenital Heart Disease

RAJAN A.G. PATEL, MD, and
D. SCOTT LIM, MD

As many as 85% of infants born with congenital heart disease can be expected to survive into adulthood.[1] In the United States, the total number of adults with congenital heart disease is increasing at a rate of about 5% per year. Now more adults have congenital heart disease than children. This number includes both unrepaired and surgically corrected patients.[2] The population of patients with congenital heart disease who reach adult life grows each year due to advances in interventional and noninvasive cardiology, cardiothoracic surgery, and intensive care. As such, a growing number of adult patients with congenital heart disease is likely to present to the general cardiologist as opposed to the uncommon subspecialty adult congenital heart disease clinics. The American College of Cardiology Task Force 1 on congenital heart disease estimated that at least 10% of patients with congenital heart disease are diagnosed as adults. Furthermore, the consensus opinion of this committee was that the number of adults with undiagnosed congenital heart disease is increasing due to the growing immigrant population.[1] A sound understanding of the hemodynamics associated with the common congenital heart disease lesions provides valuable insight into the pathophysiology of these conditions.

Our understanding of the physiology of congenital heart disease in humans was largely theoretical until the 1940s when Dexter et al.[3] published the first manuscript that described the use of right-heart catheterization to assess hemodynamics and oxygenation saturations in patients with congenital heart disease. Since then, the complete assessment of congenital heart disease has evolved to include echocardiography and magnetic resonance imaging, making reliance on diagnostic catheterization a less frequent occurrence.

This chapter will focus on lesions more commonly seen in an adult cardiologist's practice, including atrial septal defect, ventricular septal defect, coarctation of the aorta, and Ebstein's anomaly of the tricuspid valve. It will also focus on the postoperative, surgically palliated patient with tetralogy of Fallot, the patient with peripheral pulmonary artery stenosis, and the patient with Eisenmenger's syndrome.

Atrial Septal Defect

Pathophysiology

Embryologically, the atrial septum is comprised of the septum primum and secundum. The septum secundum develops to the right of the septum primum and contains the foramen ovale. The endocardial cushions fuse to form the inferior aspect of the atrial septum and the superior aspect of the ventricular septum in addition to the mitral and tricuspid valves. During normal fetal development, the septum primum functions as a valve that maintains right-to-left flow through the foramen ovale. After birth the septum primum typically prevents left-to-right blood flow between the atria, despite the foramen ovale remaining patent in the majority of newborn infants. The overall incidence of a patent foramen ovale has been estimated to be as high as 27% but has been reported to decline with increasing age.[4]

A patent foramen ovale rarely results in significant clinical sequelae and is not associated with hemodynamic abnormalities. The notable (and often debated) clinical exception is the case of a paradoxical embolus, presumed to occur via a patent foramen ovale. However, four types of interatrial communications have important clinical sequelas: (1) primum atrial septal defect, (2) secundum atrial septal defect, (3) sinus venosus defect, and (4) coronary sinus septal defect.[2] The majority of cases occur spontaneously; however, reports of inherited cases exist.[5]

The primum atrial septal defect is the third most common type of interatrial communication after patent foramen ovale and secundum atrial septal defect. It comprises up to 15% of atrial septal defects.[2] The defect is due to maldevelopment of the endocardial cushions and is associated with a cleft in the anterior mitral leaflet and mitral regurgitation.

After patent foramen ovale, the secundum atrial septal defect is the most common type of interatrial communication. It comprises up to 75% of atrial septal defects.[2] The interatrial communication may be due to a single hole or multiple fenestrations in the septum primum. In rare cases, the secundum atrial septal defect may result from an incomplete septum secundum. Leachman et al.[6] have reported an association of mitral valve prolapse with secundum atrial septal defect; in a study of 92 patients with secundum atrial septal defect, 16 had mitral valve prolapse, and 3 of those with mitral valve prolapse developed chordal rupture. The pathophysiologic manifestation of a secundum atrial septal defect is a left-to-right shunt across the atrial septum, with resultant volume overload of the right heart. Campbell's[7] natural history studies have shown that, with time, right-sided heart failure and pulmonary hypertension develop and lead to early mortality.

A sinus venosus defect occurs when the tissue between either vena cava, the right atrium, and the pulmonary veins fails to develop properly. It comprises up to 10% of atrial septal defects.[2] The most frequently encountered sinus venosus defect involves a communication between the superior vena cava/right atrial junction and the right upper pulmonary vein.[8,9] Less frequently, these defects involve other right-sided pulmonary veins and the inferior vena cava/right atrial junction. Patients with sinus venosus defects frequently have partial anomalous pulmonary venous return, with the right upper pulmonary vein draining to the superior vena cava.

The least frequently encountered atrial septal defect is the coronary sinus septal defect. The tissue that constitutes the wall between the coronary sinus and the left atrium is either completely absent or only partially developed. Therefore, the left atrium and right atrium are connected via the coronary sinus.

Hemodynamics

The hemodynamics of interatrial communications are intimately linked to the compliance of the two ventricles. Dexter[10] was among the first to suggest that the direction of blood flow was due to the increased compliance of the right ventricle relative to the left ventricle. Hemodynamically, the ventricular compliance is reflected in the end-diastolic pressure and atrial-filling pressures. The example (Figure 11-1) illustrates the elevated right atrial pressure due to poor right ventricular function from a dilated, clinically volume overloaded right ventricle. The right atrial pressure waveform morphology is also abnormal. In a normal heart the right atrial *a* wave is larger than the *v* wave, and the left atrial *v* wave is greater than the *a* wave. With a large atrial septal defect that causes right ventricular volume overload, the right atrial *v* wave may increase due to tricuspid valve regurgitation. Because the tricuspid valve apparatus is intimately related to right ventricular geometry, when the right ventricle becomes dilated, the tricuspid leaflets cannot coapt appropriately,

resulting in tricuspid regurgitation. Left ventricular compliance is, in turn, affected by the dilated right ventricle. During diastole, the ventricular septum bulges to the left, impairing left ventricular filling (Figure 11-1, *C*). The elevated left ventricular filling pressure is, in turn, reflected in the left atrial pressure tracing (Figure 11-1, *B*). Therefore, the left atrial pressure is elevated, but the waveform

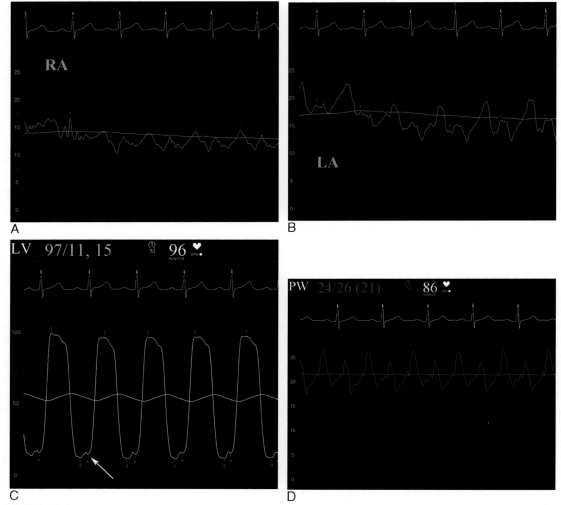

FIGURE 11-1. Hemodynamic tracings from a patient with a secundum atrial septal defect. **A,** Right atrial pressure tracing is remarkable for a more prominent *v* wave than *a* wave, likely due to tricuspid regurgitation from a dilated right ventricle from long-standing right ventricular volume overload. Also, note that the right atrial pressure is lower than left atrial pressure (see **B**), consistent with left-to-right flow across the defect. **B,** Left atrial pressure tracing with a large *v* wave relative to the *a* wave is normal for this chamber. Left atrial pressure is elevated due to decreased left ventricular compliance. **C,** Left ventricular waveform prior to atrial septal defect closure, demonstrating an end-diastolic pressure *(LVEDP)* *(arrow)* of 15 mmHg. **D,** Pulmonary capillary wedge pressure *(PW)* after the defect has been closed. LVEDP after closure has increased to 21 mmHg as a consequence of increased blood flowing from the left atrium to the left ventricle.

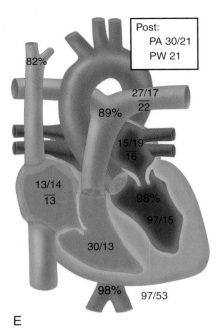

Post:
PA 30/21
PW 21

82%

89%

$\frac{27/17}{22}$

$\frac{15/19}{16}$

$\frac{13/14}{13}$

98%

97/15

30/13

98%   97/53

E

FIGURE 11-1—cont'd. **E,** Schematic of a heart illustrating the step-up in pulmonary artery saturation compared to superior vena cava saturation, suggesting a Qp/Qs of approximately 2:1. Chamber pressures before and after (see box insert) atrial septal defect closure are labeled.

morphology remains normal. After closure of the atrial septal defect, the fraction of blood that previously entered the right atrium is now directed into the left ventricle. The result of closing the "pop-off valve" is an increase in left ventricular end-diastolic pressure, particularly in patients with reduced compliance of the left ventricle (Figure 11-1, *D*). Small defects are generally considered to have a diameter of less than 0.5 cm. The ratio of pulmonary flow to systemic flow (Qp/Qs) in such patients is less than 1.5, and echocardiography demonstrates no dilatation of the right atrium or ventricle. These patients have no hemodynamic derangements and are often asymptomatic. Larger atrial septal defects frequently have a Qp/Qs ratio ≥1.5 and resultant right ventricular volume overload. Despite this, the patient frequently remains asymptomatic until the development of late right-heart failure or pulmonary hypertension. Often in adult

patients who present with a symptomatic atrial septal defect, right ventricular remodeling due to long-standing volume overload has led to decreased compliance and a decrease in the shunt. If right ventricular compliance worsens substantially relative to that of the left ventricle, right-to-left shunting may occur.[2] This physiology has been termed *Eisenmenger's syndrome* and can occur even with subsystemic pulmonary hypertension.[11] In large defects, no difference in mean pressures exists between the right and left atria, leading to the term *nonrestrictive atrial septal defect.* In the right atrium of patients with long-standing right-sided volume overload, elevated filling pressures are found. Right ventricular and pulmonary arterial systolic pressures may also be elevated, a sign of secondary pulmonary hypertension. Elevated right ventricular end-diastolic pressures, along with large right atrial *a* waves, are a sign of decreased right ventricular compliance.

The hemodynamic derangements associated with an atrial septal defect can be used to explain the physical exam findings in these patients. When right ventricular pressure and volume overload are present, a right ventricular heave may be appreciated. Fukuda et al.[12] performed phonoechocardiography on 17 patients with atrial septal defect and demonstrated that, prior to repair, the tricuspid component of the first heart sound (S1) was accentuated, and that the second heart sound had a wide and fixed split. With increased flow through the right ventricle (the systemic venous return plus the shunt flow), tricuspid valve closure was delayed. Similarly, the pulmonary valve closure is delayed with respect to the aortic valve, leading to the wide second heart sound. Equalization of interatrial pressures also leads to elimination of the respiratory variation of the second heart sound and a perceived fixed splitting.

Effects of Treatment

The majority of patients in the United States with atrial septal defect undergo either surgical or percutaneous closure during childhood. In a study of 123 patients who underwent closure at the Mayo Clinic, Murphy et al.[13] found that two factors correlated with survival after repair: (1) the age of the patient at the time of the operation ($p < .0001$) and (2) the pulmonary artery systolic pressure ($p < .0027$). Those patients who had a repair prior to age 25 had a long-term survival similar to that of the control population. However, those patients who were older than age 25 and who had a pulmonary artery pressure ≥ 40 mmHg had a shorter life expectancy than controls. At the 25-year follow-up, survival was 39% vs. 74% ($p < .0001$). The increase mortality was related to the development of congestive heart failure, atrial fibrillation, or cerebrovascular accident. Kobayashi et al.[14] demonstrated that defect closure in patients with Qp/Qs ≤ 3 with a pulmonary artery pressure ≤ 50 mmHg or with Qp/Qs ≥ 3, regardless of pulmonary artery pressure, resulted in increased exercise capacity. Gatzoulis et al.[15] found that as many as 60% of patients with atrial septal defect and atrial fibrillation continued to experience this arrhythmia after surgical closure of their defect. Murphy et al.[13] reported that of 104 patients in sinus rhythm prior to repair, 80 remained in sinus rhythm 27–32 years after the procedure.

Ventricular Septal Defect

Pathophysiology

The left and right ventricles are divided by a septum that consists of muscular and connective tissue components. The muscular ventricular septum arises from the primitive ventricle and grows in a caudal to cephalic direction, fusing with the infundibular septum and the endocardial cushions. Ventricular septal defects are commonly in the wall between the two ventricles and rarely between the left ventricle and the right atrium.[16] Anatomically, ventricular septal defects can be considered in four nonexclusive categories: (1) muscular, (2) membranous or perimembranous, (3) inlet defects, and (4) supracristal defects. Muscular defects are holes within the anterior, mid, inferior, or apical muscular septum. Membranous or perimembranous defects occur in the membranous tissue at the crux of the heart between the muscular septum and the conal septum. Defects in the inlet septum are also referred to as *atrioventricular canal defects*. Supracristal defects, also known as *outlet septal defects,* are defects in the conal septum above the supraventricular crest.[17] Twenty percent of all ventricular septal defects are muscular, 70% are membranous, 5% are inlet, and 5% are outlet.

Hemodynamics

From a hemodynamic perspective, ventricular septal defects can be classified broadly as restrictive (i.e., pressure-and flow-limiting), restrictive but with volume overload, or unrestrictive. Restrictive (pressure-and flow-limiting) defects are small or obstructed by tricuspid valve tissue, have a large pressure gradient between the left and right ventricles, and have normal pulmonary artery pressures. The Qp/Qs is <1.5. The pulmonary artery to aortic pressure ratio is <0.3. Ventricular septal defects that are pressure restrictive only may still have significant left-to-right shunt flow, as demonstrated in Figure 11-2. Right ventricular pressure will be normal, but the pulmonary arteries, the left atrium, and the left ventricle will be dilated from the volume overload. Unrestrictive ventricular septal

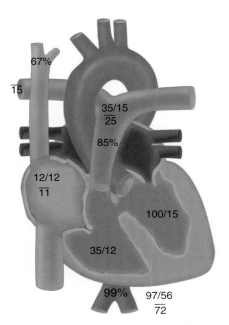

FIGURE 11-2. Schematic of a heart with a pressure-limited restrictive ventricular septal defect. The Qp/Qs of this patient prior to closure was approximately 2:1. Note the step-up in pulmonary artery saturation relative to superior vena cava saturation. Despite the communication between the two ventricles apparent with the step-up in saturation, a significant pressure differential exists between the right and left ventricles.

defects have systemic right ventricular pressures[18] (Figure 11-3). The degree of shunt across an unrestrictive ventricular septal defect is dependent upon the systolic compliance ratio of the systemic vascular bed and the pulmonary circuit (i.e., pulmonary stenosis or pulmonary hypertension).

These hemodynamics can explain the physical findings in patients with ventricular septal defects. The smaller the defect, the larger the pressure gradient across the septum. The resultant higher velocity shunt generates a higher-pitched systolic murmur. In larger defects, left-to-right flow usually occurs throughout systole, resulting in a holosystolic murmur; however, with smaller muscular defects the shunt may close as the myocardium thickens during systole. This results in a murmur that stops prior to the

end of systole. Before the onset of pulmonary hypertension, the physical exam in patients with larger but pressure-limited defects is notable for tachycardia, tachypnea, and a hyperdynamic and laterally displaced point of maximum impulse. The holosystolic murmur is often best heard at the lower left sternal border. The increased blood flow through the pulmonary circuit results in an increase in left atrial volume. The subsequent increased flow through the mitral valve may be appreciated as a mid-diastolic apical rumble. As pulmonary hypertension develops, right ventricular pressure increases. As the right and left ventricular pressures approach one another, the pressure gradient across the ventricular septal defect decreases, as does the intensity of the holosystolic murmur. Pressure and volume overload of the right ventricle may be apparent on physical exam with the presence of a heave. In unrestrictive ventricular septal defects, the murmur may be absent because the pressures between the two ventricles are equivalent. Outlet septum defects may cause one of the aortic valve leaflets to be sucked into the defect by the Venturi effect. The right coronary cusp is most often affected. While the valve leaflet reduces the size of the hole, the leaflet itself may become damaged leading to aortic valve regurgitation and an accompanying diastolic murmur.

Effect of Treatment

Restrictive defects often close spontaneously and do not result in clinically apparent hemodynamic sequelae. However, a potential risk of endocarditis exists as long as interventricular communication occurs. In patients who previously underwent closure of a ventricular septal defect, a residual shunt may persist with an accompanying high-pitched murmur.

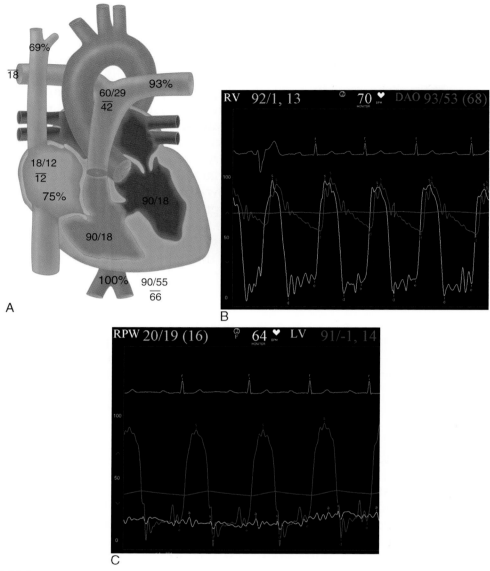

FIGURE 11-3. A, Schematic of a heart with an unrestricted ventricular septal defect and valvular pulmonic stenosis. The Qp/Qs of this patient prior to closure was approximately 2:1. Note the step-up in pulmonary artery saturation relative to superior vena cava saturation. The pressure in both ventricles is equal. **B,** Simultaneous pressure tracings from the right ventricle *(RV)* and descending aorta *(DAO).* Peak systolic pressures are equal. **C,** Simultaneous pressure tracings from a catheter wedged in the right pulmonary artery *(RPW)* and a catheter in the left ventricle *(LV).* The wedge pressure and the left ventricular end-diastolic pressures are essentially equal, suggesting that the elevated right ventricular pressure is not a consequence of pulmonary vascular obstructive disease or left-sided inflow obstruction. Additionally, the left ventricular end-diastolic pressure is elevated secondary to volume overload of the left ventricle.

Coarctation of The Aorta

Pathophysiology

Coarctation of the aorta refers to a congenital narrowing of the artery. Although it may occur in the transverse aortic arch, the distal thoracic aorta, or even rarely in the abdominal aorta, it occurs most commonly in the proximal descending aorta near the ligamentum arteriosum,

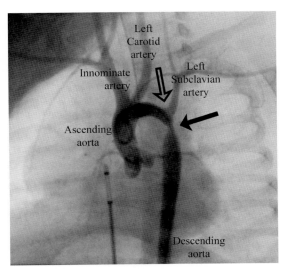

FIGURE 11-4. Angiogram from a patient with a coarctation of the aorta. Note the discrete narrowing of the aorta at the region of the ligamentum arteriosum.

the remnant of the ductus arteriosus. The most frequently observed variety consists of a discrete narrowing distal to the left subclavian artery (Figure 11-4). Additionally, cases of coarctation that consist of a long segment of hypoplastic aorta have been described. The embryologic etiology of aortic coarctation is hypothesized to be an extension of tissue from the ductus arteriosus into the aortic wall or the consequence of abnormal blood flow during development. Most cases of coarctation are sporadic. However, an association exists with Turner's syndrome.[19] The most commonly reported cardiovascular abnormality coexisting with a coarctation is a bicuspid aortic valve, which has been noted in as many as 85% of patients with coarctation. Abnormal circulation that involves collateral flow through the intercostal arteries and internal mammary arteries can be found in older patients with hemodynamically significant coarctations. Other abnormalities include Berry aneurysms in 3%–5% of patients, ventricular septal defect, aortic medial disease, and abnormalities of the innominate and left subclavian arteries.[20]

The majority of severe coarctations are discovered and treated during infancy in the United States. When the ductus arteriosus closes in an infant with a severe coarctation, shock or heart failure develops rapidly. The presentation of a coarctation in an adolescent or an adult is usually much more subtle. Symptoms are not often reported. Patients may complain of lower extremity fatigue with exertion and headaches. Physical exam may reveal upper extremity hypertension with an arm-leg blood pressure gradient, diminished lower extremity pulses, and a continuous or systolic murmur heard loudest in the back. The electrocardiogram in patients with coarctation may demonstrate left ventricular hypertrophy. Chest X-ray in older patients may demonstrate rib notching. This finding represents erosion of the inferior border of the ribs by intercostal arteries that have become enlarged from collateral flow. Additionally, dilatation of the aorta proximal and distal to the coarctation may cast a shadow that resembles the number *3* or a reversed *E* on chest X-ray.

Campbell[21] has reported that the majority of symptomatic infants with coarctation who were untreated died during the first year of life. The median survival of all untreated patients with coarctation was 31 years. Reifenstein et al.[22] reported that approximately 20% of asymptomatic children with coarctation survive to adulthood. Twenty-three percent of these patients died from aortic rupture at an average age of 27 years. Eighty percent of these were rupture of the ascending aorta. The remaining 20% experienced rupture distal to the coarctation. Of the remaining patients, 22% died from infection, including aortitis at an average age of 25 years, and 29% died from intracranial hemorrhage or congestive heart failure.

Hemodynamics

The coarctation represents a fixed obstruction to aortic flow. The hemodynamic hallmark of coarctation is a pressure gradient across the coarctation. Therefore, this diagnosis should be made by sphygmomanometry in both arms (in case of an anomalous right subclavian artery arising distal to the coarctation segment) and in one leg. A significant coarctation has been defined as a pressure in the upper extremity greater than 20 mmHg relative to the lower extremity. This measured gradient may be diminished in the presence of a large patent ductus arteriosus in a newborn or with significant aortic collaterals. Invasively measured gradients (Figure 11-5) demonstrate a wide pulse pressure proximal to the lesion and a diminished pulse pressure distally. The diminished pulse and the late or delayed pulse wave distal to the coarctation are termed *parvus* and *tardus*, respectively, similar to the pulse described in patients with severe aortic stenosis.

Effects of Treatment

Previously, traditional surgical treatment options for coarctation have included (1) coarctation excision with end-to-end anastomosis; (2) interposition graft; (3) patch aortoplasty; (4) radically extended end-to-end anastomosis; (5) bypass jump grafting; and (6) subclavian flap aortoplasty. Contemporary treatment at specialized centers now includes percutaneous balloon angioplasty and stent implantation.[23,24]

Unfortunately, after surgical or percutaneous therapy for coarctation, residual hemodynamic derangements may still occur. The mortality associated with surgery for simple coarctation repair is less than 1%. Cohen et al.[25] have reported that even after coarctation repair the mortality of these patients is elevated. In an analysis of 571 patients with repaired coarctations, the mean age of death was 38 years. Thirty-seven percent died from premature coronary artery disease. Additionally, certain types of repairs place

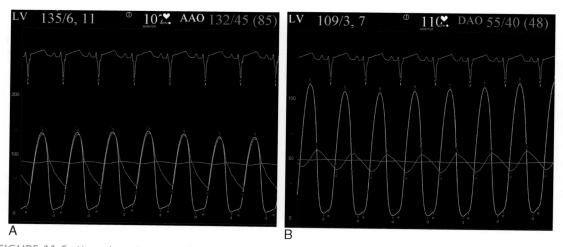

A   B

FIGURE 11-5. Hemodynamic tracings from a patient with coarctation of the aorta. **A,** Simultaneous pressure tracings from the left ventricle *(LV)* and the ascending aorta *(AAO)*. Peak systolic pressures are equal, demonstrating no valvular aortic stenosis. However, the pulse pressure of the ascending aorta is wide due to aortic valve regurgitation. **B,** Simultaneous pressure tracings from the left ventricle *(LV)* and the descending aorta *(DAO)* distal to the coarctation. A significant drop occurs in systolic pressure distal to the coarctation. The lower pulse pressure and systolic delay in the descending aorta represent the "parvus and tardus" of coarctation.

patients at increased risk for aortic aneurysm formation and rupture. Mendelsohn et al.[26] reported the incidence of aneurysm development at the site of patch repair to be as high as 30%. Patients who underwent either patch aortoplasty or balloon angioplasty should undergo screening for this complication, preferably with magnetic resonance imaging or computed tomography.[27] Finally, systemic hypertension is a residual problem for many patients with repaired coarctation, even without anatomic recoarctation. The incidence of hypertension is directly related to the age at the time of corrective operation. Ninety percent of patients who undergo surgery during childhood are normotensive at 5 years. However, of those who undergo repair after age 40, 50% will continue to experience hypertension at rest and a substantial fraction will have exercise-induced hypertension.[2] This persistent hypertension may be due, in part, to impaired aortic distensibility but also to intrinsic abnormalities of the microvasculature in these patients.[28]

Ebstein's Anomaly

Pathophysiology

Ebstein's anomaly is an eponym used to denote a syndrome in which the tricuspid valve is apically displaced with significant tricuspid regurgitation. Typically, the anterior tricuspid leaflet is enlarged and sometimes fenestrated. The septal and posterolateral leaflets are positioned below the atrioventricular grove, inside the morphologic right ventricle to varying degrees. The resultant abnormal coaptation of the tricuspid leaflets results in significant tricuspid regurgitation. However, extremely rare cases of Ebstein's anomaly with tricuspid stenosis have been reported.[29] Because the tricuspid valve is displaced apically,

part of the morphologic right ventricle has become functionally atrialized. As such, the functional right ventricle is a relatively small chamber. This results in poor compliance of the right ventricle. With severe tricuspid regurgitation, functional pulmonary atresia may develop as the right ventricle is unable to generate enough pressure to open the pulmonary valve. The majority of patients with Ebstein's anomaly have an interatrial communication, typically in the form of a stretched patent foramen ovale or a secundum atrial septal defect. Ebstein's anomaly is also associated with Wolff-Parkinson-White syndrome and atrial dysrhythmias.

The natural history of Ebstein's anomaly depends on the severity of the tricuspid regurgitation, with the spectrum varying from the severely cyanotic neonate with massive cardiomegaly to the asymptomatic adult. Patients with Ebstein's anomaly are at increased risk for endocarditis. Patients with an interatrial communication are at risk for paradoxical embolism and stroke. Adult patients may come to clinical attention after a primary care physician notices the tricuspid regurgitation murmur or after a supraventricular tachycardia develops. Newborns with severe Ebstein's anomaly may have severe cardiomegaly secondary to a massively stretched right atrium, to the point that pulmonary function can be compromised. In those neonates with functional or actual pulmonary atresia, oxygenation of venous blood may be dependent on ductal flow to the pulmonary circuit. Survival among adult patients with Ebstein's anomaly is inversely related to NYHA functional class, the severity of cyanosis, and the degree of cardiomegaly. The presence of atrial tachycardia may compromise the prognosis.

On physical exam the first heart sound is often widely split due to increased filling of the right ventricle from left-to-right flow across an interatrial communication. The tricuspid regurgitation murmur is often best appreciated at the left lower sternal border. An S3 and an S4 gallop may also be present. The degree of cyanosis is directly related to the magnitude of the right-to-left shunting.[30] An electrocardiogram of a patient with Ebstein's anomaly may demonstrate the stigmata of Wolff-Parkinson-White syndrome. As many as 20% of patients with Ebstein's anomaly have an accessory pathway. Otherwise, high-amplitude, wide *P* waves and right bundle branch block may be seen in addition to first degree AV block.[31] In severe cases, reduced pulmonary vascularity may be appreciated on chest X-ray, along with the impressive cardiomegaly.

Hemodynamics

In mild cases of Ebstein's anomaly, the only hemodynamic observation may be that of tricuspid regurgitation, elevation of right atrial pressures, and a cannon *v* wave in the right atrium (Figure 11-6). In more severe cases, right-to-left shunts may occur across the atrial septal defect due to the chronic volume overload and loss of compliance of the right ventricle, in addition to a severe tricuspid regurgitation jet. The classical hemodynamic definition of Ebstein's anomaly is a catheter measuring an atrial pressure tracing but recording a ventricular electrocardiogram from the atrialized portion of the right ventricle.

Effects of Treatment

Infants who present with severe symptoms from Ebstein's anomaly may require single ventricle palliation culminating in the Fontan procedure.[32] For adults with heart failure symptoms or

tachyarrhythmias refractory to medical therapy, closure of the interatrial communication and repair or replacement of the tricuspid valve is recommended.[33] Danielson et al.[34,35] have reported excellent results with surgical intervention, including tricuspid repair in this patient population, but results of valve repair at other centers have been less optimal. Patients with atrial tachyarrhythmias may require pharmacologic therapy or ablation.

Tetralogy of Fallot

Pathophysiology

The original description of tetralogy of Fallot was in 1888.[36] The contemporary incidence of tetralogy of Fallot is estimated at 356 cases per million live births.[37] The four components of this syndrome consist of (1) an overriding aorta, (2) an unrestricted malalignment ventricular septal defect, (3) infundibular pulmonary stenosis, and (4) right ventricular hypertrophy.[36] Embryologically, these cases are the consequence of abnormal conotruncal development. The hallmark of the lesion is anterior displacement of the conal septum, creating the ventricular septal defect, the overriding aorta, and the infundibular pulmonary stenosis. The latter leads to right ventricular hypertrophy. Several abnormalities are associated with tetralogy of Fallot frequently enough to merit comment. Twenty-five percent of patients with tetralogy of Fallot have a right-sided aortic arch.[38,39] Ten percent of patients have an associated secundum atrial septal defect.[38] Finally, 10% of patients have abnormalities of the coronary arteries.[40] An epicardial coronary artery may actually cross the right ventricular outflow tract in 5%–6% of patients.[41] This often involves the left anterior descending arising from the right coronary

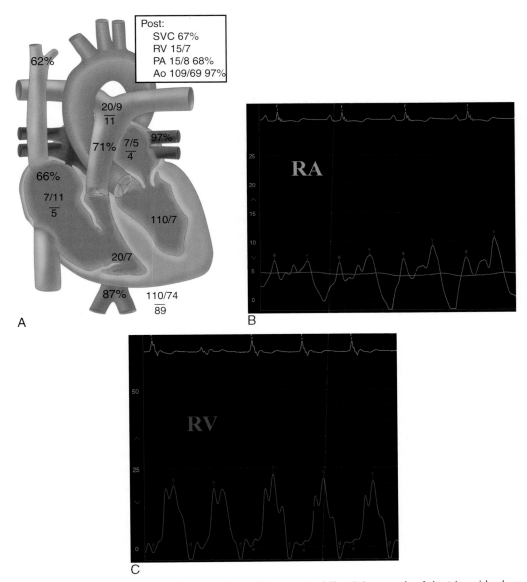

FIGURE 11-6. Hemodynamic tracings from a patient with unrepaired Ebstein's anomaly of the tricuspid valve and an atrial septal defect with cyanosis. **A,** Schematic of the patient's heart with Ebstein's anomaly. Note the apical displacement of the tricuspid valve. Bidirectional shunting exists at the atrial septum as demonstrated by the oximetry step-up from the superior vena cava to the pulmonary artery and step-down from the pulmonary vein to the aortic saturation. **A,** *(Box insert)* Note that in this patient, an atrial septal defect occlusion device was placed, resulting in resolution of the bidirectional atrial shunting, a fall in right ventricular and pulmonary artery pressures, an improvement in systemic saturation, and the resolution of cyanosis. **B,** Right atrial pressure tracing showing elevated *v* waves consistent with tricuspid regurgitation. **C,** Right ventricular pressure tracing showing normal, low pressures.

artery and crossing over the infundibular free wall before continuing in the usual location down the anterior interventricular groove. Genetic abnormalities associated with tetralogy of Fallot include DiGeorge's syndrome and chromosome 22q11 deletion in as many as 15% of patients.[42] Most cases of 22q11 deletion are spontaneous; however, tetralogy of Fallot may be transmitted in an autosomal dominant pattern by patients with the 22q11 deletion.

Patients with unrepaired tetralogy of Fallot may experience *tet spells* during which they become tachypneic and develop hyperpnea. They then experience worsening cyanosis and sometimes seizure activity, syncope, or death.[43] The mechanism of such spells is spasm of the already narrowed pulmonary infundibulum, and therefore treatment is aimed at overcoming this resistance to pulmonary blood flow with oxygen, fluid bolus, morphine (to relax the infundibular muscle), and systemic vasoconstrictors. A variant of tetralogy of Fallot involves minimal right ventricular outflow tract obstruction. These patients exhibit the hemodynamics associated with a large ventricular septal defect and pulmonary overcirculation soon after birth. However, within months they develop right ventricular outflow tract obstruction and then become cyanotic.[43] The main symptoms reported by the rare adult with unrepaired tetralogy of Fallot are cyanosis, decreased exercise tolerance, and tet spells. Complications in the adult with unrepaired tetralogy of Fallot include endocarditis, cerebral abscess, and stroke, in addition to hyperviscosity and coagulation issues related to hypoxemia.[33] Without surgery, the majority of affected patients die as children. Bertranou et al.[44] reviewed a large volume of published autopsy cases and reported that the untreated survival of tetralogy of Fallot is as follows: 66% at 1 year; 49% at 3 years; 24% at 10 years; 11% at 20 years; 6% at 30 years; and 3% at 40 years.

Patients with unrepaired tetralogy of Fallot will often have stigmata of chronic hypoxia such as digital clubbing on exam. Palpation of the chest may reveal a right ventricular heave. A systolic thrill may also be appreciated due to turbulent flow through the right ventricular outflow tract. On auscultation, a normal S1 will be heard, but S2 will be a single sound because no pulmonary component exists as the valve is severely stenotic or atretic. Instead of P2, a systolic ejection murmur may be appreciated at the left sternal border from right ventricular outflow tract obstruction. Note that, unlike aortic valve stenosis, the more severe the obstruction, the softer and shorter the murmur will be. The electrocardiogram in unrepaired adult patients with tetralogy of Fallot will have right axis deviation and demonstrate right ventricular hypertrophy. The classic shadow on a posterior-anterior chest X-ray is a boot-shaped cardiac silhouette. Furthermore, a right-sided arch may be appreciated in as many as 25% of cases.

Adult patients with surgically palliated tetralogy of Fallot frequently have remaining hemodynamic issues related to a surgical technique, using a transannular patch across the right ventricular outflow tract. This has left these patients with free pulmonary insufficiency, thereby volume loading an already dilated and dysfunctional right ventricle. Some patients also may have had a previous aortopulmonary shunt such as a Potts, Waterston, or Blalock-Taussig shunt, leaving residual branch pulmonary artery stenosis. The increased afterload of branch pulmonary artery stenosis adds a component of pressure-overload to the volume-overloaded right ventricle.

Hemodynamics

In the unrepaired state, the major determinant hemodynamic factor for patients with tetralogy of Fallot is the degree of right ventricular outflow tract obstruction. Ventricular septal defects in this condition are usually large; however, rare cases of restrictive ventricular septal defects have been reported.[45] The unrestrictive ventricular septal defect results in equalization of left and right ventricular pressures. Initially, there may still be a left-to-right shunt across the ventricular septal defect, and pulmonary overcirculation (the so-called *pink tet*). However, the infundibular pulmonary stenosis is progressive, and right-to-left shunting occurs at the ventricular septal defect, with resulting systemic cyanosis. Infundibular pulmonary stenosis provides a fixed obstruction in the right ventricular outflow tract. Therefore, resistance to right ventricular outflow via this route is essentially constant. Thus, the magnitude of the right-to-left shunt is a function of the systemic vascular resistance. Increases in systemic vascular resistance result in a decrease of right-to-left shunting. Patients with unrepaired tetralogy take advantage of this by performing maneuvers such as squatting to increase afterload, causing more venous blood to enter the pulmonary circuit. Conversely, a drop in systemic vascular resistance will result in increased right-to-left shunting and worsening cyanosis.

The hemodynamics of pregnancy in patients with unrepaired tetralogy of Fallot deserves special attention. During pregnancy, systemic vascular resistance decreases, increasing the degree of right-to-left shunting and worsening hypoxemia. Therefore, it is imperative that all patients with tetralogy of Fallot should receive counseling from an adult congenital heart disease physician prior to conception.

Effect of Treatment

In the past, several types of palliative operations were used to increase pulmonary blood flow. All involved directing blood from the aorta to the pulmonary artery. The Waterston shunt involved a direct anastomosis from the ascending aorta to the right pulmonary artery. The Potts shunt similarly involved a direct anastomosis from the descending aorta to the left pulmonary artery. Both the

Waterston and the Potts shunts were limited by pulmonary overcirculation, pulmonary hypertension, and late branch pulmonary artery stenosis. The classic Blalock-Taussig shunt involved the connection of a turned-down subclavian artery to the pulmonary artery. The modified Blalock-Taussig shunt involved routing a conduit from the subclavian or innominate artery to the pulmonary artery. Historically, complete *repair* included a transannular patch, which led to significant pulmonary insufficiency and chronic right ventricular volume overload.

Contemporary treatment involves complete surgical correction, with the avoidance of a transannular incision, if possible. However, this is unfortunately more common in actual practice (Figure 11-7). In infants, Lee et al.[46] reported <1% mortality for this procedure. However, the mortality of this procedure in

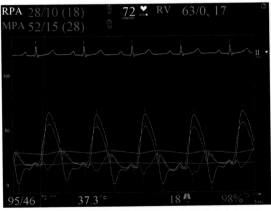

FIGURE 11-7. Hemodynamic tracings from a patient with repaired tetralogy of Fallot. This patient underwent a transannular patch of the pulmonary valve and infundibulum and was left with free pulmonary regurgitation. The right ventricular *(RV)*, main pulmonary artery *(MPA)*, and right pulmonary artery *(RPA)* tracings are shown. The right ventricular pressure is elevated but with a minimal gradient across the right ventricular outflow tract. However, branch pulmonary stenosis exists with a lower right pulmonary artery pressure. The wave form of the pulmonary artery tracing is notable for a ventricular morphology, that is, no dicrotic notch is present from pulmonary valve closure, and the end-diastolic pressures of the pulmonary artery and right ventricle are essentially equal. This is consistent with severe pulmonary insufficiency.

adults is significantly higher. Despite surgical advances, long-term survival after repair is decreased relative to age-matched controls. Murphy et al.[47] reported an 86% survival of repaired tetralogy of Fallot patients after 32 years vs. 96% in an age-matched control population. Nollert et al.[48] reported an 85% survival at 36 years. Ventricular and atrial arrhythmias are a significant cause of morbidity and mortality in this population.[49] Restoration of more normal hemodynamics may help reduce these arrhythmias.[50] Finally, replacement of the pulmonary valve to address the problem of associated pulmonary insufficiency is frequently performed in the older patient. The timing of such an operation remains controversial; however, increasing data supports the practice of performing pulmonary valve replacement before significant right ventricular dysfunction and enlargement occurs.[51]

Peripheral Pulmonary Artery Stenosis

Pathophysiology

Isolated peripheral pulmonary artery stenosis is a relatively rare disorder. More frequently, it complicates the course of other congenital heart disease, such as tetralogy of Fallot or truncus arteriosus. Valvular pulmonary stenosis is addressed in Chapter 7. The main pulmonary artery along with the right and left branches are formed from the bulbus cordis and truncus arteriosus. The peripheral arteries are formed from the ventral aspect of the sixth branchial arches and the postbranchial pulmonary vascular plexus.[52] Maternal rubella during pregnancy is a known risk factor for the development of peripheral pulmonary artery stenosis. Other conditions associated with peripheral pulmonary artery stenosis include Williams' syndrome, Noonan's syndrome, LEOPARD syndrome, and Alagille's syndrome. Peripheral pulmonary artery stenosis may also occur as a result of systemic vasculitis; however, this may represent a different pathophysiological process from congenital peripheral pulmonary artery stenosis. Patients with vasculitis and peripheral pulmonary artery stenosis have evidence of chronic inflammation, scar, and thrombosis on histology sections of segmental pulmonary arteries, whereas those with congenital peripheral pulmonary artery stenosis do not. In children, peripheral pulmonary artery stenosis may occur as isolated focal or multiple stenoses in the main pulmonary artery or left and right branches. Another reported pattern is that of multiple stenoses, involving only the peripheral pulmonary artery branches. Combinations of these two patterns have also been found. More common than these conditions is an association with complex congenital heart lesions such as tetralogy of Fallot (Figures 11-8 and 11-9) and iatrogenic peripheral pulmonary artery stenosis that occurs after various aortopulmonary shunt procedures. Another example of the latter would be patients with transposition of the great vessels who undergo an arterial switch procedure as infants. Although such surgery is necessary for survival, it may compromise the pulmonary arteries, in that one or both arteries are stretched or compressed over the posteriorly located, dilated ascending aorta.

Adults with peripheral pulmonary artery stenosis may present with dyspnea on exertion and exercise intolerance. Although the source of symptoms is often blatant in patients with a history of surgery to correct congenital cardiac problems, those with no such history are frequently given an initial diagnosis of pulmonary embolism on the basis of ventilation-perfusion scans that demonstrate decreased perfusion tracer uptake

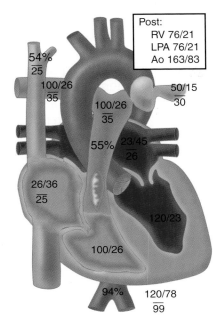

Post:
RV 76/21
LPA 76/21
Ao 163/83

54%
25

100/26
35

50/15
30

100/26
35

55%
23/45
26

26/36
25

120/23

100/26

94%
120/78
99

FIGURE 11-8. Schematic of a heart from a patient with repaired tetralogy of Fallot. The left pulmonary artery is stenotic from a prior Potts shunt, resulting in pulmonary hypertension of the right pulmonary artery. *Box insert* shows hemodynamics after placement of a covered stent into left pulmonary artery, eliminating both the stenosis and aneurysm.

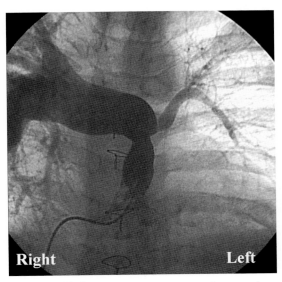

Right   Left

FIGURE 11-9. Pulmonary artery angiogram from another patient with tetralogy of Fallot and pulmonary atresia s/p repair with a right-ventricle-pulmonary-artery conduit, leaving the patient with left pulmonary artery stenosis. The patient had a hypertensive right pulmonary artery, and nonpulsatile distal left pulmonary artery pressure, with elevated right ventricular pressures.

in the pulmonary vascular territory subtended by the stenosed artery. The location and severity of peripheral pulmonary artery stenosis determine whether right ventricular hypertension develops. With right ventricular hypertension, a right ventricular heave may be present on exam. The reduced right ventricular compliance from hypertrophy may also result in an S4 gallop during atrial contraction. Sometimes a large *a* wave can be appreciated. S2 may be split with a delayed P2. In cases with severe pulmonary hypertension and an atrial communication, cyanosis may develop. Finally, Kreutzer et al.[53] report that patients with peripheral pulmonary artery stenosis may develop symptoms of right ventricular failure, including peripheral edema and hepatic congestion.

Hemodynamics

Kreutzer et al.[53] have published the largest series, describing invasively attained hemodynamics of adults with peripheral pulmonary artery stenosis and no history of cardiac surgery. Twelve patients with NYHA class II–III symptoms, no history of vasculitis and abnormal ^{99}Tc-macroaggregated albumin perfusion scans without matching ventilation defects underwent cardiac catheterization. The right ventricular pressure of these patients ranged between 40% and 200% of systemic pressure. Except in one patient who had a right ventricular pressure 200% of systemic pressure, pulmonary artery pressure was low distal to the stenoses. In addition, all 12 of these patients were noted to have elevated pulmonary artery pressures in other distal segments that were not as severely stenosed as the primary lesion.

In patients with unilateral branch pulmonary artery stenosis, the pressure in the contralateral nonstenotic pulmonary artery is frequently elevated, and a significant flow imbalance exists between the right and left lungs. Indications for therapy include contralateral pulmonary arterial hypertension, right ventricular hypertension (Figure 11-10), or significant flow imbalance, particularly in younger patients with continued growth potential of the lungs.

Effects of Treatment

If the pulmonary artery branch stenosis is proximal to the hilum, both surgical and percutaneous transcatheter therapies have been used. However, if the stenoses are multiple and distal to the hilum, percutaneous therapy is the only option. For branch stenosis lesions that are discrete, pulmonary artery balloon angioplasty may be successful (Figure 11-11). Unfortunately, if the stenosis involves a long segment or is due to a stretch lesion, angioplasty often leads to an inadequate result. Stent implantation may be useful in such situations. In addition to relief of symptoms, Kreutzer et al.[53] defined procedural success as an increase in vessel diameter by ≥50%,

with a consequent improvement in angiographic flow and a ≥30% drop in right ventricular systolic pressure. Of the aforementioned 12 patients with severe distal peripheral pulmonic stenosis, 11 underwent balloon angioplasty. One died post-procedure from pulmonary hemorrhage. One continued to experience right ventricular pressure that was greater than systemic pressure and died while waiting for transplantation. The remaining nine were reported to have sustained improvement in symptoms for 52 ± 32 months.[53]

Eisenmenger's Syndrome

Pathophysiology

Eisenmenger's syndrome is pulmonary vascular obstructive disease that develops secondary to increased pulmonary blood flow from a large left-to-right shunt, resulting in pulmonary artery pressures that approximates systemic pressures and consequent bidirectional or right-to-left shunting.[54,55] The initial vascular changes that occur with a large

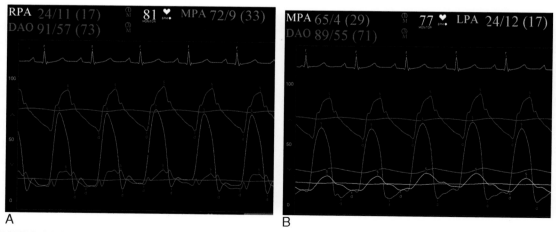

FIGURE 11-10. Hemodynamic tracings from a patient with left and right pulmonary artery stenosis after an arterial switch operation for *d*-type transposition of the great arteries. **A,** The main pulmonary artery pressure *(MPA)* is markedly elevated relative to the right pulmonary artery pressure *(RPA)* distal to the site of stenosis. *DAO,* Descending aortic pressure. **B,** The main pulmonary artery pressure is markedly elevated relative to the left pulmonary artery pressure *(LPA)* distal to the site of stenosis. Note the appearance of the main pulmonary artery pressure waveform. It appears like a ventricular waveform due to severe pulmonary insufficiency.

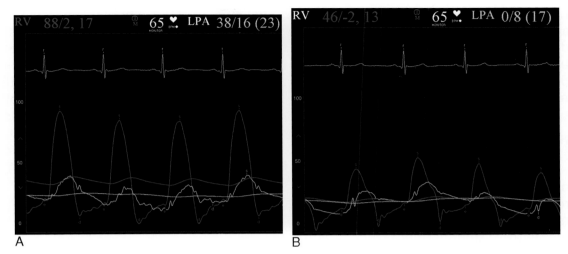

FIGURE 11-11. Hemodynamic tracings from a patient with left pulmonary artery *(LPA)* stenosis and free pulmonary regurgitation. **A,** The right ventricular *(RV)* pressure is markedly elevated (80% of systemic), and equilibration of diastolic pressures between the left pulmonary artery and the right ventricle is consistent with severe regurgitation. **B,** After balloon dilatation and stent implantation across the left pulmonary artery stenosis, the right ventricular pressure has dropped to 41% of systemic.

left-to-right shunt are potentially reversible. These changes include intimal proliferation, hypertrophy of the media, and small vessel occlusion. With time, these changes become irreversible, resulting in an elevated pulmonary vascular resistance. The majority of conditions that lead to Eisenmenger's syndrome commence in childhood and include atrial septal defect, ventricular septal defect, and patent ductus arteriosus, in addition to conotruncal abnormalities with initial left-to-right shunts. In addition, certain palliative procedures, including the Potts and Waterson shunts, can lead to Eisenmenger's syndrome. As pulmonary vascular resistance increases, right-to-left shunting increases. Eventually, patients become symptomatic with dyspnea and exercise intolerance.[56] As cyanosis develops, erythrocytosis and hyperviscosity become significant issues. Patients may experience hemoptysis as a consequence of pulmonary infarction or capillary rupture. Right-to-left shunting can result in paradoxical embolism and stroke. Patients with Eisenmenger's syndrome are also at increased risk for endocarditis.

A further problem is that of both hemorrhage and hypercoagulability due to hypoxemia.[57] In a review of the literature from 1966 to 1998, Vongpatanasin et al.[58] reported that at 10 years after diagnosis 80% of patients survived, at 15 years 77% survived, and at 25 years only 42% survived. Saha et al.[59] found that 30% of patients die of sudden death, 25% die of congestive heart failure, and 15% die of pulmonary hemorrhage.

The physical exam of a patient with Eisenmenger's syndrome is notable for cyanosis and digital clubbing in proportion to the magnitude of the right-to-left shunt. Large jugular *v* waves may be noted in the presence of significant tricuspid regurgitation. A right ventricular heave may be palpated. The P2 component of the second sound is loud due to the pulmonary hypertension. Murmurs from right-to-left shunting are soft or absent, because the pressure gradient between the pulmonary and systemic circuits is low. However, the murmurs of tricuspid regurgitation and pulmonary regurgitation may be prominent. A right-sided S4 gallop may also be heard due to the right atrium contracting against a right ventricle with decreased compliance due to hypertrophy. The electrocardiogram may show right ventricular hypertrophy, and a chest X-ray will demonstrate changes consistent with pulmonary hypertension.

Hemodynamics

As alluded to previously, the hemodynamics of Eisenmenger's syndrome are related to decreased flow through the pulmonary circuit and right-to-left shunting with systemic hypoxemia (Figure 11-12). The evaluation of patients with Eisenmenger's syndrome often includes

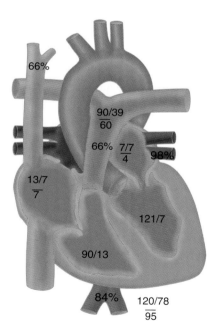

FIGURE 11-12. Schematic of a heart from a patient with Eisenmenger's physiology from a long-standing atrial septal defect. Chronic right ventricular volume overload from left-to-right shunting at the atrial septal defect has led to a severely dilated right ventricle with elevated end-diastolic pressures from decreased compliance. As shunting at the atrial septal defect is determined by the relative compliance of the two ventricles, the direction of flow across the shunt then became right-to-left, as shown by the step-down in oxygen saturations from the pulmonary vein to the aorta. Note the severely elevated pulmonary and right ventricular systolic pressures from pulmonary vascular occlusive disease.

cardiac catheterization and a vasodilator challenge to assess whether the elevated pulmonary vascular resistance is reversible. With high pulmonary vascular resistance, the right-to-left shunt serves to volume unload the right ventricle. If the pulmonary vascular resistance is not reversible and the right-to-left shunt is closed, then the right ventricle will fail, because it cannot compensate for the increased afterload of the pulmonary vascular resistance.

Effects of Treatment

Palliative treatment of Eisenmenger's syndrome includes prevention of infection with endocarditis prophylaxis and appropriate vaccinations. It also includes prevention of dehydration with volume expansion to prevent problems with hyperviscosity. Phlebotomy with volume replacement must be undertaken with care as it could reduce the oxygen carrying capacity of an already hypoxic patient.[57] Phlebotomy can also result in iron deficiency, which is problematic because iron-deficient red blood cells are less deformable, potentially obstructing the microvasculature. End-stage treatment for Eisenmenger's syndrome involves lung transplantation with repair of the underlying defect or a combined heart-lung transplantation. The 1-year survival for adults with lung transplantation and cardiac repair is 70%. At 4 years, the survival is under 50%. Combined heart-lung transplantation has a 1-year survival rate as high as 60% and a 10-year survival rate under 30%.[60]

References

1. Warnes CA, Liberthson R, Danielson GK, et al. Task force 1: The changing profile of congenital heart disease in adult life. *J Am Coll Cardiol* 2001;37(5): 1170–1175.
2. Brickner ME, Hillis LD, Lange RA. Congenital heart disease in adults. First of two parts. *N Engl J Med* 2000;342(4):256–263.

3. Dexter L, Haynes FW, Burwell CS, et al. Studies of congenital heart disease. III. Venous catheterization as a diagnostic aid in patent ductus arteriosus, tetralogy of Fallot, ventricular septal defect, and auricular septal defect. *J Clin Invest* 1947;26(3):561–576.
4. Hagen PT, Scholz DG, Edwards WD. Incidence and size of patent foramen ovale during the first 10 decades of life: An autopsy study of 965 normal hearts. *Mayo Clin Proc* 1984;59(1):17–20.
5. Lynch HT, Bachenberg K, Harris RE, Becker W. Hereditary atrial septal defect. Update of a large kindred. *Am J Dis Child* 1978;132(6):600–604.
6. Leachman RD, Cokkinos DV, Cooley DA. Association of ostium secundum atrial septal defects with mitral valve prolapse. *Am J Cardiol* 1976;38(2):167–169.
7. Campbell M. Natural history of atrial septal defect. *Br Heart J* 1970;32(6):820–826.
8. Van Praagh S, Carrera ME, Sanders SP, et al. Sinus venosus defects: Unroofing of the right pulmonary veins—anatomic and echocardiographic findings and surgical treatment. *Am Heart J* 1994;128(2):365–379.
9. Van Praagh S, Carrera ME, Sanders S, et al. Partial or total direct pulmonary venous drainage to right atrium due to malposition of septum primum. Anatomic and echocardiographic findings and surgical treatment: A study based on 36 cases. *Chest* 1995;107(6):1488–1498.
10. Dexter L. Atrial septal defect. *Br Heart J* 1956;18(2):209–225.
11. Craig RJ, Selzer A. Natural history and prognosis of atrial septal defect. *Circulation* 1968;37(5):805–815.
12. Fukuda N, Oki T, Iuchi A, et al. The first heart sound in atrial septal defect with reference to atrioventricular valve motion and hemodynamics. *Jpn Heart J* 1995;36(6):763–774.
13. Murphy JG, Gersh BJ, McGoon MD, et al. Long-term outcome after surgical repair of isolated atrial septal defect. Follow-up at 27 to 32 years. *N Engl J Med* 1990;323(24):1645–1650.
14. Kobayashi Y, Nakanishi N, Kosakai Y. Pre- and postoperative exercise capacity associated with hemodynamics in adult patients with atrial septal defect: A retrospective study. *Eur J Cardiothorac Surg* 1997;11(6):1062–1066.
15. Gatzoulis MA, Freeman MA, Siu SC, et al. Atrial arrhythmia after surgical closure of atrial septal defects in adults. *N Engl J Med* 1999;340(11):839–846.
16. Gerbode F, Hultgren H, Melrose D, Osborn J. Syndrome of left ventricular-right atrial shunt; successful surgical repair of defect in five cases, with observation of bradycardia on closure. *Ann Surg* 1958;148(3):433–446.
17. Van Praagh R, Geva T, Kreutzer J. Ventricular septal defects: How shall we describe, name and classify them? *J Am Coll Cardiol* 1989;14(5):1298–1299.
18. Therrien J, Dore A, Gersony W, et al. CCS Consensus Conference 2001 update: Recommendations for the management of adults with congenital heart disease. Part I. *Can J Cardiol* 2001;17(9):940–959.
19. Wald R, Powell AJ. Simple congenital heart lesions. *J Cardiovasc Magn Reson* 2006;8(4):619–631.
20. Roos-Hesselink JW, Scholzel BE, Heijdra RJ, et al. Aortic valve and aortic arch pathology after coarctation repair. *Heart* 2003;89(9):1074–1077.
21. Campbell M. Natural history of coarctation of the aorta. *Br Heart J* 1970;32(5):633–640.
22. Reinfenstein G, Levine S, Gross R. Coarctation of the aorta: A review of 104 autopsied cases of the "adult type." 2 years of age or older. *Am Heart J* 1947;33:146–168.
23. Hellenbrand WE, Allen HD, Golinko RJ, et al. Balloon angioplasty for aortic recoarctation: Results of Valvuloplasty and Angioplasty of Congenital Anomalies Registry. *Am J Cardiol* 1990;65(11):793–797.
24. Rao PS, Najjar HN, Mardini MK, et al. Balloon angioplasty for coarctation of the aorta: Immediate and long-term results. *Am Heart J* 1988;115(3):657–665.
25. Cohen M, Fuster V, Steele PM, et al. Coarctation of the aorta. Long-term follow-up and prediction of outcome after surgical correction. *Circulation* 1989;80(4):840–845.
26. Mendelsohn AM, Crowley DC, Lindauer A, Beekman RH III. Rapid progression of aortic aneurysms after patch aortoplasty repair of coarctation of the aorta. *J Am Coll Cardiol* 1992;20(2):381–385.
27. Therrien J, Thorne SA, Wright A, et al. Repaired coarctation: A "cost-effective" approach to identify complications in adults. *J Am Coll Cardiol* 2000;35(4):997–1002.
28. Gardiner HM, Celermajer DS, Sorensen KE, et al. Arterial reactivity is significantly impaired in normotensive young adults after successful repair of aortic coarctation in childhood. *Circulation* 1994;89(4):1745–1750.
29. Dearani JA, Danielson GK. Congenital Heart Surgery Nomenclature and Database Project: Ebstein's anomaly and tricuspid valve disease. *Ann Thorac Surg* 2000;69(4 Suppl):S106–S117.
30. Celermajer DS, Bull C, Till JA, et al. Ebstein's anomaly: Presentation and outcome from fetus to adult. *J Am Coll Cardiol* 1994;23(1):170–176.
31. Kastor JA, Goldreyer BN, Josephson ME, et al. Electrophysiologic characteristics of Ebstein's anomaly of the tricuspid valve. *Circulation* 1975;52(6):987–995.
32. van Son JA, Falk V, Black MD, et al. Conversion of complex neonatal Ebstein's anomaly into functional tricuspid or pulmonary atresia. *Eur J Cardiothorac Surg* 1998;13(3):280–284.
33. Brickner ME, Hillis LD, Lange RA. Congenital heart disease in adults. Second of two parts. *N Engl J Med* 2000;342(5):334–342.
34. Boston US, Dearani JA, O'Leary PW, et al. Tricuspid valve repair for Ebstein's anomaly in young children: A 30-year experience. *Ann Thorac Surg* 2006;81(2):690–695.
35. Danielson GK, Driscoll DJ, Mair DD, et al. Operative treatment of Ebstein's anomaly. *J Thorac Cardiovasc Surg* 1992;104(5):1195–1202.
36. Fallot A. Contribution a l'anatomie pathologique de la maladie bleue (cyanose cardiaque). *Marseille Med* 1888;25:77–93.
37. Hoffman JI, Kaplan S. The incidence of congenital heart disease. *J Am Coll Cardiol* 2002;39(12):1890–1900.
38. Rao BN, Anderson RC, Edwards JE. Anatomic variations in the tetralogy of Fallot. *Am Heart J* 1971;81(3):361–371.
39. Rowe RD, Vlad P, Keith JD. Experiences with 180 cases of tetralogy of Fallot in infants and children. *Can Med Assoc J* 1955;73(1):23–30.

40. Dabizzi RP, Teodori G, Barletta GA, et al. Associated coronary and cardiac anomalies in the tetralogy of Fallot. An angiographic study. *Eur Heart J* 1990;11(8): 692–704.
41. Need LR, Powell AJ, del Nido P, Geva T. Coronary echocardiography in tetralogy of Fallot: Diagnostic accuracy, resource utilization and surgical implications over 13 years. *J Am Coll Cardiol* 2000;36(4): 1371–1377.
42. Goldmuntz E, Clark BJ, Mitchell LE, et al. Frequency of 22q11 deletions in patients with conotruncal defects. *J Am Coll Cardiol* 1998;32(2): 492–498.
43. Morgan BC, Guntheroth WG, Bloom RS, Fyler DC. A clinical profile of paroxysmal hyperpnea in cyanotic congenital heart disease. *Circulation* 1965; 31:66–69.
44. Bertranou EG, Blackstone EH, Hazelrig JB, et al. Life expectancy without surgery in tetralogy of Fallot. *Am J Cardiol* 1978;42(3):458–466.
45. Flanagan MF, Foran RB, Van Praagh R, et al. Tetralogy of Fallot with obstruction of the ventricular septal defect: Spectrum of echocardiographic findings. *J Am Coll Cardiol* 1988;11(2):386–395.
46. Lee C, Lee CN, Kim SC, et al. Outcome after one-stage repair of tetralogy of Fallot. *J Cardiovasc Surg (Torino)* 2006;47(1):65–70.
47. Murphy JG, Gersh BJ, Mair DD, et al. Long-term outcome in patients undergoing surgical repair of tetralogy of Fallot. *N Engl J Med* 1993;329(9): 593–599.
48. Nollert G, Fischlein T, Bouterwek S, et al. Long-term results of total repair of tetralogy of Fallot in adulthood: 35 years follow-up in 104 patients corrected at the age of 18 or older. *Thorac Cardiovasc Surg* 1997;45(4):178–181.
49. Gatzoulis MA, Balaji S, Webber SA, et al. Risk factors for arrhythmia and sudden cardiac death late after repair of tetralogy of Fallot: A multicentre study. *Lancet* 2000;356(9234):975–981.
50. Oechslin EN, Harrison DA, Harris L, et al. Reoperation in adults with repair of tetralogy of Fallot: Indications and outcomes. *J Thorac Cardiovasc Surg* 1999;118(2):245–251.
51. Therrien J, Provost Y, Merchant N, et al. Optimal timing for pulmonary valve replacement in adults after tetralogy of Fallot repair. *Am J Cardiol* 2005; 95(6):779–782.
52. Hislop A, Reid L. Pulmonary arterial development during childhood: Branching pattern and structure. *Thorax* 1973;28(2):129–135.
53. Kreutzer J, Landzberg MJ, Preminger TJ, et al. Isolated peripheral pulmonary artery stenoses in the adult. *Circulation* 1996;93(7):1417–1423.
54. Wood P. The Eisenmenger syndrome or pulmonary hypertension with reversed central shunt. I. *Br Med J* 1958;2(5098):701–709.
55. Wood P. The Eisenmenger syndrome or pulmonary hypertension with reversed central shunt. *Br Med J* 1958;2(5099):755–762.
56. Daliento L, Somerville J, Presbitero P, et al. Eisenmenger syndrome. Factors relating to deterioration and death. *Eur Heart J* 1998;19(12):1845–1855.
57. Perloff JK, Rosove MH, Child JS, Wright GB. Adults with cyanotic congenital heart disease: Hematologic management. *Ann Intern Med* 1988;109(5):406–413.
58. Vongpatanasin W, Brickner ME, Hillis LD, Lange RA. The Eisenmenger syndrome in adults. *Ann Intern Med* 1998;128(9):745–755.
59. Saha A, Balakrishnan KG, Jaiswal PK, et al. Prognosis for patients with Eisenmenger syndrome of various aetiology. *Int J Cardiol* 1994;45(3):199–207.
60. Hosenpud JD, Bennett LE, Keck BM, et al. The Registry of the International Society for Heart and Lung Transplantation: Eighteenth Official Report—2001. *J Heart Lung Transplant* 2001;20(8):805–815.

CHAPTER 12

Coronary Hemodynamics

Michael Ragosta, MD

Selective coronary angiography is one of the most commonly performed procedures in the United States. In most cases, careful interpretation of the images obtained by angiography yields diagnostic information adequate for decision making. Not uncommonly, however, situations exist when angiography fails to definitively assess the nature and severity of atherosclerotic coronary disease. In such cases, hemodynamic principles applied to the coronary arteries provide valuable adjunctive data to the cardiologist, allowing greater diagnostic certainty.

At a minimum, cardiologists who perform coronary angiography must be capable of promptly recognizing abnormalities in pressure waveforms sampled from the catheter tip during selective coronary angiography. This is important for both patient safety and proper diagnosis. In addition, invasive and interventional cardiologists need to understand the more sophisticated coronary hemodynamic assessments made possible by recent technological advances allowing the invasive assessment of coronary flow reserve. These techniques serve as important adjuncts to angiography and have become indispensable to the routine practice of invasive cardiology.

Coronary Catheter Pressure Waveforms

Analysis of the pressure waveforms generated from the tip of the catheter during performance of selective coronary angiography can provide valuable information to the operator. Upon engagement of a catheter into the ostium of either the right or left coronary artery, the physician should immediately review the catheter-tip pressure tracing before proceeding with contrast injection. This tracing normally appears as a typical aortic pressure waveform. An alert angiographer seeks two abnormalities in the pressure waveform: damping and ventricularization. Recognizing these abnormalities is essential because their presence sometimes enhances the information provided by the angiogram and may help avoid potentially serious complications of selective angiography.

Pressure *damping* refers to a drop in the systolic pressure and a loss of the usual features of an arterial pressure waveform. Damping of the waveform often indicates the presence of narrowing of the coronary ostium. An example of this phenomenon is shown in Figure 12-1. In this case, the catheter pressure showed marked damping upon engagement of the left coronary artery (Figure 12-1, *A*). The angiogram showed modest narrowing of the ostium of the left main stem (Figure 12-1, *B*). Removal of the catheter from the left main stem reestablished the normal aortic pressure (Figure 12-1, *C*).

Ventricularization of the catheter-tip pressure is seen when, upon engagement of the catheter, the diastolic pressure drops and shifts appearance from the usual, arterial waveform to one with a ventricular morphology (Figure 12-2). Pure ventricularization, in which there is only a drop in diastolic pressure and not in the systolic pressure, implies a precise match between the diameters of the artery and the catheter lumen that leads to a coronary artery "wedge" pressure, reflecting left ventricular pressure (Figure 12-3). More typically, the pressure trace appears both ventricularized

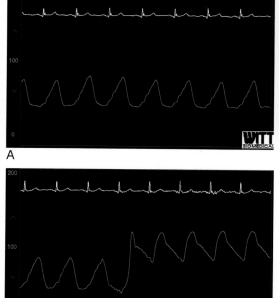

A

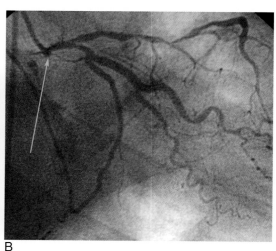

B

C

FIGURE 12-1. **A,** Example of pressure damping and ventricularization observed following engagement of the left coronary catheter. **B,** The angiogram showed at least moderate disease of the ostium of the left main coronary artery (*arrow*) as well as significant disease in the left anterior descending artery. **C,** When the catheter was withdrawn into the aorta, the pressure waveform was restored.

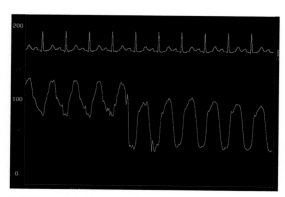

FIGURE 12-2. Example of ventricularization of the coronary catheter pressure waveform.

and damped. Both ventricularization and/or damping may be obvious; sometimes the change is subtle (Figure 12-4).

Both damping and ventricularization have similar causes (Table 12-1); both imply that the catheter tip plugs and obstructs the coronary artery lumen. The

most common causes are from obstructive disease at the coronary ostium and from selective engagement of a smaller artery such as the conus branch of the right coronary artery. Upon observing these abnormal waveforms, the angiographer should determine the cause before proceeding with coronary arteriography in the usual manner. The presence of ventricularization or damping may be the only clues to the existence of a significant ostial stenosis not appreciated by angiography. More importantly, the injection of contrast into a catheter with a damped or ventricularized pressure tracing might lead to serious complications. For instance, selective and forceful injection of a full syringe of contrast into a conus branch of the right coronary artery or into a small nondominant artery may lead to ventricular fibrillation or

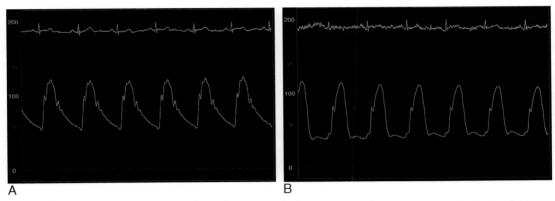

FIGURE 12-3. Example of pure ventricularization observed after engagement of a coronary catheter. **A,** The normal-appearing aortic pressure waveform **(B)** changes to a ventricular waveform with little drop in systolic pressure.

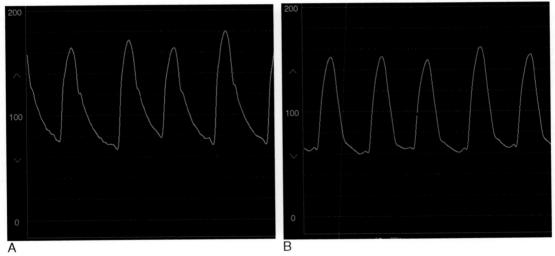

FIGURE 12-4. An example of subtle ventricularization. **A,** The catheter pressure demonstrated a normal aortic waveform prior to engagement and **(B)** showed a loss of the dicrotic notch, narrowing of the waveform, and a slight drop in diastolic pressure consistent with mild ventricularization.

TABLE 12-1.	Common Causes of Damping and/or Ventricularization of Catheter Pressure Waveform During Coronary Angiography

During Engagement of the Right Coronary Artery (RCA)
Atherosclerotic disease of the ostium of the RCA
Catheter-induced spasm of the coronary artery
Selective engagement of the conus branch of the RCA
Total occlusion of the RCA
Engagement of a small, nondominant artery

During Engagement of the Left Coronary Artery
Atherosclerotic disease of the ostium of the left main stem
Deep seating of the catheter and selective engagement of either the LAD or LCX

During Engagement of Either Coronary Artery
Presence of a small caliber artery with match in size between the diameter of the catheter and the coronary artery
Kinking of the catheter during catheter manipulation
Malposition of the catheter against the wall of the aorta
Presence of thrombus or air bubble in the catheter

LAD, Left anterior descending; *LCX,* left circumflex.

asystole. Similarly, if damping or ventricularization is caused by the presence of a small caliber coronary artery, then the naive angiographer might inject excessive contrast, causing an arrhythmia. Furthermore, if significant atherosclerotic disease is present at the ostium, a carelessly performed contrast injection into a damped catheter might dissect the proximal artery and close the vessel with potentially fatal consequences. Thus, the angiographer should be constantly vigilant for this finding. When observed, the catheter may be withdrawn into the aortic root and contrast injected into the aortic cusp to determine the presence of ostial disease. Alternatively, a very small amount of contrast may be carefully injected into the damped coronary catheter to determine the cause.

Coronary Hemodynamics

More sophisticated coronary hemodynamic measurements are now possible with recent technological advances, allowing precise flow and pressure assessments in the coronary arteries. These techniques have greatly improved our ability to understand, diagnose, and treat coronary disease. Although coronary angiography forms the basis for revascularization decisions in patients with coronary artery disease, coronary hemodynamic assessment is necessary because of the well-known limitations of angiography. Angiography provides high-quality images but is influenced by the operator's injection technique, the patient's body habitus, and the presence of overlapping vessel segments and arterial tortuosity. Particularly troublesome scenarios include eccentric lesions, diffuse disease, or lesions of intermediate stenosis severity (40%–70% narrowing). Adjunctive diagnostic testing provided by coronary hemodynamic assessment helps determine the physiologic significance of such lesions and guides revascularization decisions.

Coronary Physiology

An increase in myocardial oxygen demand, caused by an increase in wall tension, contractility, or heart rate, requires an increase in oxygen supply or else results in myocardial ischemia. Because myocardial oxygen extraction from blood is already near maximal, the only compensatory mechanism for an increase in oxygen demand is an increase in blood flow to the myocardium. Coronary blood flow is regulated by changes in coronary vascular resistance. Because the epicardial coronary arteries function primarily as conductance vessels, accounting for only 5% of total coronary vascular resistance; the small ($<300\ \mu m$), intramyocardial arterioles account for 95% of the resistance across the coronary bed and thus are the major regulators of coronary blood flow.

These small resistance vessels are influenced by multiple regulators, including endothelium-derived agents (nitrous oxide, prostaglandins, and endothelin), metabolites (adenosine, hypoxia, and hypercapnia), and neurohormonal mechanisms. The process of autoregulation provides fine control of the resistance vessels, maintaining myocardial blood flow over the relatively wide range of coronary perfusion pressures seen with physiologic changes in blood pressure. Thus, in normal individuals, myocardial perfusion is maintained when the mean aortic pressure is between 50 and 150 mmHg. Outside of this range, however, autoregulatory mechanisms fail, and coronary blood flow depends on perfusion pressure (Figure 12-5).

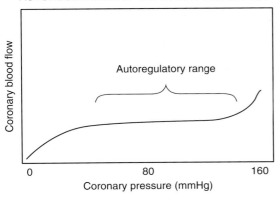

AUTOREGULATION OF CORONARY BLOOD FLOW

FIGURE 12-5. Schematic representation of the phenomenon of autoregulation, which states that coronary blood flow is maintained over the physiologic range of coronary pressure.

myocardial blood flow can be maintained over a fairly wide range of stenosis. Eventually, when stenosis severity is severe, autoregulatory mechanisms become exhausted, and myocardial blood flow decreases. During conditions of increased myocardial oxygen demand, however, autoregulatory mechanisms fail at much lower stenosis severity. Accordingly, coronary flow reserve diminishes at less severe degrees of stenosis than resting coronary blood flow. Therefore, a deficiency of coronary flow reserve implies maximal vasodilation of the resistance vessels and the presence of a hemodynamically significant stenosis.

Effects of Coronary Stenosis on Coronary Flow (Figure 12-6)

In the absence of a stenosis, coronary blood flow can increase 4–5 times above resting flow under conditions of high myocardial oxygen demand. This ability to increase blood flow over the resting state is termed *coronary flow reserve.* In the presence of a stenosis, a pressure drop will occur in a coronary artery; however, autoregulation will attempt to preserve blood flow by reducing the resistance of the small arterioles. Resting

Coronary Flow Reserve

Several different terms describe different aspects of coronary flow reserve. *Absolute flow reserve* describes the ratio of hyperemic flow in a stenotic artery to resting flow in the same artery. This is the basis of the Doppler-derived method for invasively determining coronary flow reserve. *Relative flow reserve* is the term used to describe the ratio of hyperemic flow in a stenotic artery to hyperemic flow in a normal artery. This is the primary principle upon which most noninvasive nuclear perfusion imaging techniques

FIGURE 12-6. Relation of stenosis severity to coronary blood flow. At rest, coronary blood flow is maintained despite progressive coronary stenosis until severe (>80%) stenosis occurs. During vasodilator stress, blood flow decreases from maximum flow at lesser stenosis severity. The ability to augment flow from the resting flow rates is known as flow reserve.

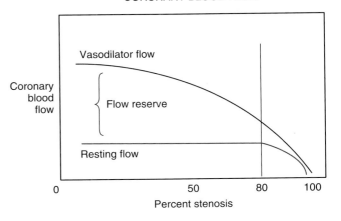

RELATION OF STENOSIS SEVERITY TO CORONARY BLOOD FLOW

are based. Importantly, relative flow reserve depends on at least one normal vascular territory; therefore, these techniques may be limited in the presence of multivessel coronary disease. Finally, *fractional flow reserve* is the term used to describe the ratio of the maximum achievable flow in the presence of a stenosis to the theoretical maximum flow in the same vessel in the absence of a stenosis.

Doppler-Derived Absolute Flow Reserve (Figure 12-7)

A 0.014-inch angioplasty guidewire outfitted with an ultrasound crystal at the tip capable of generating a Doppler signal and measuring blood flow velocity provides the means to estimate absolute flow reserve in the cardiac catheterization laboratory.[1-3] This method assumes that blood velocity is proportional to blood flow for a constant vessel area. The technique involves positioning the tip of the Doppler wire past the stenosis and obtaining a satisfactory velocity envelope. The wire tip samples blood velocity a few millimeters away from the tip, typically expressed as the average peak velocity, or APV. Normal resting APV is 15–30 cm/sec. Without moving the wire tip, hyperemia is induced either from intravenous administration of adenosine (140 µg/kg/min for at least 2–4 minutes), or from intracoronary administration of bolus adenosine (20–100 µg bolus). The average peak velocity measurement is repeated during peak hyperemia. Coronary flow reserve (or, more accurately, coronary velocity reserve) is described as the ratio of hyperemic averaged peak velocity to resting averaged peak velocity. Normal coronary velocity reserve is at least 2.0; values up to 5 may be observed. In the setting of a moderate stenosis, coronary flow reserve

less than 2.0 by the Doppler technique correlates with ischemia by nuclear perfusion techniques.[1-3] The Doppler method is rarely used for clinical purposes, mainly due to several important limitations. First, this methodology is dependent on obtaining a stable, high-quality Doppler signal, which is not always feasible, particularly in the presence of vessel tortuosity or large branches. Intermittent loss of signal due to tenuous wire position against the wall of the artery may frustrate the operator. More importantly, however, the average peak velocity varies with blood pressure and heart rate, and changes in these variables during the measurements influence the results.[4] In addition, conditions other than the status of the epicardial coronary artery affect Doppler-derived coronary flow reserve. A failure to increase the average peak velocity in response to adenosine may be due to an unresponsive microvasculature rather than the presence of a significant stenosis. Conditions associated with high resting velocities (i.e., left ventricular hypertrophy) will not augment further with adenosine. This makes the technique less useful to assess the hemodynamic significance of a stenosis in the presence of conditions associated with microvascular abnormalities such as prior myocardial infarction, heart failure, left ventricular hypertrophy, and, perhaps, diabetes mellitus.

Pressure-Derived Fractional Flow Reserve

Fractional flow reserve, or FFR, is an alternative method of assessing the hemodynamic significance of an intermediate or ambiguous coronary stenosis. This popular technique is simple to perform and is based on the measurement of the coronary pressure, using

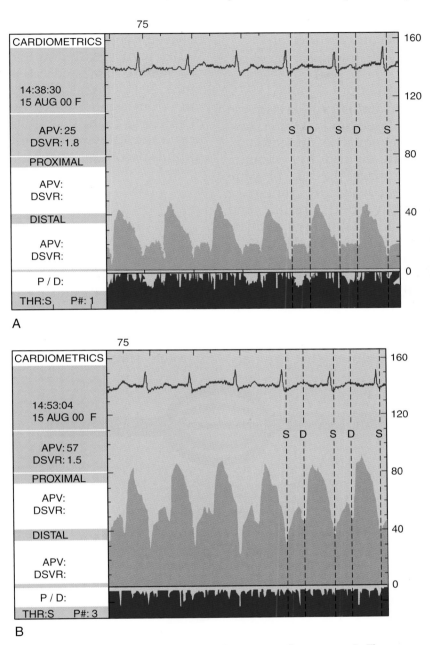

FIGURE 12-7. Example of the Doppler method of measuring coronary flow reserve. **A,** The average peak velocity at baseline was 25 cm/sec. **B,** Intravenous adenosine was infused at a rate of 140 μg/kg/min and the average peak velocity increased to 57 cm/sec.

an angioplasty guidewire outfitted with a micromanometer.

The mathematics and experimental basis of this technique have been well described.[5] The underlying concept states that fractional flow reserve is the ratio between the maximum achievable blood flow in the presence of a stenosis and the theoretical maximum flow in the absence of a stenosis (i.e., a normal artery). It can be calculated simply by the formula:

$$FFR = \frac{\text{Mean hyperemic distal intracoronary pressure}}{\text{Mean hyperemic aortic pressure}}$$

The unequivocal normal value is 1.0.

The derivation of this formula is simple (Figure 12-8). Based upon Ohm's law, coronary flow is equal to the coronary driving pressure divided by coronary resistance. Coronary driving pressure can be expressed as the difference between coronary artery pressure and coronary venous pressure (Pv), with Pv best approximated by the right atrial pressure. In the absence of a coronary stenosis, the coronary driving pressure equals the difference between the aortic pressure (Pa) and Pv. Thus, flow in the absence of a stenosis is simply (Pa – Pv)/Resistance 1. Similarly, in the presence of a coronary stenosis, the coronary driving pressure equals the difference between the pressure distal to the stenosis (Pd) and Pv, with flow in the presence of a stenosis expressed as (Pd – Pv)/Resistance 2. Fractional flow reserve is the ratio of maximum flow in the presence of a stenosis to the theoretical maximum flow if the artery were normal. Thus, the formula becomes

$$FFR = \frac{(Pd - Pv)/R_2 \text{ under maximum hyperemia}}{(Pa - Pv)/R_1 \text{ under maximum hyperemia}}$$

During maximum hyperemia, because the resistances R_1 and R_2 are very low, they will be similar and cancel out. In addition, Pv is usually very low and does not contribute significantly. The formula is usually simplified as:

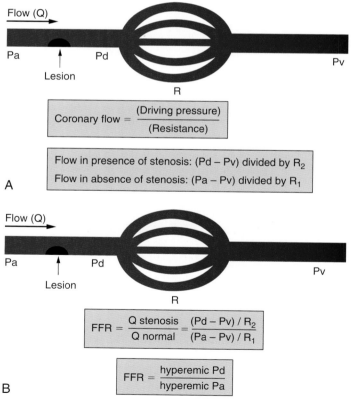

FIGURE 12-8. Derivation of fractional flow reserve. *Q*, Coronary blood flow; *Pa*, aortic pressure; *Pd*, coronary pressure distal to the stenosis; *Pv*, coronary venous pressure or right atrial pressure; *R*, resistance; *FFR*, fractional flow reserve.

$$FFR = \frac{\text{Mean hyperemic Pd}}{\text{Mean hyperemic Pa}}$$

Although the normal value of 1.0 is well accepted and has been firmly established in humans,[6] the value below which a stenosis is deemed *significant* is of some debate. Several investigations have determined the FFR value associated with ischemia on noninvasive tests.[7-9] These investigations involved patients with single vessel disease, stable chest pain syndromes, and moderate coronary lesions and excluded patients with potentially confounding conditions such as left ventricular hypertrophy or prior myocardial infarction. Based on these studies, lesions associated with ischemia have FFR <0.75. Lesions with FFR between 0.75 and 0.78 are generally recognized as *borderline* and may, in fact, represent significant lesions, particularly in the setting of left ventricular hypertrophy.

Fractional Flow Reserve Technique

Assessment of FFR is fairly straightforward to perform, using basic interventional skills (Figure 12-9). After engaging a standard angioplasty guide catheter into the coronary ostium, the pressure wire is zeroed and calibrated. Because the procedure involves instrumentation of the coronary artery, the University of Virginia Cardiac Catheterization Laboratory typically administers unfractionated heparin (50 U/kg) prior to wire passage distal to the coronary lesion. Once the operator has established that the pressures recorded from the catheter tip and the pressure wire's micromanometer are identical (Figure 12-9, B and C), the wire is advanced down the coronary artery and the transducer positioned distal to the lesion in question. The pressure waveforms are recorded at rest and during maximal hyperemia induced by one of several

methods.[10] Intracoronary adenosine is perhaps the simplest and is the most commonly used method in the University of Virginia Cardiac Catheterization Laboratories. For the left coronary artery, 80–100 µg of adenosine is injected as a bolus into the artery using a concentration of 10 µg/mL. To capture maximal hyperemia, simultaneous catheter tip (or Pa) and distal wire pressure (Pd) are recorded for 15–20 seconds. The point of maximum hyperemia is apparent at the nadir of the mean pressure typically observed several seconds after the bolus is administered. For the right coronary artery, 30–40 µg of intracoronary adenosine is usually adequate; higher doses may cause transient heart block, asystole, or bradyarrhythmias but these are transient and usually self-limiting. Alternatively, some advocate an infusion of adenosine through a large peripheral vein at 140 µg/kg/min. Intravenous administration provides a longer period of hyperemia and a more stable response but at greater cost and more potential for systemic side effects such as flushing and chest pain. Using this methodology, hyperemia is usually maximal about 1 minute into the peripheral infusion. Regardless of the method, the pressure waves are recorded during hyperemia, and FFR is simply calculated as Pd/Pa during hyperemia, as described (Figure 12-9, D). Most operators end the procedure by withdrawing the pressure transducer to the catheter tip, verifying that the pressures remain equal and confirming that transducer drift has not occurred, establishing the reliability of the measurements.

Several important considerations and potential sources of errors when making these measurements include the following:

1. The operator should be careful to note if engagement of the guide catheter causes pressure damping or ventricularization. This will falsely lower the Pa and

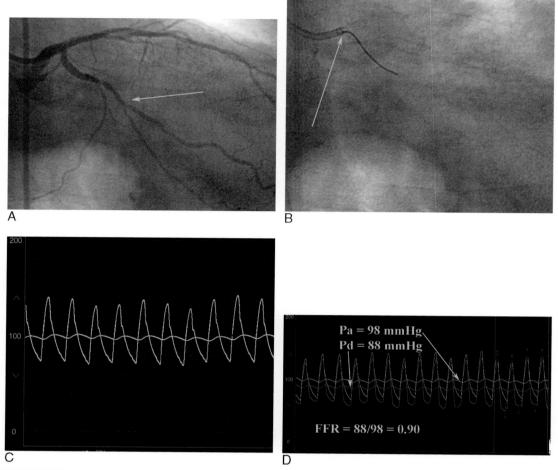

FIGURE 12-9. **A,** Example of method for measuring fractional flow reserve. A moderate lesion is seen in the mid-portion of the left circumflex artery *(arrow)*. **B,** The pressure wire is placed initially with the transducer *(arrow)* at the guide tip to ensure that **(C)** the guide pressure and wire transducer pressure are identical. The wire is then advanced with the transducer positioned past the lesion. Baseline pressures are usually sampled and then maximal hyperemia induced with adenosine. **D,** During maximal hyperemia, pressures are sampled at the catheter tip or aorta *(Pa)* and distal to the lesion *(Pd)*. In this case, the FFR = 0.90.

an erroneously high calculated FFR (Figure 12-10). Furthermore, if the intracoronary method of adenosine administration is used, the operator should avoid using a guide catheter with side-holes and be sure the catheter is selectively engaged. This ensures that the adenosine bolus actually sees the coronary circulation; otherwise, maximal hyperemia will not occur, underestimating FFR.

2. If the FFR value obtained with intracoronary adenosine is in the intermediate range (i.e., between 0.75 and 0.78), the operator should consider repeating the measurement at higher bolus doses of adenosine or by using intravenous adenosine before concluding that the lesion is not hemodynamically significant.

3. A point often not considered relates to the potential risk of guidewire instrumentation of an atherosclerotic coronary artery. Rarely, the guidewire results in disruption or dissection of the atherosclerotic plaque and abrupt vessel closure. Therefore, if the lesion in question is not amenable to percutaneous interventional techniques, FFR should not be performed.

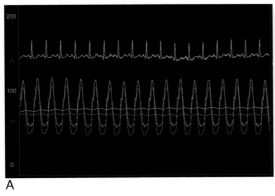
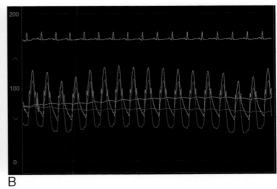

A   B

FIGURE 12-10. Example of a potential source of error during FFR measurement. **A,** A subtle ventricularization of the guide catheter, resulting in a falsely low Pa pressure (74 mmHg) with a Pd pressure of 68 mmHg and a calculated FFR of 0.92, suggesting that this lesion is not significant. **B,** However, when the guide catheter is repositioned into the aorta, the Pa pressure rises to 86 mmHg with a Pd of 64 and a calculated FFR of 0.75, suggesting that the lesion is, in fact, a significant one.

4. Finally, transducer pressure drift can occur during the performance of the procedure. For this reason, confirmation that the catheter-tip pressure and the pressure wire transducers are the same at the conclusion of the case provides the operator great confidence in the FFR measurement obtained.

Clinical Applications of Fractional Flow Reserve

Coronary hemodynamic assessment is indispensable in the current practice of interventional cardiology. Application to common clinical scenarios includes evaluation of moderate or ambiguous coronary lesions, left main stem disease, multivessel disease, diffuse disease and tandem lesions, as well as for post-coronary intervention assessment.

Fractional flow reserve is most commonly used to assess lesions that appear only modestly narrowed. Angiography alone is notoriously misleading in this subset. Not only are experienced interventional cardiologists unable to discriminate significant from nonflow limiting lesions by angiography alone, but also they completely disagree regarding the significance of the same lesions![11]

Figure 12-11 is an example of the value of FFR in a 52-year-old woman with peripheral vascular disease and a remote history of a coronary intervention on the right coronary artery now presenting with a stable anginal syndrome. Angiography revealed total occlusion of a small right coronary artery and normal-appearing left main stem and left circumflex arteries. The left anterior descending artery had a stenosis of moderate severity at the bifurcation of a diagonal branch (Figure 12-11, *A*). Despite imaging in multiple views, the lesion did not appear particularly worrisome or severe. However, FFR assessment demonstrated that this lesion was hemodynamically significant with an FFR calculated at 0.71 (Figure 12-11, *B*).

Another common indication for FFR is for the assessment of ambiguous lesions, that is, coronary disease not well visualized by angiography either because of overlapping segments, vessel tortuosity, or lesion eccentricity. Fractional flow reserve assessment is especially valuable when the patient's clinical symptoms are atypical. The FFR measurement can be extremely valuable to the cardiologist who wishes to reconcile the clinical syndrome and the angiogram. If the ambiguous lesion is not significant, it is unlikely

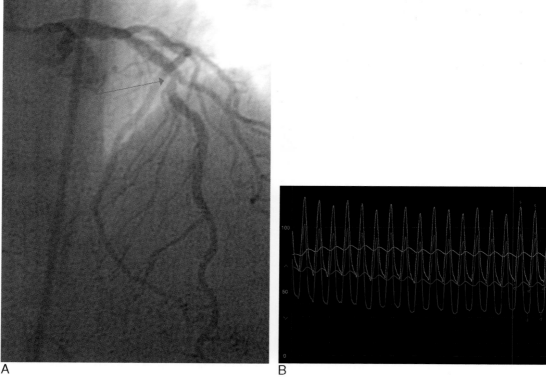

A   B

FIGURE 12-11. **A,** Example of the value of FFR in determining the significance of a moderate stenosis of the left anterior descending artery in a 52-year-old woman. **B,** FFR was calculated at 0.71 consistent with a hemodynamically significant stenosis.

that the patient's atypical symptoms are due to the stenosis or that the condition will improve if revascularized. Alternatively, the angiogram may underrepresent an important stenosis, causing the practitioner to erroneously dismiss the symptoms as noncardiac.

The angiogram shown in Figure 12-12 reveals an ambiguous lesion in the proximal left anterior descending artery in a 55-year-old morbidly obese woman with dyspnea on exertion and an abnormal but nondiagnostic noninvasive study. Left ventricular function was normal and no atherosclerotic disease was found in the right coronary and circumflex arteries. In this case, a complex array of branches emanated from the proximal segment of the left anterior descending artery, overlapping the area in question. In addition, the patient's body habitus limited the

range of angiographic angles, preventing optimal visualization of the area. An FFR of 0.94 confirmed that this lesion was not significant and therefore not responsible for the clinical syndrome.

It is important for the cardiologist to understand the natural history of patients with either ambiguous lesions or lesions of moderate severity in whom revascularization is deferred based on the presence of a nonischemic FFR. This was the focus of several studies summarized in Table 12-2. The 12-month rate of major adverse events (cardiac death, nonfatal myocardial infarction, or target vessel revascularization), ranging from 8%–14%, was surprisingly consistent across all studies.[12–17] The few events during follow-up were nearly all due to target vessel revascularization; the rates of death or nonfatal infarction were very low. These data

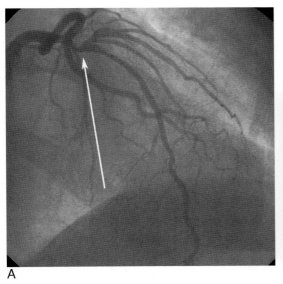

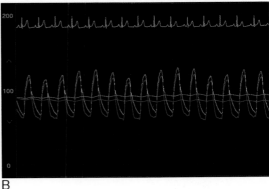

A   B

FIGURE 12-12. **A,** Example of an ambiguous lesion in the proximal left anterior descending artery. Note the complex array of vessels that surround the lesion, making it difficult to see by angiography. **B,** FFR was 0.94, confirming that this lesion was not significant.

TABLE 12-2.	Outcome of Patients with Fractional Flow Reserve Greater than 0.75 in Whom Revascularization Is Deferred		
AUTHOR	**PTS**	**FOLLOW-UP**	**EVENT RATE**
Bech et al., 1998[12]	100	18 months	10%
Bech et al., 2001[13]	91	12 months	8%
Chamuleau et al., 2002[14]	92	12 months	11%
Rieber et al., 2002[15]	59	12 months	11%
Mates et al., 2005[16]	85	24 months	13%
Fischer et al., 2006[17]	111	12 months	14%

reassures the practitioner and the patient that revascularization is not necessary for lesions that appear moderately narrowed on angiography with an FFR >0.75. However, important caveats to these studies exist. They consist primarily of patients with stable coronary disease as these studies typically exclude patients with acute coronary syndromes. The pathobiology of a moderate stenosis seen in the setting of an acute coronary syndrome may be different and associated with a higher event rate. Furthermore, there is little information on unselected, "real world" patients in whom FFR is routinely used

to make decisions. In addition, non-U.S. patients constitute the bulk of the published studies; in the United States, there may be different patient expectations and referral physician demands that lead to higher rates of revascularization during follow-up.

Significant atherosclerotic narrowing of the left main coronary artery is a potentially life-threatening condition that may not always be easily imaged by coronary angiography, which is particularly true for lesions that involve the ostium, an area commonly obscured from clear view. Such lesions are ideal for assessment by FFR, allowing the physician fewer sleepless nights worrying about a decision based solely on the angiogram. This topic has been explored, and several studies have demonstrated the safety of deferring revascularization of ambiguous left main stem lesions with FFR >0.75.[18,19] An example of an ambiguous left main lesion assessed by FFR is shown in Figure 12-13.

Patients with multivessel disease represent another challenging subset. The choice of revascularization (i.e., surgery

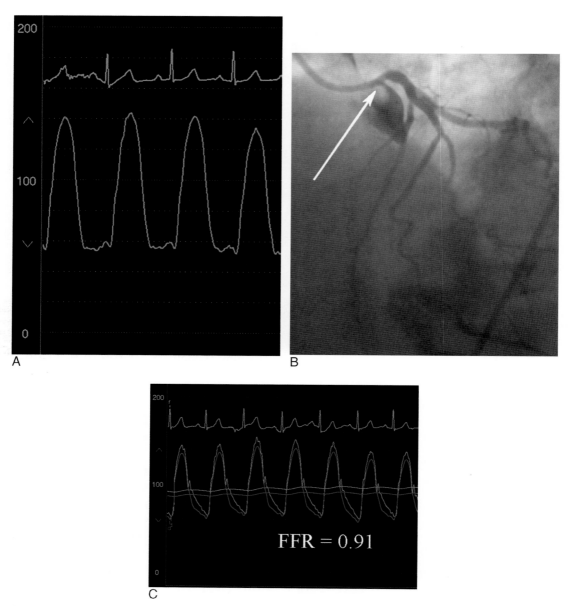

FIGURE 12-13. Example of the role of FFR determination in assessment of an ambiguous left main lesion. **A,** The catheter pressure waveform ventricularized and damped. **B,** Angiography identified an ostial narrowing of moderate severity of the left main artery *(arrow).* **C,** Coronary pressure measurement determined the FFR at 0.91.

vs. percutaneous intervention) is often based on the angiogram. While a "culprit" lesion is often readily apparent, the significance of disease in other arteries may be difficult to discern. Myocardial perfusion imaging, based on the concept of relative flow reserve, may be entirely normal despite severe three-vessel disease because of "balanced" ischemia.[20,21] Again, in

such scenarios, FFR can allow the physician to make revascularization decisions with great confidence (Figure 12-14).

Diffuse coronary disease and tandem, or serial, lesions represent unique subsets difficult to assess by angiography alone. Coronary hemodynamic assessment can prove extremely valuable in these settings. Recall that coronary angiography

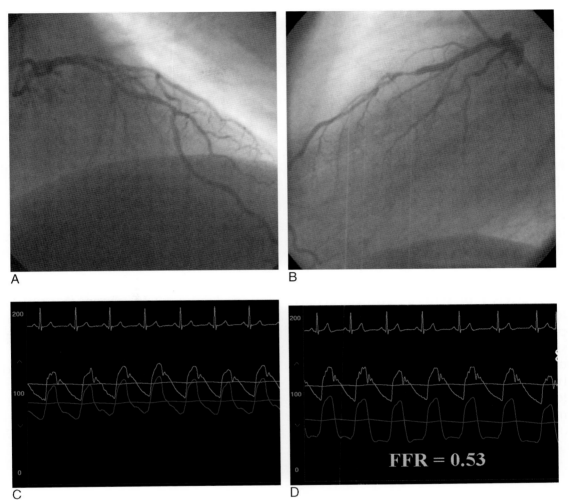

FIGURE 12-14. Example of use of FFR for assessment of multivessel coronary disease. A 60-year-old man with classic angina pectoris undergoes a stress test that reveals inferior ischemia. Coronary angiography confirmed a severe narrowing of the right coronary artery. **A–B,** However, the left coronary angiogram showed moderate narrowing of the mid-portion of left anterior descending artery. **C,** The lesion was crossed with a pressure wire demonstrating a large gradient at rest; **(D)** following administration of 80 µg of intracoronary adenosine, the FFR = 0.53 and thus represents a hemodynamically significant lesion.

represents only the arterial lumen. Angiography accurately identifies and characterizes coronary artery disease only in the presence of a normal *reference* segment. Atherosclerosis may involve the entire artery, however, making it difficult to appreciate the extent of arterial narrowing by angiography alone. Coronary hemodynamic assessment has the potential of detecting disease not apparent on angiography. In a study of patients with angiographic coronary disease in one artery, a significant pressure gradient existed between the aorta and the distal coronary artery of another, angiographic "normal" artery in 57% of arteries; in 8% of such normal arteries, the FFR was <0.75, demonstrating the truly diffuse nature of coronary disease.[22]

A modification in the technique for FFR assessment is required in the setting of diffuse coronary disease. Because there is no specific, focal lesion, the pressure transducer is positioned in the distal artery and slowly pulled back during hyperemia. This technique requires sustained hyperemia that mandates the use of an intravenous infusion of adenosine at 140 µg/kg/min. The duration of hyperemia induced by intracoronary adenosine is too brief and will likely dissipate during the course of the pullback. Typically, the lowest FFR value is at the most distal site, and a slow, progressive rise in the FFR occurs as the pressure wire is withdrawn toward the guide catheter (Figure 12-15). Occasionally, the operator may note an abrupt step-up in the hyperemic pressure gradient, suggesting a more focal area of disease treatable with stenting.

Determination of the significance of tandem, or serial, lesions within the same artery represents a significant challenge to the operator. One cannot simply calculate hyperemic Pd/Pa at each site because significant interaction occurs between the two lesions. With two lesions in tandem, FFR of the distal lesion is influenced by both the proximal and distal stenosis. Similarly, FFR of the proximal stenosis is affected by

the presence of the distal stenosis. Flow through the first stenosis will be submaximal, leading to a falsely high FFR, potentially misclassifying a hemodynamically significant stenosis. Equations for the calculation of FFR for sequential stenosis have been described but are cumbersome and not suitable for application to routine clinical practice.[23,24] Probably the most practical method is to simply measure the FFR across the distal stenosis. This will determine if the serial lesions together constitute a significant stenosis. If FFR <0.75, then the operator can either treat both lesions or treat the most severe lesion and repeat FFR of the remaining single lesion. Figure 12-16 shows the use of FFR in a case of sequential stenoses that involves the left anterior descending artery.

Fractional flow reserve has been used to assess the results of coronary stenting. Ideally, the operator strives for an FFR >0.95 following coronary stent placement because an FFR value of >0.94–0.96

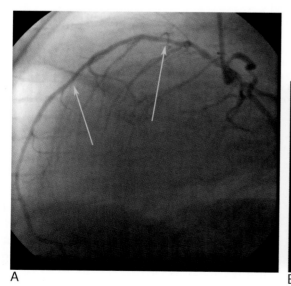
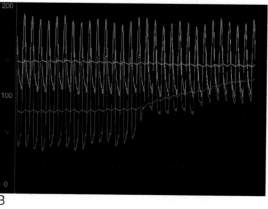

A   B

FIGURE 12-15. An example of diffuse disease that involves the left anterior descending artery. **A,** The angiogram showed only moderate, diffuse disease that involves the proximal to mid-portion of the artery *(arrows).* **B,** With the wire positioned distally, and under conditions of sustained, maximal hyperemia with intravenous adenosine, FFR was determined to be 0.59. The wire was slowly pulled back with a slow, progressive rise in distal pressure noted all the way to the proximal segment of the artery.

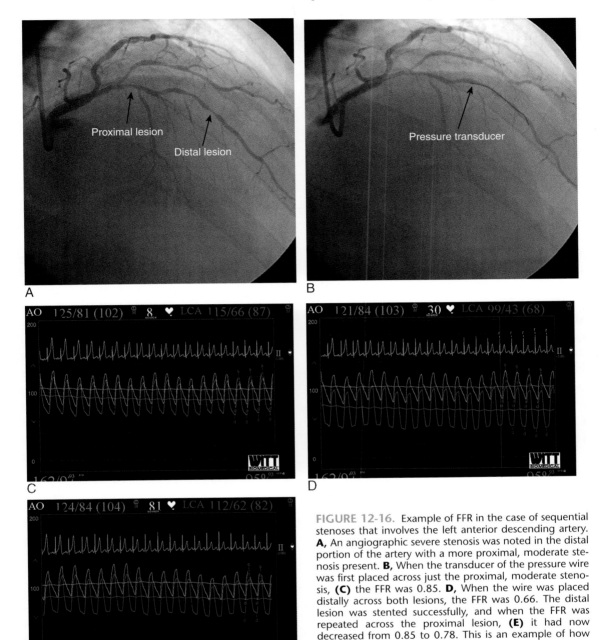

FIGURE 12-16. Example of FFR in the case of sequential stenoses that involves the left anterior descending artery. **A,** An angiographic severe stenosis was noted in the distal portion of the artery with a more proximal, moderate stenosis present. **B,** When the transducer of the pressure wire was first placed across just the proximal, moderate stenosis, **(C)** the FFR was 0.85. **D,** When the wire was placed distally across both lesions, the FFR was 0.66. The distal lesion was stented successfully, and when the FFR was repeated across the proximal lesion, **(E)** it had now decreased from 0.85 to 0.78. This is an example of how a distal lesion may falsely raise the FFR of the more proximal lesion and exemplifies the complexity of FFR assessment in the setting of tandem lesions.

correlates with optimal stent deployment by intravascular ultrasound.[25,26] More importantly, the post-stent FFR correlates with outcome. A large, multicenter registry, performed in the bare metal stent era, found a 6-month major adverse cardiac event rate of only 5%–6% if the FFR measured >0.90 post-stenting compared to a rate of adverse events of 21% if post-stent FFR measured <0.90 (Figure 12-17).[27] Importantly, however, it may not always be possible to achieve

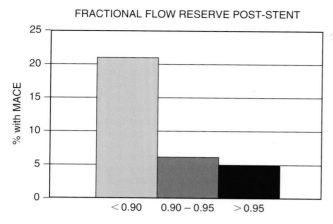

FRACTIONAL FLOW RESERVE POST-STENT

FIGURE 12-17. Relationship between post-stent FFR and major adverse cardiac events *(MACE)* during follow-up. (Adapted from Pijls NH, Klauss V, Siebert U, et al. Coronary pressure measurement after stenting predicts adverse events at follow-up. A multicenter registry. *Circulation* 2002;105:2950–2954.)

such high FFR values post-stenting. The post-stent FFR does not solely reflect the status of the stent deployment or degree of residual stenosis at the stent site. The presence of unappreciated disease proximal to the stent is a common alternate explanation for a suboptimal FFR after stent deployment.

Criticisms of Fractional Flow Reserve Theory

Fractional flow reserve assessment has become an established adjunctive to angiography, and FFR values <0.75 are generally accepted as hemodynamically significant or *ischemic*. Nevertheless, several important limitations and criticisms exist of the theory behind FFR assessment.[28] First, some critics question the validity of FFR in conditions associated with abnormal microvasculature such as extensive myocardial infarction and left ventricular hypertrophy. Second, some of the underlying assumptions of FFR theory may be in error. For example, myocardial resistance may not be constant or uniform during hyperemia. In fact, microvascular resistance may increase from rest to hyperemia in the presence of a stenosis. Thus, cancelling resistance may overestimate the true FFR. A common shortcut is to ignore venous pressure; however, this

may not be appropriate. This may be particularly true if the FFR is the so-called *indeterminate* or *gray* zone of 0.75–0.78. Consider the following example. If, during maximum hyperemia, the Pa = 105 mmHg and the Pd = 80 mmHg, and the right atrial pressure is ignored, then FFR = 0.78 and the lesion is classified as *nonsignificant*. If right atrial pressure were taken into consideration and measured only 5 mmHg, then the corrected FFR would not change the designation of the lesion (FFR = 0.77). If, however, the right atrial pressure were elevated at 25 mmHg, then the FFR would now calculate to 0.71, changing the lesion designation. Therefore, it might make sense to consider measuring right atrial pressure when lesions are in the gray zone of 0.75–0.78. The third criticism is that FFR theory idealizes many of the relationships between pressure and flow; however, in reality, a nonlinear relationship exists between flow and pressure and there are complex fluid dynamics due to viscosity, post-stenotic pressure loss, etc. involved, thus undermining the idealized relationship.

Future Directions

Important future directions for coronary hemodynamics include the ability to simultaneously measure both FFR and CFR. This would help discern the role of the microvasculature versus the epicardial coronary artery in various clinical syndromes such as anginal pain in the presence of *nonischemic* FFR or as a method of detecting subclinical disease in certain patient subsets. Thus, hemodynamic coronary assessment is likely to achieve a greater level of sophistication than at present, providing greater refinement in our understanding of coronary artery disease.

References

1. Joye JD, Schulman DS, Lasorda D, et al. Intracoronary Doppler guide wire versus stress single-photon emission computed tomographic thallium-201 imaging in assessment of intermediate coronary stenoses. *J Am Coll Cardiol* 1994;24:940–947.
2. Miller DD, Donohue TJ, Younis LT, et al. Correlation of pharmacological Tc-sestamibi myocardial perfusion imaging with poststenotic coronary flow reserve in patients with angiographically intermediate coronary artery stenoses. *Circulation* 1994;89:2150–2160.
3. Donohue TJ, Miller DD, Bach RG, et al. Correlation of poststenotic hyperemic coronary flow velocity and pressure with abnormal stress myocardial perfusion imaging in coronary artery disease. *Am J Cardiol* 1996;77:948–954.
4. Gould KL, KirKeeide RL, Buchi M. Coronary flow reserve as a physiologic measure of stenosis severity. *J Am Coll Cardiol* 1990;15:459–474.
5. Pijls NHJ, van Son JAM, Kirkeeide RL, et al. Experimental basis of determining maximum coronary, myocardial, and collateral blood flow by pressure measurements for assessing functional stenosis severity before and after percutaneous transluminal coronary angioplasty. *Circulation* 1993;87:1354–1367.
6. Pijls NHJ, Van Gelder B, Van der Voort P, et al. Fractional flow reserve: A useful index to evaluate the influence of an epicardial coronary stenosis on myocardial blood flow. *Circulation* 1995;92:3183–3193.
7. De Bruyne B, Baudhuin T, Melin JA, et al. Coronary flow reserve calculated from pressure measurements in humans: Validation with positron emission tomography. *Circulation* 1994;89:1013–1022.
8. De Bruyne B, Bartunek J, Sys SU, Heyndrickx GR. Relation between myocardial fractional flow reserve calculated from coronary pressure measurements and exercise-induced myocardial ischemia. *Circulation* 1995;92:39–46.
9. Pijls NHJ, De Bruyne B, Peels K, et al. Measurement of fractional flow reserve to assess the functional severity of coronary-artery stenoses. *N Engl J Med* 1996;334:1703–1708.
10. Casella G, Leibig M, Schiele TM, et al. Are high doses of intracoronary adenosine an alternative to standard intravenous adenosine for the assessment of fractional flow reserve? *Am Heart J* 2004;148:590–595.
11. Fischer JJ, Samady H, McPherson JA, et al. Comparison between visual assessment and quantitative angiography versus fractional flow reserve for native coronary narrowings of moderate severity. *Am J Cardiol* 2002;90:210–215.
12. Bech GJW, DeBruyne B, Bonnier HJRM, et al. Long-term follow-up after deferral of percutaneous transluminal coronary angioplasty of intermediate stenosis on the basis of coronary pressure measurement. *J Am Coll Cardiol* 1998;31:841–847.
13. Bech GJ, De Bruyne B, Pijls NH, et al. Fractional flow reserve to determine the appropriateness of angioplasty in moderate coronary stenosis: A randomized trial. *Circulation* 2001;103:2928–2934.
14. Chamuleau SA, Meuwissen M, Koch KT, et al. Usefulness of fractional flow reserve for risk stratification of patients with multivessel coronary artery disease and an intermediate stenosis. *Am J Cardiol* 2002;89:377–380.
15. Rieber J, Schiele TM, Koenig A, et al. Long-term safety of therapy stratification in patients with intermediate coronary lesions based on intracoronary pressure measurements. *Am J Cardiol* 2002;90:1160–1164.
16. Mates M, Hrabos V, Hajek P, et al. Long-term follow-up after deferral of coronary intervention based on myocardial fractional flow reserve measurement. *Coron Artery Dis* 2005;16:169–174.
17. Fischer JJ, Wang XQ, Samady H, et al. Outcome of patients with acute coronary syndromes and moderate coronary lesions undergoing deferral of revascularization based on fractional flow reserve assessment. *Catheter Cardiovasc Interv* 2006;68(4):544–548.
18. Bech GJ, Droste H, Pijls NH, et al. Value of fractional flow reserve in making decisions about bypass surgery for equivocal left main coronary artery disease. *Heart* 2001;86:547–552.
19. Vasti V, Ivan E, Yalamanchili V, et al. Correlations between fractional flow reserve and intravascular ultrasound in patients with an ambiguous left main coronary artery stenosis. *Circulation* 2004;110:2831–2836.
20. Lima RS, Watson DD, Goode AR, et al. Incremental value of combined perfusion and function over perfusion alone by gated SPECT myocardial perfusion imaging for detection of severe three vessel coronary artery disease. *J Am Coll Cardiol* 2003;42:64–70.
21. Aarnoudse WH, Botman KJ, Pijls NH. False-negative myocardial scintigraphy in balanced three-vessel disease, revealed by coronary pressure measurement. *Int J Cardiovasc Interv* 2003;5:67–71.
22. DeBruyne B, Hersbach F, Pijls NH, et al. Abnormal epicardial coronary resistance in patients with diffuse atherosclerosis but "normal" coronary angiography. *Circulation* 2001;104:2401–2406.
23. DeBruyne B, Pijls NH, Heyndrickx GR, et al. Pressure-derived fractional flow reserve to assess serial epicardial stenoses. Theoretical basis and animal validation. *Circulation* 2000;101:1840–1847.
24. Pijls NH, De Bruyne B, Bech GJ, et al. Coronary pressure measurement to assess the hemodynamic significance of serial stenoses within one coronary artery. Validation in humans. *Circulation* 2000;102:2371–2377.
25. Hanekamp C, Koolen JJ, Pijls NH, et al. Comparison of quantitative coronary angiography, intravascular

ultrasound and pressure-derived fractional flow reserve to assess optimal stent deployment. *Circulation* 2004;99:1015–1021.

26. Fearon WF, Luna J, Samady H, et al. Fractional flow reserve compared with intravascular ultrasound guidance for optimizing stent deployment. *Circulation* 2001;104:1917–1922.

27. Pijls NH, Klauss V, Siebert U, et al. Coronary pressure measurement after stenting predicts adverse events at follow-up. A multicenter registry. *Circulation* 2002;105:2950–2954.

28. Bishop AH, Samady H. Fractional flow reserve: Critical review of an important physiologic adjunct to angiography. *Am Heart J* 2004;147:792–802.

Chapter 13

Advanced Hemodynamic Assessment of Ventricular Function

D. Scott Lim, MD, and
Howard P. Gutgesell, MD

Commonly, ventricular function assessment is performed by relatively crude and inaccurate methods that are load-dependent. Angiographically assessed left ventricular (LV) ejection fraction is a frequently performed index of LV systolic function but is based on certain assumptions about geometric symmetry and is affected by both preload and afterload.[1-3] Left ventricular end-diastolic pressure is also commonly cited as an index of LV diastolic performance[4] but is also similarly affected by both volume and pressure-loading conditions.[5] In the earlier days of cardiology, investigators focused on isolated nonhuman cardiac muscle preparations to elucidate the underlying mechanisms of ventricular performance, and these observations were applied to the cardiac patient at the bedside by clinicians. However, up until recently, these advanced measurements were neither practical nor sufficiently real-time to be applied clinically.

In this chapter, we will cover the principles of the invasively measured indices derived from commercially available pressure-volume loop recordings. Examples are shown from patients with congenital heart disease recorded in real-time, both prior to and after transcatheter intervention.

Equipment

Commercially available equipment (CD Leycom, Zoetermeer, The Netherlands) has been developed to determine the real-time volume of the LV by means of the conductance catheter technique.[6,7] This principle uses a low-energy electric field between two poles on the catheter, and a series of electrodes located in between those two poles measures the conductance of the electrical field. As the volume of blood that separates the electrical field changes, the conductance of the electrical field also changes, and thus the change in volume of the surrounding blood pool can be rapidly inferred. Our laboratory uses either of two commercially available conductance catheters (Millar Instruments, Houston, or Sentron, Zoetermeer, the Netherlands), placed either retrograde into the left ventricle or by transvenous approach into the systemic ventricle (Figure 13-1). Both types of catheters have at least one high-fidelity pressure sensor for simultaneous pressure measurements.

To differentiate between the conductance of the ventricular blood pool and the surrounding tissue, parallel conductance (Vc) correction is performed by injecting 10 milliliters of hypertonic (3%) saline in a pulmonary artery catheter.[8] The hypertonic saline bolus transiently changes the conductance of the blood pool, allowing differentiation between it and the static conductance of the surrounding tissues. For exact volume measurements, α correction is performed by calibration with stroke volume (measured either by thermodilution cardiac output measurement or the Fick principle, divided by the heart rate). After positioning the conductance catheter in the ventricle of interest, it is then connected to a CFL-512 Cardiac Function Computer (CD Leycom).

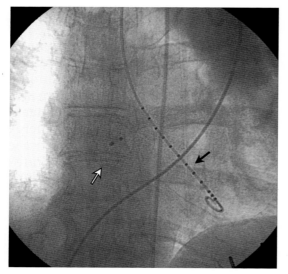

FIGURE 13-1. Cineradiogram of retrograde placement of conductance catheter in the left ventricle. The *closed black arrow* indicates the conductance catheter positioned from a retrograde approach into the body of the left ventricle. The *white arrow* is an atrial septal defect occluder. Stable position during measurements is confirmed both by loop analysis and by fluoroscopic markers.

Other laboratories have also used the Sigma5 conductance computer (CD Leycom). Both types of catheters have a high-fidelity pressure sensor at the tip. Either will allow the real-time measurement of the pressure-volume relationship.

The Pressure-Volume Loop

The real-time recorded relationship between ventricular pressure and volume is plotted and shown in Figure 13-2. As the data are acquired in the ventricle, a counterclockwise loop is created. This direction of the loop is important in distinguishing between ventricular and aortic positioning of the catheter; in the latter case, a clockwise loop is created. Figure 13-3 shows the relationship between chamber volume and time. Note that in the aorta, pressure rises with systole and the aorta distends, increasing the volume. This relationship is in contrast to the ventricle, in which the rising pressure during systole is associated with a decrease in chamber volume. The volume measurements are divided into a series of discs based upon the number of conductance sensors in the catheter. If a superior segment of the volume measurement, plotted against the simultaneous pressure measurements, changes from a counterclockwise loop to a clockwise loop, it means that the catheter position has migrated out of the ventricle with ventricular contraction. Our laboratory uses both this technique as well as fluoroscopic

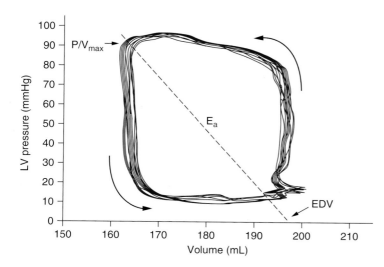

FIGURE 13-2. The pressure-volume loop. This diagram was taken from measurements at baseline in a patient prior to percutaneous closure of an atrial septal defect. The *open arrow* demonstrates the point of end-diastole, coincident with the R wave on the electrocardiogram. The loop, starting at end-diastole (referenced from the *QRS* on the electrocardiogram) proceeds in a counterclockwise direction through isovolumic contraction, to the ejection phase, which ends in end-systole. End-systole *(closed arrow)* is determined by the maximum P/V ratio, which then starts the isovolumic relaxation phase. Afterload is measured as the slope of the line (E_a) from end-systole to the end-diastolic volume at zero pressure *(EDV)*.

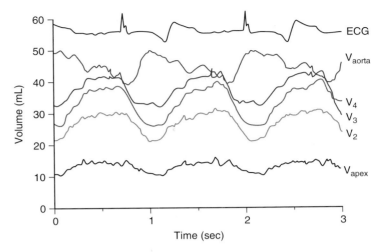

FIGURE 13-3. Catheter positioning by volume measurements. The first four volume segments, from V_{apex} to V_4, are located within the ventricle as demonstrated by the simultaneous decrease in volumes during systole and increase during diastole. The most superior segment, V_{aorta}, is showing the expected volume rise as the aorta distends with systolic ventricular contraction and the reverse during diastole.

landmarks to maintain a consistent position of the catheter within the ventricle to generate reproducible measurements.

Methods of Recording

Derivatives of the high-fidelity pressure recordings are used to determine several indices of ventricular function. These measurements are affected by noise in the recording system, and, frequently, curve-smoothing algorithms are used as well as multiple beat averaging to record a stable pressure-volume loop. Additionally, measurements are taken with breath-hold at end-expiration. Often, the currently available catheters are without a lumen and therefore are difficult to manipulate in a retrograde fashion across abnormal aortic valves without damage to the catheter. To solve this problem, our laboratory first positions a long sheath retrograde across the aortic valve to the LV apex, through which we can then advance the conductance catheter. The long sheath is then pulled back, exposing the conductance catheter to the left ventricle.

Indices Measured

The ultimate measurement of ventricular function is the load-independent indices of elastance, or end-systolic pressure-volume relationship,[9] and compliance, or end-diastolic pressure volume relationship (Figure 13-4).[10] Elastance is determined by the slope of the end-systolic points of the pressure-volume loop obtained under changing of the loading conditions.[11] Preload and afterload can be changed by one of several methods: (1) acute volume challenge, (2) inferior vena caval occlusion using a balloon, and (3) phenylephrine infusion. End-systole is defined as the point of maximum pressure/volume ratio.[4] The end-systolic pressure-volume relationship, as the ultimate load-independent index of ventricular systolic function, is particularly useful in the evaluation of interventions that may affect ventricular function as well as loading conditions. Our laboratory has used this index in evaluation of percutaneous repair of large atrial septal defects, in which the repair acutely volume loads the left ventricle, to determine whether the occlusion device may also adversely affect cardiac mechanics. In 28 patients studied, we found that, as expected, the preload-dependent indices showed the expected alterations, but that elastance also increased, possibly related to improved LV geometry.[12]

End-diastole is defined as coincident with the electrocardiographic T wave.

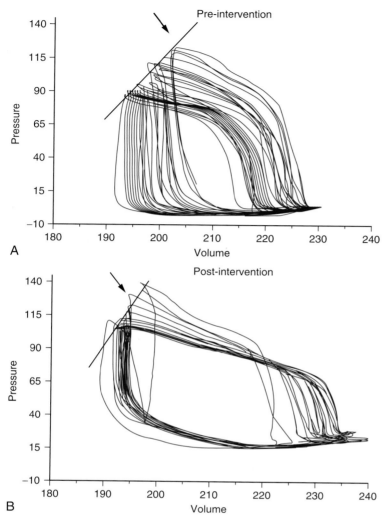

A

B

FIGURE 13-4. Elastance pre-intervention and post-intervention. **A,** From a stable pressure-volume loop recording, loading conditions are changed with phenylephrine and saline bolus (to augment afterload and preload, respectively), and the series of end-systolic points is plotted in the graph. The slope of this line *(closed black arrow)* yields the value of elastance, or the end-systolic pressure-volume relationship, which is a load-independent index of ventricular systolic function. **B,** After the intervention is performed (in this case, closure of an atrial septal defect), elastance is remeasured.

Compliance is similarly determined by the slope of the end-diastolic points of the pressure-volume loop under changing of the loading conditions. However, preliminary data suggest that the slope of the end-diastolic pressure-volume relationship may not be linear, and further work is needed to clarify this.[10,13]

Specific indices of ventricular function have been determined from the first derivatives of the change in pressure. Although these indices derived from the pressure waveform are affected by loading conditions, they have some use in defining ventricular function.

When the slope of the change in pressure with respect to the change in time is plotted (Figure 13-5), the maximal and minimum values become apparent. The peak maximal value, $+dP/dt_{max}$, is a preload-dependent index of ventricular function.[14] *In vivo*, it has been shown to be relatively afterload-independent,[15] and the degree of preload-dependence is generally less than 10%.[15–17] However, the range of normal values appears to

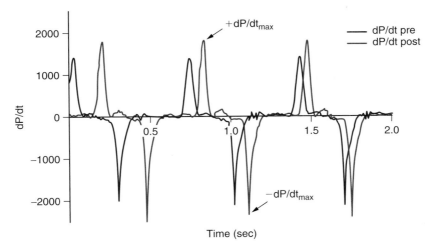

FIGURE 13-5. Measurement of dP/dt pre-intervention and post-intervention. The first derivative of the change in ventricular pressure with respect to time is plotted, and maximum and minimum values become clear.

be between 1350 and 2144 mmHg/sec for the left ventricle, and given the smaller muscle mass of the normal right ventricle, normal values in the right ventricle are 233–296 mmHg/sec. [15,16,18] As such, its value is in intrapatient assessment of ventricular function before and after an intervention that does not markedly change volume-loading conditions. However, due to its ease in measurement, this index is one of the more commonly measured, particularly because it may also be derived from easily measured noninvasive Doppler methods.

Attempts have been made to account for the preload-dependence of $+dP/dt_{max}$, by correcting it using the developed isovolumic pressure (dP/dt/IP). This index has been shown to be preload and afterload independent in the isolated canine model[19] but has not been validated in humans.

Similarly, the peak minimal value, or $-dP/dt_{min}$, has also been shown to be affected by inotropic agents and is thought to be a relatively crude assessment of diastolic function.[20,21] While normal ranges have been established (1581–2661 mmHg/sec),[22,23] it has been shown to be exquisitely sensitive to preload and afterload conditions,[21,24]

rendering this index less useful as an invasive assessment of diastolic function.

Another index derived from the changing ventricular pressure signal is tau (τ), also known as the time constant of isovolumic relaxation.[25] Tau has been shown to be a preload-independent measure of ventricular diastolic function.[26] This measure is derived from the time it takes for the pressure to fall from the point of $-dP/dt_{min}$ to the inverse natural log of that pressure, and is expressed in milliseconds. Given that there remains some uncertainty with measurement of compliance, and that the other indices of diastolic function are significantly preload dependent, tau is the most reliable assessment of diastolic function currently available. Although normal values have not been determined, its value has been correlated with postoperative outcomes in single ventricle patients.[27] It may be measured in real-time by commercially available software (CD Leycom).

Limitations of the Technique

In vivo human use of these techniques is now possible using commercially available and FDA-approved equipment. The cost of the equipment and lack of third-party reimbursement limit its usage primarily to research endeavors. Additionally, to make accurate and reliable volumetric measurements, the conductance catheter technique relies on calibration to cardiac output (α correlation). The frequently used techniques (thermodilution or Fick method) have a significant degree of variability. Therefore, our laboratory has found that the conductance catheter technique is most reliable for intrapatient assessment, particularly before and after interventions that may affect either ventricular function or loading conditions. However, we have not been as confident with interpatient assessment and the value of absolute values of these indices of ventricular function.

Future Directions

The high cost of the equipment precludes its general clinical usage. With future evolution of this technology to lower cost equipment, it is possible that this will supplant the currently used, relatively crude assessments, such as angiographic ejection fraction and cardiac output measurement, which are highly dependent on loading conditions. Additionally, as MRI-guided catheter interventions develop, real-time assessment of volume measurements in combination with invasive pressure recordings will afford a similar hybrid approach to ventricular function analysis.

References

1. Eckberg DL, Gault JH, Bouchard RL, et al. Mechanics of left ventricular contraction in chronic severe mitral regurgitation. *Circulation* 1973;47(6):1252–1259.
2. Krayenbuhl HP, Bussmann WD, Turina M, et al. Is the ejection fraction an index of myocardial contractility? *Cardiologia* 1968;53(1):1–10.
3. MacGregor DC, Covell JW, Mahler F, et al. Relations between afterload, stroke volume, and descending limb of Starling's curve. *Am J Physiol* 1974;227(4):884–890.
4. Yang SS, Bentivoglio LG, Maranhao V, et al. *From Cardiac Catheterization Data to Hemodynamic Parameters*, 3rd ed. Philadelpha: F. A. Davis, 1988.
5. Braunwald E, Brockenbrough EC, Frahm CJ. Left atrial and left ventricular pressures in subjects without cardiovascular disease. *Circulation* 1961;24:267.
6. Cassidy SC, Teitel DF. The conductance volume catheter technique for measurement of left ventricular volume in young piglets. *Pediatr Res* 1992;31(1):85–90.
7. Teitel DF, Klautz RJ, Cassidy SC, et al. The end-systolic pressure-volume relationship in young animals using the conductance technique. *Eur Heart J* 1992;13(Suppl E):40–46.
8. Baan J, van der Velde ET, de Bruin HG, et al. Continuous measurement of left ventricular volume in animals and humans by conductance catheter. *Circulation* 1984;70(5):812–823.
9. Taylor RR, Covell JW, Ross J Jr. Volume-tension diagrams of ejecting and isovolumic contractions in left ventricle. *Am J Physiol* 1969;216(5):1097–1102.
10. Diamond G, Forrester JS, Hargis J, et al. Diastolic pressure-volume relationship in the canine left ventricle. *Circ Res* 1971;29(3):267–275.
11. Suga H, Sagawa K, Shoukas AA. Load independence of the instantaneous pressure-volume ratio of the canine left ventricle and effects of epinephrine and heart rate on the ratio. *Circ Res* 1973;32(3):314–322.
12. Lim DS, Gutgesell HP, Rocchini AP. Left ventricular function by pressure-volume loop analysis before and after percutaneous repair of large atrial septal defects. *Catheter Cardiovasc Interv* 2006;67(5):788–838.
13. Glantz SA, Kernoff RS. Muscle stiffness determined from canine left ventricular pressure-volume curves. *Circ Res* 1975;37(6):787–794.
14. Reeves TJ, Hefner LL, Jones WB, et al. The hemodynamic determinants of the rate of change in pressure in the left ventricle during isometric contraction. *Am Heart J* 1960;60:745–761.
15. Quinones MA, Gaasch WH, Alexander JK. Influence of acute changes in preload, afterload, contractile state and heart rate on ejection and isovolumic indices of myocardial contractility in man. *Circulation* 1976;53(2):293–302.
16. Grossman W, Haynes F, Paraskos JA, et al. Alterations in preload and myocardial mechanics in the dog and in man. *Circ Res* 1972;31(1):83–94.
17. Mehmel H, Krayenbuehl HP, Rutishauser W. Peak measured velocity of shortening in the canine left ventricle. *J Appl Physiol* 1970;29(5):637–645.
18. Gleason WL, Braunwald E. Studies on the first derivative of the ventricular pressure pulse in man. *J Clin Invest* 1962;41:80–91.
19. Stein PD, McBride GG, Sabbah HN. The fractional rate of change of ventricular power during isovolumic contraction. Derivation of haemodynamic terms and studies in dogs. *Cardiovasc Res* 1975;9(4):456–467.
20. Kreulen TH, Bove AA, McDonough MT, et al. The evaluation of left ventricular function in man. A comparison of methods. *Circulation* 1975;51(4):677–688.

21. Weisfeldt ML, Scully HE, Frederiksen J, et al. Hemodynamic determinants of maximum negative dP-dt and periods of diastole. *Am J Physiol* 1974;227(3):613–621.
22. McLaurin LP, Rolett EL, Grossman W. Impaired left ventricular relaxation during pacing-induced ischemia. *Am J Cardiol* 1973;32(6):751–757.
23. Reale A, Gioffre PA, Nigri A. Maximum rate of pressure decline in the normal, hypertrophied, and dilated left ventricle in man. *Am J Cardiol* 1972;29:286.
24. Cohn PF, Liedtke AJ, Serur J, et al. Maximal rate of pressure fall (peak negative dP-dt) during ventricular relaxation. *Cardiovasc Res* 1972;6(3):263–267.
25. Weiss JL, Frederiksen JW, Weisfeldt ML. Hemodynamic determinants of the time-course of fall in canine left ventricular pressure. *J Clin Invest* 1976;58(3):751–760.
26. Gaasch WH, Blaustein AS, Andrias CW, et al. Myocardial relaxation. II. Hemodynamic determinants of rate of left ventricular isovolumic pressure decline. *Am J Physiol* 1980;239(1):H1–H6.
27. Border WL, Syed AU, Michelfelder EC, et al. Impaired systemic ventricular relaxation affects postoperative short-term outcome in Fontan patients. *J Thorac Cardiovasc Surg* 2003;126(6):1760–1764.

CHAPTER 14

Miscellaneous Hemodynamic Conditions

MICHAEL RAGOSTA, MD

Physicians often become confused by unusual findings on pressure waveforms. Some of these are easily explained by one of several well-known artifacts. Many, however, are due to distortion from the effects of an arrhythmia. If not recognized or understood, the hemodynamic data may be misinterpreted, leading to errors in diagnosis or management. In addition, several commonly occurring clinical conditions such as obesity, lung disease, and pulmonary embolism have important and interesting hemodynamic effects. Finally, physicians have applied hemodynamic techniques and principles to the invasive evaluation of peripheral arterial disease. The hemodynamic effect of these miscellaneous conditions will be discussed in this chapter.

Effect of Arrhythmia on Hemodynamic Measurements

The cardiac rhythm determines the events responsible for generation of the pressure waveforms during the cardiac cycle, and disturbances of the cardiac rhythm are often reflected in the waveforms. Perhaps the simplest and most commonly observed rhythm abnormality is the premature ventricular beat, or PVC. The premature beat produces a systole with a contraction that may be too weak to open the aortic valve. This may be apparent hemodynamically as absence of the arterial pressure wave

that causes the "skipped beat" reported by many patients (Figure 14-1, A). More often, however, the premature beat is associated with reduced aortic pressure (Figure 14-1, B). Because of the lower pressures of the right heart, right ventricular contraction associated with a premature beat is usually adequate to open the pulmonic valve and generate a weakened pulmonary artery pressure wave. This does create the scenario, however, in which one ventricle ejects (the right ventricle) while the other does not (left ventricle) and may explain the symptoms of "fullness" and dyspnea accompanying PVCs in some patients.

A normal beat after a PVC follows a compensatory pause and is typically a beat with stronger contraction due to enhanced filling and increased contractility.[1] This may manifest as an increased systolic pressure on the aortic or left ventricular pressure wave compared to the usual sinus beats (Figure 14-2). Most normal hearts do not exhibit this behavior and it is more readily apparent in patients with left ventricular dysfunction in whom the greater contractile force of the post-PVC beat has more impact on the cardiac output. The phenomenon of extrasystolic potentiation assists in the diagnosis of hypertrophic obstructive cardiomyopathy. The increased contractility of the post-PVC beat increases the degree of obstruction, raising the pressure gradient between the aorta and the left ventricle but lowering the pulse pressure on the aortic pressure waveform (Figure 14-3). Compare this to the patient with valvular aortic stenosis where the degree of obstruction is fixed and the post-PVC beat raises the gradient but also raises both left ventricular and aortic systolic pressure; the pulse pressure on the aortic waveform consequently increases (Figure 14-4).

Atrial premature beats may be inapparent on the electrocardiogram but

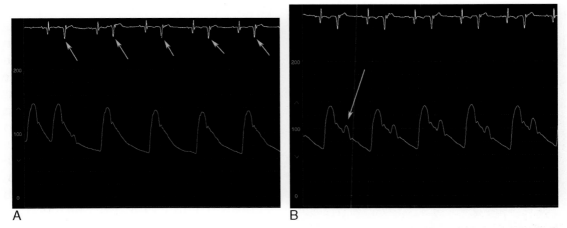

FIGURE 14-1. An example of an aortic pressure waveform obtained in a patient with ventricular bigeminy. **A,** In the first panel, the premature ventricular beats *(arrows)* are unable to generate enough force to open the aortic valve and there is no associated aortic pressure waveform. **B,** In the second panel, each premature beat is associated with a diminished aortic pressure *(arrow)*.

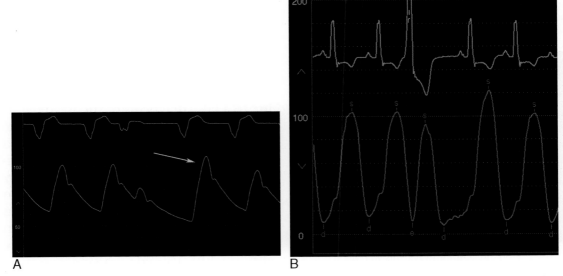

FIGURE 14-2. The beat following a premature ventricular contraction typically has greater contractile force and may have a higher systolic pressure. **A,** Depiction of finding on aortic pressure trace. **B,** Depiction of finding on a left ventricular tracing.

significantly affect the hemodynamic waveforms and may lead to errors in interpretation. A classic example is shown in Figure 14-5, where the aortic pressure appears to show pulsus alternans. Upon close inspection of the monitoring lead, however, an atrial bigeminal pattern is apparent. This finding has deceived experienced cardiologists since the 1960s, when it was also described with sinus arrhythmia.[2]

Atrial fibrillation is a very common dysrhythmia with important effects on the hemodynamics. On the right and left atrial waveforms, the absence of atrial systole is apparent by the absence

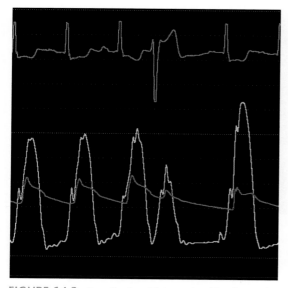

FIGURE 14-3. In patients with hypertrophic obstructive cardiomyopathy, the beat following a premature ventricular contraction is associated with greater obstruction, an increase in the outflow tract gradient, and a *drop* in aortic pulse pressure known as the Brockenbrough sign.

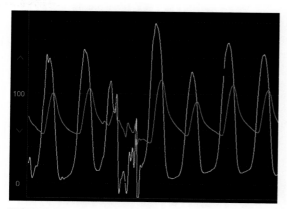

FIGURE 14-4. In contrast to patients with hypertrophic obstructive cardiomyopathy, the augmented post-premature beat results in an increase in the transvalvular gradient and an *increase* in aortic pulse pressure in patients with valvular aortic stenosis.

of an *a* wave. The *x* descent, however, may still be evident because this is caused by downward excursion of the tricuspid or mitral annulus during ventricular systole (Figure 14-6). In atrial flutter, atrial systole occurs, albeit at a very rapid rate, and this translates to clearly notable systolic waves on the atrial pressure tracing (Figure 14-7). The varying R-R intervals in atrial fibrillation cause varying degrees of ventricular filling with each beat and result in a wide variation in the systolic pressure peaks (Figure 14-8). This may be confused as a pulsus paradox. Furthermore, this same phenomenon results in beat-to-beat variations in the transvalvular gradients that impact valve area calculations in patients with aortic or mitral stenosis (Figures 14-8 and 14-9). It is for this reason that data from at least 10 consecutive beats are averaged in patients with atrial fibrillation when calculating the valve area invasively.

Complete heart block results in loss of AV synchrony. Contraction of the atrium against a closed valve causes a marked increase in atrial pressure, particularly if this chamber is not compliant. This can be appreciated on a right atrial waveform as a *cannon wave* and may be confused with prominent *v* waves, leading to a false diagnosis of tricuspid regurgitation (Figure 14-10). The importance of AV synchrony in patients with reduced left ventricular function and a ventricular pacemaker can be appreciated by the increase in systolic pressure when the atria contracts compared to beats where there is just ventricular contraction (Figure 14-11). Additional hemodynamic abnormalities caused by pacemakers have been reviewed.[3] First-degree AV block causes the *c* wave to become more obvious since the *c* wave follows the *a* wave by the same time as the PR interval on the electrocardiogram (Figure 14-12).

Effect of Obesity on Hemodynamic Measurements

Obtaining accurate hemodynamic measurements in morbidly obese patients

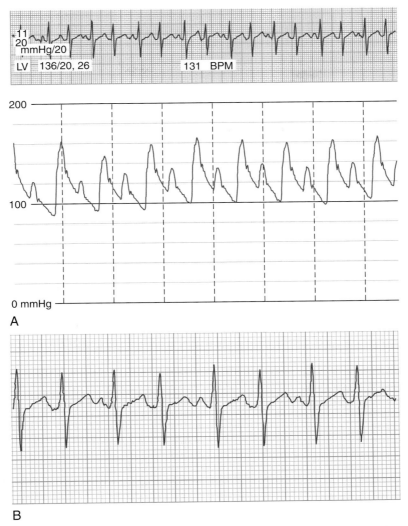

FIGURE 14-5. **A,** Upon initial observation, the aortic waveform on this tracing appears to show pulsus alternans. **B,** Close inspection of the rhythm strip reveals atrial bigeminy.

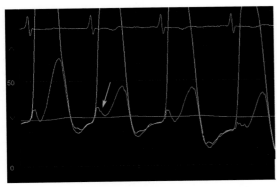

FIGURE 14-6. Atrial fibrillation distorts the atrial pressure waveform. Because atrial systole is not present, the a wave is absent. However, an x descent may be seen due to downward displacement of the mitral or tricuspid annulus *(arrow).*

can be challenging. The *zero* level is often erroneously set to the same level as more svelte patients, causing erroneous measurements of diastolic pressures. Importantly, patients with morbid obesity generate tremendous negative inspiratory forces during respiratory efforts and are readily apparent on right-heart pressure tracings; the end-expiratory values should be used in such cases (Figure 14-13). A pulsus paradoxus becomes more prominent and is often erroneously attributed to other conditions such as pericardial effusion. The right

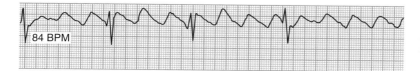

FIGURE 14-7. In contrast to atrial fibrillation, atrial systoles are generated with atrial flutter as shown.

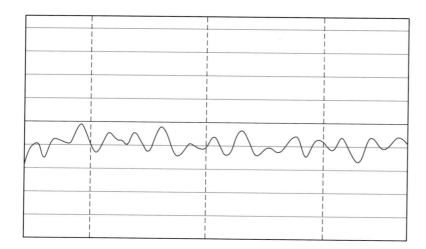

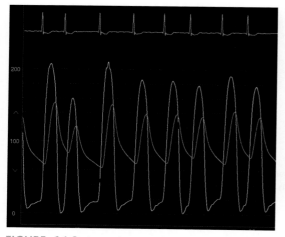

FIGURE 14-8. In patients with atrial fibrillation, the varying R-R intervals will result in different pressure gradients with each beat in patients with aortic stenosis. In addition, systolic pressure will vary and may lead to a false diagnosis of pulsus paradoxus.

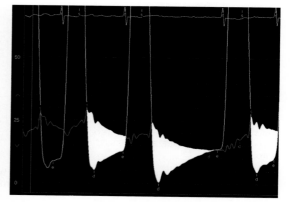

FIGURE 14-9. The varying R-R intervals seen in a patient with atrial fibrillation and mitral stenosis will result in different transvalvular pressure gradients. Long R-R intervals will reach diastasis, whereas short intervals are associated with the greatest gradient.

atrial, right ventricular diastolic, and pulmonary artery pressures may be modestly elevated in severe obesity. One study found approximately one third of obese individuals to have pulmonary artery systolic pressure <35 mmHg.[4] In addition, obesity is commonly associated with obstructive sleep apnea that also causes pulmonary hypertension.[5]

Effect of Pulmonary Disease on Hemodynamics

Pulmonary diseases may profoundly impact right-heart hemodynamics. This

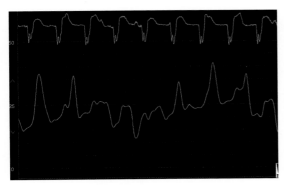

FIGURE 14-10. Cannon *a* waves associated with complete AV block in a patient with a pacemaker.

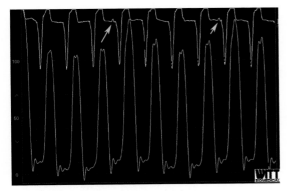

FIGURE 14-11. This patient with known severe left ventricular dysfunction has a permanent pacemaker with only a ventricular lead and underlying severe sinus node dysfunction with complete heart block. Occasional sinus beats *(arrows)* allow for AV synchrony and result in increased cardiac output, as evidenced by the increase in systolic pressure.

has been understood for many years and, in fact, patients with chronic obstructive pulmonary disease were among the first individuals to undergo systematic right-heart catheterization studies to further understand the effect of lung disease on cardiac hemodynamics.[6]

Alveolar hypoxia increases pulmonary vascular resistance. Initially, the reason is vasoconstriction, but, over time, elevations in pulmonary vascular resistance are caused by chronic, structural changes in the pulmonary vasculature. Pulmonary hypertension ensues and leads to right ventricular hypertrophy. *Cor pulmonale* is the term used to describe right-heart failure on the basis of pulmonary disease and the associated pulmonary hypertension.

The hemodynamic abnormalities observed in chronic lung disease vary widely depending on the nature and extent of parenchymal damage and whether or not there is involvement of the pulmonary vasculature. Pure emphysema generally requires extensive parenchymal destruction before pulmonary pressures are elevated. The pulmonary artery pressures may be entirely normal despite advanced lung disease.[6] When pulmonary pressures are elevated, they generally reach modest levels that do not usually exceed systolic pressures of 40–50 mmHg.[7] Right atrial and right ventricular diastolic pressures are typically in the normal range. Because of an associated increased inspiratory effort, there may be more prominent pressure changes due to respiration than normally observed, and a pulsus paradoxus of 12–15 mmHg is not unusual. Patients who develop cor pulmonale, however, exhibit more profound hemodynamic abnormalities with marked elevations in pulmonary artery pressure. Elevations of both right atrial and right ventricular diastolic pressures reflect right-heart failure similar to those with pulmonary hypertension from other causes (see Chapter 7).

Hemodynamics of Pulmonary Embolism

The hemodynamic consequences of acute pulmonary embolism depend upon both the size of the embolism and the presence of co-existing heart or lung disease. Simple mechanical obstruction of the pulmonary artery fails to explain the generation of elevated pulmonary artery pressures in pulmonary embolism. In fact, interestingly, one of the earliest

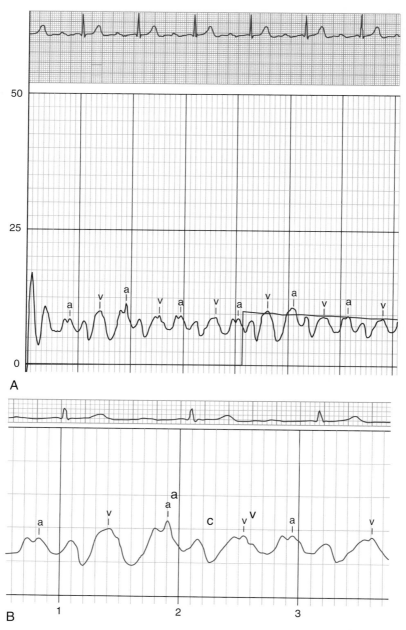

FIGURE 14-12. **A,** First-degree AV block accentuates the c wave on the right atrial waveform, as shown. **B,** Individual waves are labeled.

reports regarding the hemodynamic consequences of pulmonary embolism observed that an entire side of the lung could be removed without raising pulmonary artery pressures above normal.[6] This suggests that neurohumoral effects and hypoxic vasoconstriction are important factors conspiring to elevate the pulmonary vascular resistance.[7,8]

Pulmonary hypertension is observed in up to 80% of individuals with pulmonary embolism, ranging from mild-to-moderate elevations (mean pulmonary pressure of 20–39 mmHg) in about

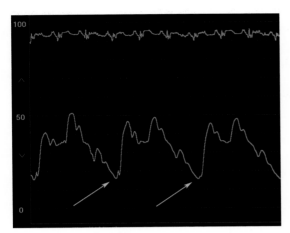

FIGURE 14-13. Marked respiratory variation on a pulmonary artery pressure waveform in a patient with morbid obesity. The large negative inspiratory forces are apparent *(arrows)*.

one-third of patients to very severe levels (>60 mmHg) in about 20%.[9] The highest levels of pulmonary hypertension are seen in patients with prior cardiopulmonary disease. Approximately 70% of patients with pulmonary embolism and no prior heart or lung disease have mean pulmonary artery pressures >20 mmHg; however, severe pulmonary hypertension (pulmonary artery mean pressures >40 mmHg) is not seen in this group even when extensive pulmonary embolism is present.[10,11] Likely, a normal right ventricle is unable to acutely generate very high pressures compared to one already hypertrophied from underlying cardiac or pulmonary disease. It requires a fairly sizable embolism (obstructing >25% total pulmonary blood flow) to raise the pulmonary pressure in an otherwise normal individual, and the larger the embolism the greater the elevation in pulmonary pressure. Cardiac output is reduced in nearly all patients with prior cardiopulmonary disease, whereas those without prior heart or lung disease only had decreased cardiac output in the setting of massive pulmonary embolism.[11]

Other hemodynamic findings associated with pulmonary embolism included tricuspid regurgitation from acute dilatation of the right ventricle and both Kussmaul's sign (elevation of right atrial pressure with inspiration) and pulsus paradoxus (inspiratory decrease in systolic aortic pressure >12 mmHg).[12,13] These abnormalities may be transient. Kussmaul's sign is likely due to obstruction to right ventricular outflow that prevents the forward passage of the augmented volume of blood entering the right atrium and ventricle with inspiration, thus elevating jugular venous and right atrial pressures. This same process bows the ventricular septum to the left, impairing left ventricular filling and resulting in a more prominent pulsus paradoxus.

Use of Hemodynamic Measurements During the Evaluation of Peripheral Arterial Disease

Angiography forms the basis of most decisions regarding revascularization in patients with peripheral arterial disease. This approach is entirely adequate when the artery under investigation appears normal or severely stenosed. Not uncommonly, however, ambiguous-appearing lesions on the angiogram with moderate (50%–70%) narrowing leads to difficult angiographic interpretation and decision making. In such cases, measurement of a translesional pressure gradient provides useful information regarding the hemodynamic impact of the lesion.

A translesional pressure gradient can be measured at the time of angiography by one of several techniques. The simplest method samples pressure from the tip of a small caliber (4 French) catheter while the catheter is pulled back

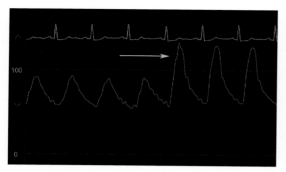

FIGURE 14-14. An example of obtaining a pullback pressure gradient by using a 4-French catheter placed distal to a subclavian stenosis *(left side)*. When the catheter is withdrawn across the lesion, the systolic pressure is noted to rise by about 40 mmHg *(arrow)*.

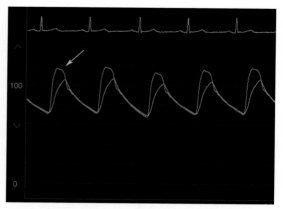

FIGURE 14-15. These tracings were obtained in a patient with a right iliac stenosis. One catheter was positioned in the descending aorta via the left femoral artery to measure aortic pressure *(arrow)* while another catheter was placed below the stenosis in the common femoral artery. A 20-mmHg systolic pressure gradient is noted. Observe also the damped appearance and delayed upstroke on the femoral artery pressure wave consistent with a significant stenosis.

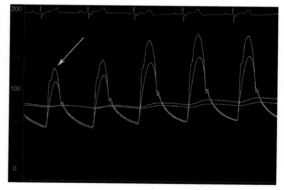

FIGURE 14-16. These pressure tracings were obtained to assess the pressure gradient across a renal artery of moderate severity. Simultaneous pressure measurements were obtained from a catheter in the aorta *(arrow)* and from a 0.014-inch pressure wire. The gradient is 20–30 mmHg. Note also the variability in the systolic pressure because of the respiratory cycle. For this reason, pullback pressures are suboptimal compared to simultaneous pressures.

across the stenosis (Figure 14-14). This method, however, is not ideal because the pullback technique is subject to beat-to-beat fluctuations in pressure from arrhythmia or the respiratory cycle. A better method involves the measurement of simultaneous pressures from two catheters positioned on either side of the stenosis. While more accurate than the pullback technique, note that the use of even a small-caliber catheter placed across the stenosis to measure a pressure gradient should be interpreted with care because the profile of the catheter across the lesion contributes to luminal obstruction, falsely elevating the gradient. Methods that avoid this problem include the positioning of two catheters on either side of the stenosis by obtaining an additional arterial access site (Figure 14-15), or use of a very small diameter (0.014-inch) wire outfitted with a pressure transducer near the catheter tip (i.e., a pressure wire). This arrangement is particularly useful for assessment of renal artery lesions (Figure 14-16). The waveform appearance of the pressure distal to a stenosis typically appears damped with a diminished peak systolic pressure and a delayed upstroke (see Figure 14-15).

Despite the widespread incorporation of translesional pressure gradients as an adjunct to angiography for decision making, the actual *cutoff* value that constitutes a hemodynamically significant stenosis is not known and is of some debate. No consensus is available regarding the choice of the absolute systolic gradient, the mean gradient or a hyperemic pressure gradient. Recently published guidelines regarding management of peripheral vascular disease suggest that a mean gradient of 10 mmHg before or after vasodilators or a peak systolic gradient of 10–20 mmHg should be considered a significant gradient.[14] Realize that this is based on little to no data.

Hemodynamic assessment is probably most helpful in the assessment of arteries that appear only moderately narrowed on angiography. One early study that correlated angiography and hemodynamics found pressure gradients >20 mmHg across most lesions narrowed >75% by angiography but not across lesions narrowed <50%.[15] Arterial lesions that narrowed the lumen by 50%–75% had a wide spectrum of pressure gradients, indicating that hemodynamic assessment is most valuable in this group. Measurement of pressure gradients helps not only with diagnosing a significant stenosis but also with determining the success of balloon angioplasty or stent implantation (Figure 14-17). In a study of balloon angioplasty of the iliac arteries, despite the appearance of a less-than-perfect angiographic result, the average peak systolic pressure gradient decreased from 44 mmHg to 7 mmHg after successful balloon dilatation and resulted in clinical improvement.[16]

In patients with peripheral arterial disease, the translesional pressure gradient at rest may not be entirely indicative of the hemodynamic consequences of the lesion during exercise when blood flow is greatly increased. This situation should be suspected when luminal narrowing is only moderate by angiography and the pressure gradient at rest is less than 20 mmHg, but the patient has convincing symptoms with exertion. In such cases, use of a vasodilator such as nitroglycerin may prove useful, as exemplified in the published case of a patient with only moderate narrowing of the common iliac artery on angiography with a resting gradient increasing from 6 mmHg to 22 mmHg with intra-arterial nitroglycerin.[17]

Pressure gradient determination has been most commonly applied to the evaluation of renal artery lesions (Figure 14-18). Early studies used 4-French catheters to measure the translesional pressure gradients in renal arteries. However, this technique is clearly problematic in the smaller caliber renal arteries because the catheter profile contributes to obstruction. One study that used both 4-French catheters and the unobtrusive 0.014-inch pressure wire to measure pressure gradients in the same arterial lesions found an average systolic pressure gradient of

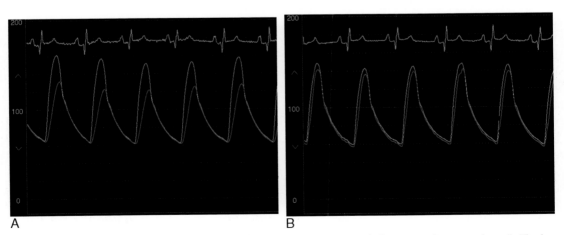

A   B

FIGURE 14-17. Example of a hemodynamic assessment of the results of a subclavian stenting procedure. **A,** The baseline peak systolic pressure gradient was about 40 mmHg and **(B)** reduced to about 5 mmHg after stenting.

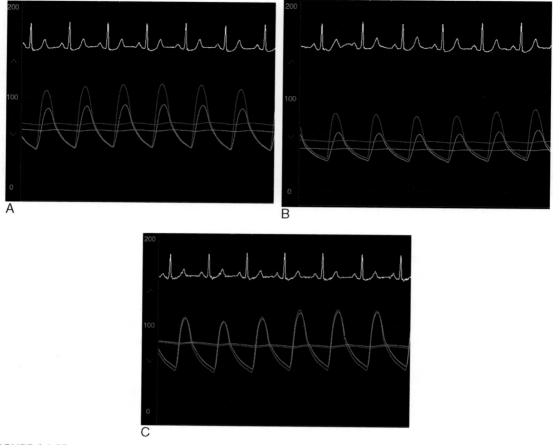

FIGURE 14-18. These tracings demonstrate the use of a pressure guidewire to assess a renal artery lesion and the result of an intervention. **A,** Simultaneous pressure measurements were obtained from a catheter in the aorta and from a 0.014-inch pressure wire and demonstrates a 30-mmHg peak systolic gradient. **B,** Intrarenal nitroglycerin was administered and lowered systolic pressure but did not change the peak systolic gradient. **C,** Following treatment of the lesion with a stent, the gradient was eliminated.

40 + 46 mmHg by pressure wire compared with 71 + 52 mmHg by 4-French catheter, thus clearly overestimating the systolic gradient, suggesting that the pressure wire is a superior technique for measuring transluminal pressure gradients.[18] Some have advocated the use of intrarenal vasodilator agents to augment the pressure gradient, although one study did not find an advantage to use of intrarenal nitroglycerin.[19] Similar to other peripheral vascular beds, no general consensus is available on the optimal translesional pressure gradient that constitutes a "hemodynamically significant" renal artery lesion.[20] An elegant study by

De Bruyne et al.[21] analyzed the hemodynamics of varying degrees of renal artery obstruction created by partial balloon inflation in the renal artery following a renal artery stenting procedure. With a pressure wire, the ratio of pressure distal to the stenosis created by the partially inflated balloon (Pd) to pressure in the aorta (Pa) was compared to renin levels sampled from the renal vein. Renin levels rose above normal at a Pd/Pa <0.9 and correlated with the degree of obstruction. This valuable information provides some of the first data that help define a hemodynamically significant renal artery lesion.

The fractional flow reserve concept, used to assess coronary lesions, has been applied to renal artery lesions.[22] Renal fractional flow reserve is calculated as the ratio of the mean pressure distal to the stenosis to mean pressure in the aorta during maximal hyperemia. Unlike the coronary vascular bed, adenosine causes vasoconstriction in the renal vascular bed, so this agent cannot be used. Instead, selective administration of intrarenal papaverine (24–32 mg) appears safe and effective for this purpose.[22] In a preliminary study of moderate renal artery lesions, the procedure was safe and the mean pressure gradient assessed with a pressure wire averaged 6 mmHg at baseline and increased to an average of 18 mmHg. The renal fractional flow reserve ranged from 0.58–0.95 and correlated poorly with the degree of angiographic stenosis but correlated well with both baseline and hyperemic gradients. The cutoff value that represents a significant renal fractional flow reserve is unknown and remains to be determined.

References

1. Kern MJ, Donohue T, Bach R, Aguirre F. Interpretation of cardiac pathophysiology from pressure waveform analysis: Cardiac arrhythmias. *Cathet Cardiovasc Diagn* 1992;27:223–227.
2. Ferrer MI, Harvey RM. Some hemodynamic aspects of cardiac arrhythmias in man. A clinico-physiologic correlation. *Am Heart J* 1964;68:153–165.
3. Kern MJ, Deligonul U. Interpretation of cardiac pathophysiology from pressure waveform analysis: Pacemaker hemodynamics. *Cathet Cardiovasc Diagn* 1991;24:22–27.
4. Weyman AE, Davidoff R, Gardin J, et al. Echocardiographic evaluation of pulmonary artery pressure with clinical correlates in predominantly obese adults. *J Am Soc Echocardiogr* 2002;15:454–462.
5. Tourkohoriti G, Kakouros S, Kosmas E, et al. Daytime pulmonary hypertension in patients with obstructive sleep apnea: The effect of continuous positive airway pressure on pulmonary hemodynamics. *Respiration* 2001;68:566–572.
6. Bloomfield RA, Lauson HD, Cournand A, et al. Recording of right heart pressures in normal subjects and in patients with chronic pulmonary disease and various types of cardio-circulatory disease. *J Clin Invest* 1946;25(4):639–664.
7. McLaughlin VV, McGoon MD. Pulmonary arterial hypertension. *Circulation* 2006;114:1417–1431.
8. Goldhaber SZ, Elliott CG. Acute pulmonary embolism: Part I: Epidemiology, pathophysiology and diagnosis. *Circulation* 2003;108:2726–2729.
9. Sasahara AA, Cannilla JE, Morse RL, et al. Clinical and physiologic studies in pulmonary thromboembolism. *Am J Cardiol* 1967;20:10–20.
10. McIntyre KM, Sasahara AA. The hemodynamic response to pulmonary embolism in patients without prior cardiopulmonary disease. *Am J Cardiol* 1971;28:288–294.
11. McIntyre KM, Sasahara AA. Hemodynamic and ventilatory responses to pulmonary embolism. *Prog Cardiovasc Dis* 1974;17:175–190.
12. Burdine JA, Wallace JM. Pulsus paradoxus and Kussmaul's sign in massive pulmonary embolism. *Am J Cardiol* 1965;15:413–415.
13. Cohen SI, Kupersmith J, Aroesty J, Rowe JW. Pulsus paradoxus and Kussmaul's sign in acute pulmonary embolism. *Am J Cardiol* 1973;32:271–275.
14. Hirsch AT, Haskal ZJ, Hertzer NR, et al. ACC/AHA 2005 Guidelines for the Management of Patients with Peripheral Arterial Disease. *J Am Coll Cardiol* 2006;47:1–192.
15. Udoff EJ, Barth KH, Harrington DP, et al. Hemodynamic significance of iliac artery stenosis: Pressure measurements during angiography. *Radiology* 1979;132:289–293.
16. Kaufman SL, Barth KH, Kadir S, et al. Hemodynamic measurements in the evaluation and follow-up of transluminal angioplasty of the iliac and femoral arteries. *Radiology* 1982;142:329–336.
17. Goldberg LR, Stouffer GA. Iliac artery stress test. *Circulation* 2004;109:1802–1803.
18. Colyer WR, Cooper CJ, Burket MW, Thomas WJ. Utility of a 0.014″ pressure-sensing guidewire to assess renal artery translesional systolic pressure gradients. *Catheter Cardiovasc Interv* 2003;59:372–377.
19. Gross CM, Kramer J, Weingartner O, et al. Determination of renal arterial stenosis severity: Comparison of pressure gradient and vessel diameter. *Radiology* 2001;220:751–756.
20. Martin LG, Rundback JH, Sacks D, et al. for the SIR Standards of Practice Committee. *J Vasc Interv Radiol* 2002;13:1069–1083.
21. De Bruyne B, Manoharan G, Pijls NH, et al. Assessment of renal artery stenosis severity by pressure gradient measurements. *J Am Coll Cardiol* 2006;48:1851–1855.
22. Subramanian R, White CJ, Rosenfield K, et al. Renal fractional flow reserve: A hemodynamic evaluation of moderate renal artery stenosis. *Catheter Cardiovasc Interv* 2005;64:480–486.

Index

Note: Page numbers followed by 'f' indicate figures; 't' indicate tables.